FIFTH EDITION

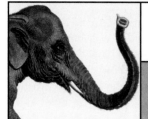

APPLETON & LANGE

REVIEW FOR THE

SURGICAL TECHNOLOGY EXAMINATION

Nancy M. Allmers, RN, BA, MA
Formerly Director, Surgical Technology Program
Associate Professor, Science and Health Division
Bergen Community College
Paramus, New Jersey

Joan Ann Verderame, RN, BA, MA
Director, Surgical Technology Program
Associate Professor, Science and Health Division
Bergen Community College
Paramus, New Jersey

Appleton & Lange Reviews/McGraw-Hill
Medical Publishing Division

New York   Chicago   San Francisco   Lisbon   London   Madrid   Mexico City   Milan
New Delhi   San Juan   Seoul   Singapore   Sydney   Toronto

Appleton & Lange Review for the Surgical Technology Examination, Fifth Edition

13 14 15 CUS/CUS 0 9

ISBN 0-07-138550-9

Notice

Medicine is an ever-changing science. As new research and clinical experience broaden our knowledge, changes in treatment and drug therapy are required. The authors and the publisher of this work have checked with sources believed to be reliable in their efforts to provide information that is complete and generally in accord with the standards accepted at the time of publication. However, in view of the possibility of human error or changes in medical sciences, neither the authors nor the publisher nor any other party who has been involved in the preparation or publication of this work warrants that the information contained herein is in every respect accurate or complete, and they disclaim all responsibility for any errors or omissions or for the results obtained from use of the information contained in this work. Readers are encouraged to confirm the information contained herein with other sources. For example and in particular, readers are advised to check the product information sheet included in the package of each drug they plan to administer to be certain that the information contained in this work is accurate and that changes have not been made in the recommended dose or in the contraindications for administration. This recommendation is of particular importance in connection with new or infrequently used drugs.

This book was set in Palatino by Circle Graphics.
The editors were Michael J. Brown and Christie Naglieri.
The production supervisor was Sherri Souffrance.
Project management was provided by Columbia Publishing Services.
Von Hoffmann Graphics was the printer and binder.

This book is printed on acid-free paper.

Library of Congress Cataloging-in-Publication Data

Allmers, Nancy M.
    Appleton & Lange review for the surgical technology examination / Nancy M. Allmers,
Joan Ann Verderame.—5th ed.
        p. ; cm.
    Includes bibliographical references.
    ISBN 0-07-138550-9 (softcover)
    1. Surgical technology—Examinations, questions, etc. I. Title: Appleton and Lange
review for the surgical technology examination. II. Title: Review for the surgical
technology examination. III. Title: Surgical technology examination. IV. Verderame, Joan
Ann. V. Title.
    [DNLM: 1. Operating Room Technicians—Examination Questions. 2. Technology,
Medical—Examination Questions. WY 18.2 A439a 2003]
RD32.3.A45 2003
617'.91'0076—dc21
                                                                2003054181

Please tell the author and publisher what you think of this book by sending your comments to surgtech@mcgraw-hill.com. Please put the author and title of the book in the subject line.

Dedicated to

Our students—past, present, and future

Contents

Part 3. INTRAOPERATIVE AND POSTOPERATIVE PROCEDURES

The questions for Part 3 include the following topics for each surgical area: indications for surgery; instrumentation; equipment; maintenance of sterile field; care, handling, and use of intraoperative supplies; and terminal disinfection.

Part 4. TECHNOLOGICAL SCIENCES FOR THE OPERATING ROOM

Part 5. PRACTICE TEST

Preface

Appleton & Lange Review for the Surgical Technology Examination, Fifth Edition, has been designed to assist technicians planning to take the National Certification Exam for Surgical Technologists, which is given every March and September. Although unable to guarantee a perfect score, a study guide can provide a good deal of assistance in test preparation by enabling the student to review relevant material while becoming familiar with the type of questions that will be encountered on the exam.

The ever-growing body of knowledge necessary to prepare the surgical technologist for a professional role in the operating room requires that competency be measured by an exam that tests both constant and technologically up-to-date information. With this in mind, the authors have prepared a fifth edition of the review book that has been extensively revised and updated to include those advances in technology that have emerged in the last 4 years.

The book contains over 1500 questions that closely correlate in percentage the amount prescribed in the Study Guide for Certification provided by the Liaison Council of the Association of Surgical Technologists. The text is divided into four areas of concentration. Each section is further divided into subsections. Each question has one answer, a full-length explanation, and a reference note for further study in the area. Difficulty in a single area indicates a need for individual study emphasis. On completion of the review, you are encouraged to take the Practice Test, which closely parallels the national exam. The exam questions are randomly selected to provide the student with a composite of questions that may appear on an actual exam. Although the questions are not from an actual certifying exam, they typify the type and style of question that may appear on the test.

ACKNOWLEDGMENTS

A very sincere thank you goes to Pilling Surgical, and specifically to Mr. Lee Wimer, for permission to reproduce the instruments from their catalogs.

Introduction

ORGANIZATION OF THE BOOK

The book is organized into four major sections, which are the major topic areas covered on the Certifying Examination for Surgical Technologists.

1. Fundamental Knowledge (including Terminology, Anatomy and Physiology, Microbiology, Pharmacology and Anesthesia, Infection Control, Concepts of Patient Care, and Occupational Hazards)
2. Preoperative Preparation (including Physical Environment of the Operating Room, Patient-Related Procedures, and Scrub Tasks)
3. Intraoperative and Postoperative Procedures (including Indications for Surgery, Instrumentation, Equipment, Maintenance of Sterile Field, Care, Handling, and Use of Supplies and Medications, Counts, Emergency Measures, and Terminal Disinfection)
4. Technological Sciences For the Operating Room (including sections on Computer Use, Surgical Application of Electricity, The Relationship between Physics and Medicine, and Surgical Robots)

Each section is designed to facilitate your review of the major content areas of surgical technology. In each section, you are given ample practice at honing your question-taking skills. In addition, because each group of questions is preceded by a heading that identifies the particular subspecialty area (e.g., Basic Sciences—Terminology), you are able to test your current knowledge in each of these areas.

Finally, each section ends with detailed explanations of each question for reinforcement of knowledge. Each of these explanations is referenced to a specific text where the information can be found so that you can supplement your study with further reading. After all the individual review sections, there is an integrated Practice Test, which will enable you to assess your areas of strength and weakness under simulated exam conditions.

HOW TO ANSWER A QUESTION INTELLIGENTLY

Unlike many examinations, which are a composite of several multiple-choice question types, the National Certification Exam for Surgical Technologists uses only one major type of question. Each question will have a "stem," which presents a problem or asks a question. The stem is then followed by four choices, only one of which is entirely correct. "Distractors," which are the choices other than the correct answer, may be partially correct; however, there can only be one best answer.

Although the question type is constant within the exam, the degree of difficulty may vary. Some questions require rote memory, some require problem solving, and others require evaluation and judgment. When the stem of the question takes on a negative aspect, the words "not" or "except," is in capital letters to catch your eye and remind you that the correct answer will be the exception to the statement in the stem of the question.

Sample Question 1

A left subcostal incision indicates surgery of the

- (A) gallbladder
- (B) pancreas
- (C) spleen
- (D) common bile duct

This question could be answered from rote memory, placing the term "subcostal" with the anatomic structure "spleen." It is more likely that the student will conjure up a picture of the human abdomen and discount gallbladder (choice A) and common bile duct (choice D) immediately because they are located on the right side of the abdominal cavity. Thus, two choices are ruled out as possible answers, improving the odds of selecting the correct answer from 25 to 50%. Although the tail of the pancreas reaches over to the left side of the body and is adjacent to the spleen, spleen is clearly the best choice and the only correct answer.

Sample Question 2

An elderly female, sleeping soundly, arrives in the OR via stretcher with siderails in place and safety strap intact. She is placed alone outside her assigned OR. The woman awakes, climbs off the stretcher, and, falling, receives a deep scalp laceration. The circulating nurse

- (A) can be charged with abandonment
- (B) can be charged with simple assault
- (C) can be charged with battery
- (D) cannot be charged because safety devices were in place

This question is more difficult. Although we clearly see choices B and C as incorrect because the nurse had no physical part in the injury to the patient, the difficulty is now in choosing between the remaining answers. Choice D may seem correct because the stem of the questions tells us that all safety devices were intact. It is only with knowledge of the legal aspect of OR procedure that we know that the key word *alone* signifies culpability on the part of the nurse. Standard OR procedures claim that one is guilty of abandonment if a patient is left *alone* at any time when in the care of OR personnel and may be charged as such in a court of law.

HOW TO USE THE BOOK

It will probably be the most efficient use of your time to follow the book from front to back, chapter to chapter, answering questions and noting difficult areas after completion of a section or subsection. Continual notation in this book or on a small notepad (which you should keep with your review book) of general areas as well as subspecialty areas, will provide you with a quick review at the end of the chapter. This will help you determine those areas that require the most emphasis for study and those areas that require only cursory review. Specific page references are provided at the end of each explanation. Jot down the references most commonly cited in that chapter. Most of the references are texts that are readily available at your nearest library. When you have completed the review and any necessary additional study, you will be ready for the 250-question Practice Test located on page 203. The Practice Test is a unique feature of this book because it provides you with an assessment of your readiness in all sections covered by the actual National Certifying Exam.

Table 1. STRATEGIES FOR ANSWERING QUESTIONS*

1. Remember that only one choice can be the correct answer.
2. Read the question carefully to be sure that you understand what is being asked.
3. Quickly read each choice for familiarity. (This important step is often not done by test takers.)
4. Go back and consider each choice individually.
5. If a choice is partially correct, tentatively consider it to be incorrect. (This step will help you lessen your choices and increase your odds of choosing the correct choice/answer.)
6. Consider the remaining choices, and select the one you think is the answer. At this point, you may want to quickly scan the stem to be sure you understand the question and your answer.
7. Fill in the appropriate circle on the answer sheet. (Even if you do not know the answer, you should at least guess—you are scored on the number of correct answers, so do not leave any blanks.)

*Note that steps 2 through 7 should take an average of 45 to 55 seconds total. The actual examination is timed for an average of 45 to 55 seconds per question.

As you may already know, the Certifying Exam integrates subtopics; i.e., the questions are not separated into discrete categories. Thus, you can use the Practice Test to acclimate yourself to taking this heterogeneous mixture of question topics. In addition, the Practice Test will give you practice answering a large number of questions over an extended period of time (3 hours).

When you have completed the entire Practice Test, you can check off your incorrect answers in the answer section. A 75% (188 questions correct) should be considered the minimum acceptable score on this test. In addition, you should check your answers against those given on the Practice Test Subject Listing on page 239. If you get less than 75% correct in any of the subject areas, you may want to supplement your studying with the references provided. The official source of applications for and information about the surgical technology exam can be obtained from the following:

Liaison Council on Certification for the Surgical Technologist
128 South Tejon Street
Suite 301
Colorado Springs, CO 80903
Telephone: (719) 328-0800
Toll-free: (800) 707-0057
Fax: (719) 328-0801
E-mail: mail@lcc-st.org

PART 1

Fundamental Knowledge
Questions

DIRECTIONS (Questions 1 through 393): Each of the numbered items or incomplete statements in this section is followed by answers or by completions of the statement. Select the ONE lettered answer or completion that is BEST in each case. Check your answers with the correct answers at the end of the chapter.

I. BASIC SCIENCES

A. Terminology

1. Adnexa refers to

   (A) adrenal glands
   (B) sympathetic nerve fibers
   (C) outer most layer
   (D) accessory organs

2. A drop is denoted by the abbreviation

   (A) gt
   (B) g
   (C) cc
   (D) mL

3. The abbreviation ung refers to

   (A) tincture
   (B) ointment
   (C) as directed
   (D) spirits

4. Proximal is a term that indicates a point

   (A) nearer to the body
   (B) farther away from the body
   (C) in the center of the body
   (D) toward the head

5. Adduction means

   (A) movement away from median plane
   (B) movement toward median plane
   (C) movement superiorly
   (D) movement inferiorly

6. Ischemic can be defined as

   (A) a decreased supply of oxygenated blood to a body part or organ
   (B) a sharp posterior bony projection of the pelvis
   (C) a painful sensation
   (D) the transmission of pain impulses to the hip bone

7. A cystocele is

   (A) a herniation of the urinary bladder
   (B) an accumulation of fluid in any sac-like cavity
   (C) a congenital herniation of intra-abdominal viscera through a defect in the abdominal wall
   (D) a dilatation in the spermatic cord

8. Nulli is a prefix that means

   (A) many
   (B) few
   (C) one
   (D) none

9. False is indicated by the prefix

   (A) non
   (B) meso
   (C) pseudo
   (D) exo

10. Tiny red or purple spots on the skin appearing as a result of small hemorrhages within the dermal or submucosal layers are called

(A) petechiae
(B) peyronies
(C) purigos
(D) pityriasis rosea

11. Kerato refers to

(A) tubular
(B) round
(C) horny
(D) spherical

12. The suffix lysis means

(A) removal
(B) activation
(C) breaking down
(D) adding

13. The left eye is indicated by the following letters

(A) OD
(B) OU
(C) OS
(D) LE

14. Tissue death is called

(A) necrosis
(B) necatoriasis
(C) nematodiasis
(D) neoteny

15. The secretion of excessive sweat is also known as

(A) diaphyseal aclasis
(B) hypercalcemic
(C) hypercapnea
(D) diaphoresis

B. Anatomy and Physiology

16. Which radiographic procedure has the ability to make images in multiple planes?

(A) PET
(B) CT
(C) MRI
(D) Ultrasound

17. The absence of a normal body opening, duct, or canal is called

(A) atrophia
(B) atrichia
(C) ataxia
(D) atresia

18. Epistaxis can be defined as

(A) gene interaction
(B) bleeding from the nose
(C) congenital urethral defect
(D) extrachromosomal replication

19. Blood gas analysis is called

(A) BGA
(B) SAT rate
(C) ABG
(D) ABO

20. A ganglion is a

(A) chemical substance secreted by the ova
(B) necrotic death of tissue
(C) missing segment
(D) collection of nerve endings

21. The lungs are covered in a serous membranous sac called the

(A) bronchial pleura
(B) pulmonary pleura
(C) visceral pleura
(D) parietal pleura

22. The passageway for foods and liquids into the digestive system, and for air into the respiratory system, is the

(A) trachea
(B) larynx
(C) epiglottis
(D) pharynx

23. The vocal cords are located in the

(A) larynx
(B) pharynx
(C) windpipe
(D) trachea

24. The function of the trachea is to

(A) conduct air into the larynx
(B) serve as a pathway for food into the esophagus
(C) serve as a resonating chamber for speech
(D) conduct air to and from the lungs

25. The nasal cavity is divided into two portions by the

(A) concha
(B) septum
(C) ethmoid
(D) vomer

26. The bones of the palm of the hand are referred to as

(A) phalanges
(B) carpals
(C) metacarpals
(D) calcaneus

27. The muscles important in respiration are

(A) trapezius
(B) latissimus dorsi
(C) pectoralis major
(D) intercostal

28. The thick, fan-shaped muscle that lies on the anterior chest is the

(A) latissimus dorsi
(B) serratus anterior
(C) pectoralis major
(D) teres major

29. The triangular muscle of the shoulder that abducts the arm is the

(A) biceps brachii
(B) deltoid
(C) triceps brachii
(D) serratus anterior

30. Which of the abdominal muscles originates at the pubic bone and ends in the ribs?

(A) rectus abdominis
(B) transversus abdominis
(C) external oblique
(D) internal oblique

31. One of the principal muscles of the pelvic floor is the

(A) sartorius
(B) levator ani
(C) internal oblique
(D) rectus abdominis

32. The gastrocnemius is the chief muscle of the

(A) calf of the leg
(B) stomach
(C) stomach's greater curvature
(D) thigh

33. A connective tissue band that holds bones together is called

(A) cartilage
(B) tendon
(C) joint
(D) ligament

34. The two bones that form the side walls and the roof of the cranium are the

(A) parietal bones
(B) frontal bones
(C) occipital bones
(D) temporal bones

35. The sternocleidomastoid muscle is located

(A) along the side of the neck
(B) above and near the ear
(C) under the tongue
(D) in the back of the neck

36. The medial bone of the forearm, which is located on the small-finger side of the hand, is called the

(A) ulna
(B) radius
(C) humerus
(D) fibula

37. The bone that is shaped like a butterfly and forms the anterior portion of the base of the cranium is the

(A) temporal
(B) sphenoid
(C) ethmoid
(D) parietal

38. The bone that forms the posterior portion of the skull is the

   (A) parietal
   (B) occipital
   (C) temporal
   (D) frontal

39. The lower jawbone is the

   (A) maxilla
   (B) mandible
   (C) mastoid
   (D) zygoma

40. The bone located in the neck between the mandible and the larynx, which supports the tongue and provides attachment for some of its muscles, is the

   (A) palatine bone
   (B) vomer
   (C) pterygoid hamulus
   (D) hyoid bone

41. The adult vertebral column has

   (A) 33 bones
   (B) 28 bones
   (C) 26 bones
   (D) 32 bones

42. How many cervical vertebrae are there?

   (A) 7
   (B) 12
   (C) 5
   (D) 4

43. The bone in the axial skeleton that does not articulate with any other bone is the

   (A) sternum
   (B) trochlea
   (C) talus
   (D) hyoid

44. The number of pairs of ribs is

   (A) 12
   (B) 10
   (C) 8
   (D) 7

45. A slender, rodlike bone that is located at the base of the neck and runs horizontally is the

   (A) scapula
   (B) shoulder blade
   (C) clavicle
   (D) sternum

46. The nucleus pulposus is the

   (A) cushioning mass within an intervertebral disk
   (B) result of a ruptured disk
   (C) outer layer of fibrocartilage within a disk
   (D) covering of the intervertebral disk

47. The upper, flaring portion of hipbone is the

   (A) ischium
   (B) pubis
   (C) ilium
   (D) femoral head

48. A large opening at the base of the skull through which the spinal cord passes is the

   (A) ossicle
   (B) hypoglossal canal
   (C) foramen ovale
   (D) foramen magnum

49. The larger, weight-bearing bone of the lower leg is the

   (A) humerus
   (B) talus
   (C) fibula
   (D) tibia

50. The bone that fits into the acetabulum, forming a joint, is the

   (A) tibia
   (B) femur
   (C) fibula
   (D) patella

51. Another name for the kneecap is

   (A) patella
   (B) tibia
   (C) fibula
   (D) phalange

52. The membranes that line closed cavities within the body are called

  (A) mucous membranes
  (B) serous membranes
  (C) fascial membranes
  (D) skeletal membranes

53. The longest bone in the body is the

  (A) femur
  (B) fibula
  (C) tibia
  (D) humerus

54. A rounded protuberance found at a point of articulation with another bone is called a

  (A) trochanter
  (B) trochlea
  (C) tubercle
  (D) condyle

55. An infection of the bone is

  (A) osteoarthritis
  (B) osteomyelitis
  (C) osteoporosis
  (D) osteomalacia

56. The epiphyses are the

  (A) ends of long bones
  (B) shafts of long bones
  (C) bone-forming cells
  (D) marrow-filled cavities within bone

57. Oil glands of the skin are called

  (A) sudoriferous
  (B) ceruminous
  (C) sebaceous
  (D) hypochlorous

58. The periosteum is

  (A) the membrane that covers bone
  (B) the membrane that surrounds a joint
  (C) the covering of the internal and external organs of the body and the lining of vessels
  (D) a fibrous connective tissue sheath

59. A transparent structure that permits the eye to focus rays to form an image on the retina is the

  (A) sclera
  (B) retina
  (C) cornea
  (D) lens

60. The purpose of the iris is to

  (A) regulate the amount of light entering the eye
  (B) protect the iris
  (C) supply the choroid with nourishment
  (D) receive images

61. The structure that is seen from the outside as the colored portion of the eye is the

  (A) cornea
  (B) pupil
  (C) retina
  (D) iris

62. The nerve that carries visual impulses to the brain is the

  (A) ophthalmic nerve
  (B) optic nerve
  (C) oculomotor nerve
  (D) trochlear nerve

63. The white outer layer of the eyeball is the

  (A) conjunctiva
  (B) sclera
  (C) choroid
  (D) retina

64. A jelly-like substance in the eye's posterior cavity is called

  (A) choroid
  (B) palpebra
  (C) vitreous humor
  (D) aqueous humor

65. The structure that connects the middle ear and the throat, allowing the eardrum to vibrate freely, is the

  (A) membranous canal
  (B) external auditory canal
  (C) eustachian tube
  (D) semicircular canal

66. The conjunctiva is the

    (A) colored membrane of the eye
    (B) covering of the anterior globe except the cornea
    (C) gland that secretes tears
    (D) membrane lining the socket

67. The number of pairs of spinal nerves is

    (A) 12
    (B) 28
    (C) 30
    (D) 31

68. The great sensory nerve of the face and head is the

    (A) trochlear
    (B) oculomotor
    (C) hypoglossal
    (D) trigeminal

69. The cranial nerve that contains special sense fibers for hearing as well as for balance is

    (A) II
    (B) V
    (C) VIII
    (D) XII

70. The part of the brain responsible for maintenance of balance and muscle tone, as well as coordination of voluntary muscle, is the

    (A) cerebellum
    (B) cerebrum
    (C) midbrain
    (D) pons

71. The frontal, temporal, parietal, and occipital lobes are divisions of the

    (A) midbrain
    (B) interbrain
    (C) cerebellum
    (D) cerebrum

72. The area of the brain that controls the respiratory center is the

    (A) cerebellum
    (B) interbrain
    (C) pons
    (D) medulla oblongata

73. The largest part of the brain is the

    (A) brain stem
    (B) cerebrum
    (C) diencephalon
    (D) cerebellum

74. The outermost covering of the brain and spinal cord is the

    (A) pia mater
    (B) dura mater
    (C) arachnoid
    (D) choroid

75. Cerebrospinal fluid circulates freely in the

    (A) subarachnoid space
    (B) arachnoid space
    (C) pia mater
    (D) subdural space

76. The brain contains four fluid-filled spaces called the

    (A) auricles
    (B) ventricles
    (C) fissures
    (D) sulci

77. Which of the following structures transmits sound vibrations to the inner ear?

    (A) external auditory canal
    (B) tympanic membrane
    (C) semicircular canal
    (D) stapes

78. The winding, cone-shaped tube of the inner ear is the

    (A) vestibule
    (B) semicircular canal
    (C) labyrinth
    (D) cochlea

79. Which of the following is not an auditory ossicle?

    (A) cochlea
    (B) stapes
    (C) incus
    (D) malleus

80. Cross-matching of blood

    (A) determines patient's blood type
    (B) determines Rh factor of both patient and donor
    (C) determines suitability of donor by mixing donor RBC's with recipient serum
    (D) determines blood group of donor

81. The highly specialized blood cell whose function is oxygen transportation is

    (A) red blood cell
    (B) white blood cell
    (C) blood plasma
    (D) fibrinogen

82. A differential count provides an estimate of

    (A) the amount of hemoglobin
    (B) the volume percentage of red cells
    (C) the percentage of each type of white cell
    (D) electrolyte percentages

83. Mixing of incompatible bloods may result in

    (A) agglutination
    (B) infectious hepatitis
    (C) leukocytosis
    (D) hyperglycemia

84. Platelets are essential for

    (A) coagulation of blood
    (B) controlling of infection
    (C) carrying oxygen
    (D) combating histamine effect

85. In the normal adult, the average number of leukocytes per cubic millimeter of circulating blood is

    (A) 1000–4000
    (B) 3000–8000
    (C) 5000–10,000
    (D) 10,000–15,000

86. A large superficial vein in the lower extremity, which begins in the foot and extends up the medial side of the leg, the knee, and the thigh, is called the

    (A) femoral
    (B) greater saphenous
    (C) iliac
    (D) popliteal

87. The vein in the bend of the elbow that is commonly used as a site for venipuncture is the

    (A) subclavian vein
    (B) cephalic vein
    (C) median cubital vein
    (D) basilic vein

88. The artery at the back of the knee is the

    (A) popliteal
    (B) femoral
    (C) iliac
    (D) celiac

89. The superior and inferior mesenteric arteries supply the

    (A) stomach
    (B) intestines
    (C) spleen
    (D) kidney

90. The vein that drains the veins of the chest wall and empties into the superior vena cava is the

    (A) azygos
    (B) hepatic
    (C) cephalic
    (D) basilic

91. The veins of the head and neck are drained by the

    (A) basilic vein
    (B) cephalic veins
    (C) azygos vein
    (D) jugular veins

92. Which arteries supply the heart?

    (A) pulmonary
    (B) aortic
    (C) coronary
    (D) common carotid

93. The atrioventricular (A-V) node causes

    (A) auricular relaxation
    (B) ventricular contraction
    (C) ventricular dilation
    (D) auricular contraction

94. Why would an aspirated foreign body be more likely to enter the right bronchus rather than the left bronchus?

    (A) the right bronchus is more vertical, shorter, and wider than the left
    (B) the division of the right bronchus is wider
    (C) the right bronchus is longer
    (D) the left bronchus is not in line with the trachea

95. The spleen filters

    (A) antibodies
    (B) tissue fluid
    (C) lymph
    (D) blood

96. Circulation that is established through an anastomosis between two vessels supplying or draining two adjacent structures is called

    (A) portal circulation
    (B) collateral circulation
    (C) systemic circulation
    (D) pulmonary circulation

97. Which artery supplies the head and neck?

    (A) subclavian
    (B) carotid
    (C) brachiocephalic
    (D) aortic arch

98. The serous membrane that covers the heart is the

    (A) pericardium
    (B) myocardium
    (C) epicardium
    (D) endocardium

99. The circle of Willis is located

    (A) in the axillary region
    (B) posterior to the ear

    (C) at the base of the brain
    (D) at the base of the neck

100. The branch of the external iliac artery that is located in the thigh is called the

    (A) tibial artery
    (B) femoral artery
    (C) popliteal artery
    (D) celiac artery

101. The descending aorta terminates at the level of the fourth lumbar vertebra, dividing into

    (A) two saphenous arteries
    (B) two femoral arteries
    (C) internal and external iliac arteries
    (D) two common iliac arteries

102. The contractions of the heart are synchronized and regulated by the pacemaker of the heart, called the

    (A) sinoatrial node
    (B) atrioventricular node
    (C) atrioventricular bundle
    (D) Purkinje fibers

103. Tiny blood vessels that permeate and nourish tissue are called

    (A) veins
    (B) venules
    (C) arterioles
    (D) capillaries

104. The wall or partition dividing the heart into right and left sides is called the

    (A) semilunar valve
    (B) mitral valve
    (C) chordae tendineae
    (D) septum

105. The heart valve that closes at the time the right ventricle begins pumping, preventing blood from returning to the right atrium, is the

    (A) aortic semilunar
    (B) pulmonary semilunar
    (C) bicuspid
    (D) tricuspid

106. The inner lining of the heart, composed of smooth, delicate membrane, is called the

   (A) pericardium
   (B) endocardium
   (C) epicardium
   (D) myocardium

107. The spleen is located

   (A) in the left hypochondriac region
   (B) behind the liver
   (C) behind the left kidney
   (D) behind the right kidney

108. All of the following are parts of the lymphatic system EXCEPT the

   (A) thyroid
   (B) tonsils
   (C) spleen
   (D) thymus

109. The s-shaped bend in the lower colon is called the

   (A) hepatic flexure
   (B) splenic flexure
   (C) rectum
   (D) sigmoid

110. The reabsorption of water and electrolytes is the main function of the

   (A) sigmoid colon
   (B) large intestine
   (C) small intestine
   (D) liver

111. The terminal portion of the large intestine is the

   (A) sigmoid
   (B) rectum
   (C) anus
   (D) anal canal

112. Which structure lies retroperitoneally?

   (A) sigmoid colon
   (B) spleen
   (C) liver
   (D) kidney

113. The first portion of the large intestine is the

   (A) sigmoid
   (B) cecum
   (C) colon
   (D) ileum

114. The appendix is attached to the

   (A) ascending colon
   (B) transverse colon
   (C) cecum
   (D) descending colon

115. The primary function of the gallbladder is

   (A) storage of bile
   (B) production of bile
   (C) digestion of fats
   (D) drainage of the liver

116. When the gallbladder contracts, bile is ejected into the

   (A) liver
   (B) duodenum
   (C) jejunum
   (D) pancreas

117. The area in the duodenum where the common bile duct and the pancreatic duct empty is called

   (A) the duct of Santorini
   (B) the ampulla of Vater
   (C) Wirsung's duct
   (D) the islet of Langerhans

118. Which structure is also known as the "fatty apron"?

   (A) greater omentum
   (B) lesser omentum
   (C) mesentery
   (D) falciform ligament

119. The common bile duct is the union of the

   (A) cystic duct and cystic artery
   (B) cystic duct and hepatic duct
   (C) cystic artery and hepatic duct
   (D) hepatic vein and cystic duct

120. The yellow tinge in the skin symptomatic of obstructive jaundice is caused by the accumulation of what substance in the blood and tissue?

   (A) cholesterol
   (B) bile salts
   (C) enzymes
   (D) bilirubin

121. The head of the pancreas is located

   (A) in the curve of the duodenum
   (B) by the spleen
   (C) on the undersurface of the liver
   (D) in the curve of the descending colon

122. The sphincter at the junction of the small and large intestines is the

   (A) sphincter of Oddi
   (B) ileocecal sphincter
   (C) pyloric sphincter
   (D) duodenal sphincter

123. The portion of the small intestine that receives secretions from the pancreas and the liver is the

   (A) ileum
   (B) jejunum
   (C) duodenum
   (D) pylorus

124. The region of the stomach that connects to the duodenum is the

   (A) fundus
   (B) body
   (C) pylorus
   (D) cardia

125. The mesentery is

   (A) a double-layered peritoneal structure shaped like a fan
   (B) a word synonymous with "fatty apron"
   (C) the membrane covering the surface of most abdominal organs
   (D) a structure that supports the sigmoid colon

126. The large central portion of the stomach is called the

   (A) pylorus
   (B) body
   (C) fundus
   (D) cardia

127. The muscle serving as a valve to prevent regurgitation of food from the intestine back into the stomach is known as the

   (A) sphincter of Oddi
   (B) ileocecal sphincter
   (C) cardiac sphincter
   (D) pyloric sphincter

128. The digestive passageway that begins at the pharynx and terminates in the stomach is the

   (A) larynx
   (B) trachea
   (C) windpipe
   (D) esophagus

129. The point at which the esophagus penetrates the diaphragm is called the

   (A) hiatus
   (B) meatus
   (C) sphincter
   (D) fundus

130. Adenoids are also called

   (A) palatine tonsils
   (B) pharyngeal tonsils
   (C) lingual tonsils
   (D) uvula

131. The function of the molar teeth is to

   (A) tear and crush food
   (B) crush and grind food
   (C) cut food
   (D) manipulate food

132. Mumps occur in the

   (A) sublingual glands
   (B) submandibular glands
   (C) parotid glands
   (D) thyroid gland

133. The salivary glands located under the tongue are the

(A) subungual
(B) sublingual
(C) submaxillary
(D) parotid

134. The liver has

(A) two lobes
(B) three lobes
(C) four lobes
(D) five lobes

135. The glomerulus is a

(A) tiny coiled tube
(B) tubelike extension into the renal pelvis
(C) double-walled cup
(D) cluster of capillaries

136. The tubes or cuplike extensions that project from the renal pelvis are called

(A) glomeruli
(B) convoluted tubules
(C) Bowman's capsules
(D) calyces

137. Urine is transported along the ureters to the bladder by

(A) gravity flow
(B) contraction of the renal pelvis
(C) peristaltic waves
(D) muscle relaxation

138. The smooth, triangular area at the bottom of the bladder that contains three openings is called the

(A) internal sphincter
(B) urinary meatus
(C) trigone
(D) external os

139. The kidneys are positioned

(A) intraperitoneally
(B) retroperitoneally
(C) in front of the parietal peritoneum
(D) in back of the visceral peritoneum

140. The kidney structure that filters blood, returns useful substances to blood, and removes substances from blood that are not needed is the

(A) nephron
(B) glomerulus
(C) medulla
(D) cortex

141. Blood is supplied to the kidney by means of the renal artery, which arises from the

(A) thoracic aorta
(B) aortic arch
(C) abdominal aorta
(D) pulmonary artery

142. The indentation in the kidney through which all structures must pass as they enter or leave the kidney is the

(A) hilus
(B) renal pelvis
(C) renal capsule
(D) cortex

143. The outer layer of the kidney is known as the

(A) medulla
(B) glomerulus
(C) nephron
(D) cortex

144. The portion of the male urethra that passes through the pelvic floor is called the

(A) prostatic portion
(B) cavernous portion
(C) membranous portion
(D) penile portion

145. A lack of voluntary control over micturition is called

(A) retention
(B) urination
(C) incontinence
(D) suppression

146. Urine empties from the bladder through a tube called the

(A) urethra
(B) urinary meatus
(C) urethral meatus
(D) external urethral sphincter

147. Fertilization occurs in the

(A) fallopian tubes
(B) uterus
(C) ovary
(D) gonads

148. The perineum is

(A) a thin tissue stretching across the vagina
(B) the region anterior to the clitoris
(C) the lower portion of the uterus
(D) the area between the vagina and the anus

149. The small, sensitive structure of the female homologous to the male penis is the

(A) hymen
(B) clitoris
(C) perineum
(D) vestibule

150. Ova are swept into the fallopian tubes by small, fringelike extensions on the distal ends of the tubes called

(A) ostium
(B) fimbriae
(C) oviducts
(D) stroma

151. The inner lining of the uterus is called the

(A) endometrium
(B) serosa
(C) myometrium
(D) oocyte

152. The ligament that attaches the ovaries to the pelvic wall is the

(A) mesovarian
(B) ovarian
(C) suspensory
(D) broad

153. The supporting structure of the male reproductive system is the

(A) inguinal canal
(B) cremaster muscle
(C) vas deferens
(D) spermatic cord

154. The loose skin covering the glans penis like a sheath is called the

(A) crura
(B) prepuce
(C) bulb
(D) tunica albuginea

155. The distal end of the penis is slightly enlarged and is called the

(A) glans penis
(B) prepuce
(C) foreskin
(D) corpora cavernosa penis

156. In a male, the structure surrounding the entrance to the urethra just below the urinary bladder is

(A) Cowper's gland
(B) the prostate gland
(C) the bulbourethral gland
(D) the seminal vesicle

157. Which structure is not a portion of the male urethra?

(A) membranous
(B) prostatic
(C) vas
(D) penile

158. This structure stores sperm and propels them toward the urethra during ejaculation

(A) vas deferens
(B) ejaculatory duct
(C) spermatic cord
(D) epididymis

159. The long, coiled tube in which sperm mature is the

(A) vas deferens
(B) epididymis

(C) ejaculatory duct
(D) seminal vesicle

C. Microbiology

160. The English surgeon who began the age of chemical control of the atmosphere was

(A) Ehrlich
(B) Madame Curie
(C) Alexander
(D) Lister

161. Passage of fluid through a cell membrane is called

(A) metosis
(B) miosis
(C) osmosis
(D) symbiosis

162. Oxygen-dependent bacteria are said to be

(A) anaerobic
(B) bacillic
(C) antibiotic
(D) aerobic

163. The destruction of bacteria by white cells during the inflammatory process is called

(A) symbiosis
(B) mitosis
(C) lymphocytosis
(D) phagocytosis

164. Bacteriostatic means

(A) to inhibit growth of microorganisms
(B) to destroy microorganisms
(C) to control microorganisms
(D) to inactivate microorganisms

165. *Staphylococcus aureus* would most likely be transmitted by

(A) urine
(B) feces
(C) nose and mouth
(D) sex organs

166. Microbial death occurs when an organism is

(A) reproducing at a slower rate
(B) reduced in population

(C) no longer capable of reproduction
(D) exposed to heat

167. What immune protection is available to the fetus?

(A) natural active
(B) natural passive
(C) active artificial
(D) passive artificial

168. The clinical syndrome characterized by microbial invasion of the bloodstream is

(A) superinfection
(B) septicemia
(C) cross-infection
(D) cellulitis

169. A toxoid is

(A) an inactivated toxin
(B) a substance that elicits an immune response
(C) a poison produced by an infectious agent
(D) a substance that the body recognizes as foreign, thus evoking an immune response

170. Inflammatory exudate that is thick and yellow is termed

(A) suppurative
(B) fibrinous
(C) serous
(D) mucous

171. The body's first line of defense against the invasion of pathogens is

(A) the immune response
(B) skin and mucous membrane linings
(C) cellular and chemical responses
(D) phagocytosis

172. Rodlike shaped bacteria are identified microscopically as

(A) bacilli
(B) cocci
(C) spirilla
(D) spirochetes

173. A procedure used to remove damaged tissue that provides growth conditions for pathogens is called

    (A) incision and drainage
    (B) dessication
    (C) lysis of adhesions
    (D) debridement

174. Herpes simplex is commonly called

    (A) cold sore
    (B) shingles
    (C) smallpox
    (D) chicken pox

175. All of the following descriptors refer to the inflammatory process EXCEPT

    (A) heat
    (B) pain
    (C) vasoconstriction
    (D) edema

176. *Clostridium tetani* causes

    (A) gangrene
    (B) nosocomial infection
    (C) lockjaw
    (D) malaria

177. A laboratory procedure useful in classifying bacteria using a staining procedure is

    (A) Gram stain
    (B) iodine stain
    (C) acid fast stain
    (D) differential stain

178. A fulminating infection arising from necrotic tissue and spreading rapidly is

    (A) rabies
    (B) gas gangrene
    (C) pasteurellosis
    (D) tetanus

179. Which bacteria is commonly found in soil?

    (A) *Clostridium tetani*
    (B) *Trypanosoma brucei*
    (C) *Pediculus vestimenti*
    (D) *Yersinia pestis*

180. The bacteria that causes rheumatic fever is

    (A) *Escherichia coli*
    (B) *Streptococcus*
    (C) *Pseudomonas*
    (D) *Staphylococcus*

181. A severe allergic reaction possibly resulting in death is called

    (A) arthus reaction
    (B) hypersensibility
    (C) anaphylactic shock
    (D) autoimmune disease

182. What organism is responsible for a boil?

    (A) *Staphylococcus aureus*
    (B) *Clostridium perfringens*
    (C) *Escherichia coli*
    (D) *Neisseria*

183. The organism most frequently found in burns is

    (A) *Clostridium perfringens*
    (B) *Pseudomonas aeruginosa*
    (C) *Clostridium tetani*
    (D) hemolytic streptococci

184. A bacterial pathogen most frequently invading damaged skin is

    (A) *Staphylococcus aureus*
    (B) *Clostridium tetani*
    (C) *Pseudomonas septica*
    (D) *Candida albicans*

185. Which type of wound would favor the development of gas gangrene?

    (A) moist
    (B) necrotic
    (C) dry
    (D) warm

186. Gas gangrene is caused by

    (A) *Fusobacterium*
    (B) *Clostridium tetani*
    (C) *Pseudomonas aeruginosa*
    (D) *Clostridium perfringens*

187. The bacteria highly resistant to sterilization and disinfection is

(A) spores
(B) fungus
(C) Gram-positive
(D) *Pseudomonas*

188. A bacteria found in the intestinal tract is

(A) *Escherichia coli*
(B) *Bordetella pertussis*
(C) *Franciscella tularensis*
(D) *Neisseria gonorrhoeae*

189. The burn classification that is characterized by a dry, pearly white, or charred-appearing surface is

(A) first
(B) second
(C) third
(D) fourth

190. OSHA is a governmental regulating agency whose aim is to

(A) provide guidelines to prevent transmission of blood-borne infections
(B) execute requirements designed to prevent transmission of blood-borne pathogens in the work environment
(C) require that communicable diseases be reported to a public health agency
(D) train employees how to recognize and execute safe practices

191. Inflammation is characterized by pain, redness, heat, swelling, and loss of function. The redness can be attributed to

(A) serum brought into the area
(B) constriction of capillaries
(C) vasodilation bringing more blood to the area
(D) heat from metabolic reaction

192. Removal of contaminated debris from a wound is called

(A) decontamination
(B) debridement
(C) dehiscence
(D) desiccation

193. The space caused by separation of wound edges is called

(A) lag phase
(B) evisceration
(C) fibrous scarring
(D) dead space

194. If tissue is approximated too tightly it can cause

(A) ischemia
(B) excessive scar tissue
(C) keloids
(D) adhesions

195. Tensile strength of a wound refers to

(A) the suture strength
(B) ability of tissue to resist rupture
(C) wound contraction
(D) tissue approximation

196. The substance that unites with thrombin to form fibrin, the basic structural material of blood clots is

(A) fibrinogen
(B) prothrombin
(C) fibrin
(D) thrombin

197. A cicatrix is

(A) an abscess
(B) a scar
(C) pus
(D) a wound

198. Keloids are

(A) a form of abscess
(B) an adhered serous membrane
(C) a raised, thickened scar
(D) a benign tumor

199. A wound that is infected or one in which there is excessive loss of tissue heals by

(A) primary intention
(B) secondary intention
(C) third intention
(D) fourth intention

200. A CDC guideline that addresses the care of "sharps" includes all of the following EXCEPT

(A) needles should always be recapped
(B) needles should not be bent or broken by hand
(C) needles should not be removed from disposable syringes
(D) needles should be discarded in puncture-resistant containers for disposal

201. The type of wound healing that requires debridement is

(A) first
(B) second
(C) third
(D) fourth

202. To promote healing, a surgical wound must have all of the following requisites EXCEPT

(A) suture closure of dead space
(B) drains to remove fluid or air
(C) a moderately tight dressing
(D) tight sutures to create tension

203. Wound healing that employs a technique allowing the wound to heal from the bottom up is called

(A) interrupted intention
(B) first intention
(C) second intention
(D) third intention

204. Which body fluid is least likely to transmit HIV?

(A) blood
(B) semen
(C) saliva
(D) spinal fluid

205. A band of scar tissue that binds together two anatomical surfaces that are normally separate from each other is called

(A) keloid
(B) adhesion
(C) cicatrix
(D) dehiscence

D. Pharmacology and Anesthesia

206. A drug that interferes with the blood-clotting mechanism is

(A) lidocaine
(B) fentanyl
(C) heparin
(D) cefazolin

207. An mg is a measurement of

(A) length
(B) weight
(C) volume
(D) temperature

208. The solutions used intravenously to replace plasma when plasma is not available is

(A) 0.9% NaCl
(B) Dextrose 5% in water
(C) Lactated Ringer's solution
(D) Dextran

209. An inch equals

(A) 2.2 cm
(B) 2.54 cm
(C) 4.4 cm
(D) 10 cm

210. How many milliliters are in 1 ounce?

(A) 10
(B) 30
(C) 75
(D) 100

211. One gram equals

(A) 100 mg
(B) 1000 mg
(C) 100 mL
(D) 1000 mL

212. A drug used to increase blood pressure is

(A) Avitene
(B) epinephrine
(C) heparin
(D) mannitol

213. The action of an anticholinergic drug is to reduce

   (A) heart rate
   (B) anxiety
   (C) nausea
   (D) secretions

214. The total volume in a 30-cc syringe is

   (A) 1 ounce
   (B) 2 ounces
   (C) 3 ounces
   (D) 4 ounces

215. Naloxone (Narcan) is an example of a/an

   (A) narcotic antagonist
   (B) mydriatic
   (C) histamine
   (D) diuretic

216. Avitene is

   (A) hemostatic
   (B) adrenergic
   (C) cycloplegic
   (D) mydriatic

217. An absorbable gelatin hemostatic agent that is often soaked in thrombin or epinephrine solution is

   (A) Avitene
   (B) Oxycel
   (C) Nu-knit
   (D) Gelfoam

218. Each of the following agents must be applied using dry gloves or instruments EXCEPT

   (A) Gelfoam
   (B) Collastat
   (C) Avitene
   (D) Helistat

219. An anticoagulant given subcutaneously, intravenously, or as a flush is

   (A) nitroglycerin
   (B) dextran
   (C) heparin
   (D) thrombin

220. A drug that decreases the tendency of blood platelets to clot is

   (A) warfarin sodium
   (B) Diazepam
   (C) lorazepam
   (D) midazolam HCl

221. An antibiotic used intraoperatively is

   (A) Diazepam
   (B) Ketoralac
   (C) Cyclogyl
   (D) Gentamicin

222. A topical antibiotic is

   (A) Bacitracin
   (B) ephedrine
   (C) Ancef
   (D) Keflex

223. Which item is used on cut edges of bone to seal off oozing of blood?

   (A) electrocautery
   (B) silver nitrate
   (C) bone wax
   (D) epinephrine

224. The most common diuretic is

   (A) Lasix
   (B) Pronestyl
   (C) Esoptin
   (D) Cefadyl

225. An osmotic diuretic agent used to decrease cerebral edema and intraocular edema is

   (A) Diuril
   (B) Fluosemide
   (C) papaverine
   (D) mannitol

226. A systemic agent used to control uterine hemorrhage is

   (A) protamine
   (B) pitocin
   (C) procainamide HCl
   (D) phenylephrine

227. Steroids are used for

    (A) reduction of fluid in body
    (B) reduction of body's need for oxygen
    (C) reduction of tissue inflammation and swelling
    (D) reduction of uterine constriction and contraction

228. Solu-Medrol is a(n)

    (A) antibiotic
    (B) myotic
    (C) mydriatic
    (D) anti-inflammatory

229. Tubal patency may be tested by the installation of _____ into the uterine cavity.

    (A) balanced salt solution
    (B) Chymar
    (C) methylene blue
    (D) gentian violet

230. A mydriatic drug, Neo-Synephrine, is used to

    (A) constrict the pupil
    (B) dilate the pupil
    (C) anesthetize the eye
    (D) lower intra-ocular pressure

231. Immobility of the eye, along with lowered intra-ocular pressure is facilitated by the use of

    (A) Diprivan block
    (B) Versed block
    (C) Xylocaine block
    (D) Retrobulbar block

232. Miochol is a(n)

    (A) antihistamine
    (B) blood thinner
    (C) miotic
    (D) anti-inflammatory

233. An agent that keeps the cornea moist during surgery and is used for irrigation as well is

    (A) Mannitol
    (B) Miochol
    (C) Chymar
    (D) BSS

234. An artificial plasma-volume expander is

    (A) mannitol
    (B) dextran
    (C) Ringer's solution
    (D) Uromatic

235. An anticoagulant used in vascular surgery is

    (A) protamine sulfate
    (B) heparin
    (C) adrenalin
    (D) papavarine

236. Heparin effects are reversed by

    (A) pitocin
    (B) phenylephrine
    (C) protamine sulfate
    (D) procainamide Hcl

237. The universal donor blood that may be given in extreme emergencies until the patient can be typed and crossmatched is

    (A) A
    (B) B
    (C) O
    (D) AB

238. Normal saline is used for laparotomy pack moistening and for intraperitoneal irrigation because it is

    (A) hypotonic
    (B) isotonic
    (C) hypertonic
    (D) hyperkalemic

239. Levophed

    (A) increases cardiac output
    (B) decreases venous return to the heart
    (C) increases urine secretion
    (D) restores and maintains blood pressure

240. A drug used to treat metabolic acidosis is

    (A) Inderal
    (B) Pronestyl
    (C) sodium bicarbonate
    (D) Isuprel

241. The last sensation to leave the patient during general anesthesia induction is

(A) hearing
(B) sight
(C) feeling
(D) smell

242. An ultrashort acting drug useful during intubation to produce paralysis and also to produce muscle relaxation when used in a dilute solution is

(A) Sublimaze
(B) Valium
(C) Versed
(D) Anectine

243. Neuroleptoanalgesia combines

(A) a narcotic and an anticholinergic
(B) a tranquilizer and narcotic
(C) an anti-inflammatory and a tranquilizer
(D) a muscle relaxant and a tranquilizer

244. A sedative-tranquilizer used to reduce anxiety and apprehension of the pre-op patient and as an adjunct to general anesthesia to reduce the amount and concentration of other more potent agents is

(A) Valium
(B) Marzicon
(C) Anectine
(D) Demerol

245. An antimuscarinic

(A) controls pain
(B) prevents nausea
(C) limits salivation
(D) reverses muscle relaxation

246. Anesthesia given in a combination of several agents to obtain optimum results is called

(A) regional anesthesia
(B) general anesthesia
(C) conduction anesthesia
(D) balanced anesthesia

247. A bolus is

(A) a small, intermittent dose intravenously
(B) a dose injected intramuscularly
(C) a rapid dose, subcutaneously
(D) a dose injected all at once, intravenously

248. A drug used to soothe and relieve anxiety is a(n)

(A) cholinergic
(B) analgesic
(C) sedative
(D) narcotic

249. A Bier block provides

(A) anesthesia to a distal portion of an extremity
(B) anesthesia below the diaphragm
(C) anesthetic block surrounding a peripheral nerve
(D) anesthetic block to a nerve group

250. Which inhalation agent is used for short procedures requiring no muscle relaxation?

(A) nitrous oxide
(B) halothane
(C) ethrane
(D) forane

251. The most frequently used barbiturate for intravenous anesthesia is

(A) ketamine
(B) Anectine
(C) Sublimaze
(D) pentothal

252. Halothane is also called

(A) Ethrane
(B) Penthrane
(C) Forane
(D) Fluothane

253. A method of anesthesia in which medication is injected into the subarachnoid space, affecting a portion of the spinal cord, is called a

   (A) Bier block
   (B) field block
   (C) nerve block
   (D) spinal block

254. The indication for an epidural would be

   (A) anorectal, vaginal, perineal, and obstetric procedures
   (B) lower intestinal procedures
   (C) upper gastrointestinal procedures
   (D) above-the-waist procedures

255. Compazine is

   (A) an antiemetic
   (B) a sedative
   (C) a tranquilizer
   (D) an anticholinergic

256. Pontocaine is

   (A) Carbocaine
   (B) tetracaine HCl
   (C) Marcaine
   (D) prilocaine HCl

257. Which technique can be employed to prevent pain during an operative procedure or to relieve chronic pain?

   (A) local infiltration
   (B) Bier block
   (C) nerve block
   (D) field block

258. The most widely used local anesthetic is

   (A) Carbocaine
   (B) Marcaine
   (C) prilocaine
   (D) lidocaine

259. Another name for adrenalin is

   (A) ephedrine
   (B) epinephrine
   (C) lidocaine
   (D) Levophed

260. A vasoconstrictor that, when added to a local anesthetic agent, extends its life is

   (A) ephedrine
   (B) epinephrine
   (C) aramine
   (D) ethrane

261. The purpose of an LMA is

   (A) to establish and maintain a patent airway
   (B) to provide patient cooling
   (C) to monitor body temperature
   (D) to evaluate cardiac and venous status

262. A drug used to reverse hypotension is

   (A) Isuprel
   (B) Inderal
   (C) Pronestyl
   (D) Levophed

263. Blood or fluid can be quickly delivered to a patient via

   (A) rapid infusion pump
   (B) SARA
   (C) Bair Hugger
   (D) Doppler

264. Blood oxygenation can be monitored during surgery by means of a(n)

   (A) blood pressure monitor
   (B) arterial catheter
   (C) pulse oximeter
   (D) CVP catheter

265. A drug that could be used to reverse the effect of muscle relaxants is

   (A) Narcan
   (B) protamine sulfate
   (C) Prostigmin
   (D) Valium

266. Arterial blood gases (ABGs) are commonly obtained by accessing the

   (A) femoral artery
   (B) carotid artery
   (C) radial artery
   (D) renal artery

267. Which piece of equipment is of extreme importance when anesthesia induction begins?

     (A) oximeter
     (B) blood pressure apparatus
     (C) oxygen
     (D) suction

II. INFECTION CONTROL

A. Aseptic Technique

268. The minimum distance a nonsterile person should remain from a sterile field is

     (A) 6 inches
     (B) 1 foot
     (C) 2 feet
     (D) 3 feet

269. Identify which of the following is <u>not</u> safe practice

     (A) discard opened sterile bottles
     (B) sterile persons drape first toward themselves, than away
     (C) sterile persons face sterile areas
     (D) sterile tables may be covered for later use

270. Tables are considered sterile

     (A) on the top and 2 inches below the table level
     (B) up to 2 feet off the ground
     (C) on the top and in the area that has been pulled close to the sterile field
     (D) only on the top

271. At the end of the case, drapes should be

     (A) pulled off and placed in a hamper
     (B) rolled off and placed on the floor so they can be checked for instruments
     (C) rolled off and placed in a hamper
     (D) checked for instruments, rolled off, and placed in a hamper

272. If a solution soaks through a sterile drape

     (A) discard drape and replace it
     (B) cover wet area with impervious sterile drape or towel

     (C) cover wet area with at least two layers of fabric
     (D) fill out an incident report at the end of the case

B. Sterilization and Disinfection

273. The pounds of pressure necessary in a steam sterilizer set at 250°F is

     (A) 15–17
     (B) 20–22
     (C) 22–25
     (D) 25–27

274. Positive assurance that sterilization conditions have been achieved can only be obtained through

     (A) biologic control test
     (B) heat-sensitive tape
     (C) color change monitor
     (D) mechanical indicator

275. A wrapped tray of instruments is sterilized in a gravity displacement sterilizer at 250°F for

     (A) 10 minutes
     (B) 15 minutes
     (C) 30 minutes
     (D) 40 minutes

276. The minimum exposure time for unwrapped instruments in a flash sterilizer that is set at 270°F (132°C) is

     (A) 2 minutes
     (B) 3 minutes
     (C) 5 minutes
     (D) 7 minutes

277. When steam is used to sterilize a rubber tubing or catheter

     (A) the lumen must be dried thoroughly before the process begins
     (B) a rubber band may be placed around it so it does not unwind
     (C) it should be fan-folded before wrapping
     (D) a residual of distilled water should be left inside the lumen

278. To be sterilized effectively, a linen pack must not weigh more than

    (A) 12 pounds
    (B) 14 pounds
    (C) 16 pounds
    (D) 18 pounds

279. Gravity displacement utilizes _____ to destroy microorganisms

    (A) gas
    (B) radiation
    (C) gamma rays
    (D) steam

280. The process called cavitation occurs in the

    (A) moist heat sterilizer
    (B) ultrasonic cleaner
    (C) high-speed pressure sterilizer
    (D) washer–sterilizer

281. All of the following statements regarding instrument sets are true EXCEPT

    (A) instruments must be placed in perforated trays
    (B) heavy instruments are placed on the bottom
    (C) all instruments must be closed
    (D) all detachable parts must be disassembled

282. All of the following statements regarding steam sterilization are true EXCEPT

    (A) flat packages are placed on the shelf on edge
    (B) small packages, placed one on top of the other, are criss-crossed
    (C) basins are placed on their sides
    (D) solutions may be autoclaved along with other items as long as they are on a shelf alone

283. Wrapped basin sets may be sterilized by steam under pressure at 250°F for a minimum of

    (A) 5 minutes
    (B) 10 minutes
    (C) 15 minutes
    (D) 20 minutes

284. Which of the following statements regarding the sterilization of basin sets is true?

    (A) basins must be separated by a porous material if they are nested
    (B) sponges and linen may be packaged inside the basin to be sterilized
    (C) basins are placed flat in the autoclave
    (D) basins must always be placed on the top shelf of the autoclave in a combined load

285. Why would gas sterilization be chosen over steam sterilization?

    (A) it is less expensive
    (B) it is less damaging to items
    (C) it is faster
    (D) it is more effective

286. The chemical agent used in gas sterilization is

    (A) ethylene glycol
    (B) ethacrynate sodium
    (C) ethyl chloride
    (D) ethylene oxide

287. What chemical system uses peracetic acid as the sterilant?

    (A) ozone gas sterilization
    (B) steris
    (C) sterrad
    (D) vapor phase sterilizer

288. The lumen of a tubing undergoing ethylene oxide (EO) sterilization is

    (A) well lubricated
    (B) dried thoroughly
    (C) prepared with a residual of distilled water
    (D) prepared with a NaCl flush

289. Why is ethylene oxide diluted with an inert gas such as chlorofluorocarbon?

    (A) it provides flame retardation
    (B) it increases effectiveness
    (C) it adds convenience and speed
    (D) it adds humidity

290. The commercial name for glutaraldehyde is

   (A) peracetic acid
   (B) phenol
   (C) Quats
   (D) Cidex

291. A 30 minute, single use, sterilization system useful for endoscopes is

   (A) Steris
   (B) ETO
   (C) steam under pressure
   (D) cold sterilization

292. Which of the following is essential when using activated glutaraldehyde for sterilization?

   (A) items must be rinsed thoroughly in sterile water before use
   (B) the solution must be heated in order to be effective
   (C) the items must be thoroughly moistened before placement in solution
   (D) the item must be air dried before use

293. What is the shelf life of Cidex?

   (A) between 14 and 28 days
   (B) 7 days
   (C) 1 month
   (D) indefinite

294. In which procedure would the use of a high-level disinfectant be acceptable instrument preparation?

   (A) suction lipectomy
   (B) tracheotomy
   (C) cystoscopy
   (D) mediastinoscopy

295. In a high-speed flash sterilizer, unwrapped instruments are exposed for a minimum of

   (A) 1 minute
   (B) 3 minutes
   (C) 5 minutes
   (D) 10 minutes

296. To kill spores, an item must be immersed in a 2% aqueous solution of glutaraldehyde for

   (A) 20 minutes
   (B) 2 hours
   (C) 10 hours
   (D) 24 hours

297. When placing tubing in an activated glutaraldehyde solution, one should

   (A) use a shallow container
   (B) be certain that the interior of the tubing is completely filled
   (C) moisten it thoroughly before submersion
   (D) B and C

298. What is the role of moisture in EO sterilization?

   (A) the items will dry out during the process if no humidity is added
   (B) the sterilizer will deteriorate from gas over a period of time if no moisture is added
   (C) dried spores are resistant to the gas, so they must be hydrated
   (D) moisture is not an essential element in gas sterilization

299. "Slow exhaust" in a gravity displacement steam sterilizer is used for

   (A) plastics
   (B) solutions
   (C) rubber
   (D) drape packs

300. Oil is best sterilized by

   (A) ethylene oxide
   (B) STERIS
   (C) convection hot air
   (D) steam

301. What is the function of an aerator in EO sterilization?

   (A) it is used to aerate items before sterilization
   (B) it is a separate unit used to decrease the aeration time
   (C) it is the last cycle in the EO sterilizer, which helps exhaust the gas and add air
   (D) it adds air to the cycle, which is essential for obtaining item sterility

302. Ethylene oxide destroys cells by

    (A) interfering with the normal metabolism of the protein and reproductive processes
    (B) coagulating cell protein
    (C) converting ions to thermal and chemical energy causing cell death
    (D) shrinking the cell

303. Activated glutaraldehyde is used to disinfect endoscopes for

    (A) 5 minutes
    (B) 10 minutes
    (C) 20 minutes
    (D) 60 minutes

304. When using a high-level disinfectant, always

    (A) submerge items while wet
    (B) rinse items with sterile distilled water before using
    (C) soak items in saline before using
    (D) add hot diluent to activated agent

305. The chemical sterilant used in the STERIS method of sterilizing is

    (A) formaldehyde
    (B) Cidex
    (C) ethylene oxide
    (D) peracetic acid

306. The Endoflush system

    (A) flushes out a vessel interior
    (B) initially cleans reusable channeled instruments
    (C) flushes debris from bladder
    (D) cleans and sterilizes endoscopes

C. Packaging and Dispensing Supplies

307. Which of the following is not an acceptable wrapper for gas sterilization?

    (A) nylon
    (B) muslin
    (C) paper
    (D) plastic

308. Which of the following is the only acceptable plastic that can be used for a steam sterilization wrapper?

    (A) polyethylene
    (B) polypropylene
    (C) polyamide
    (D) polyvinyl chloride

309. All of the following statements regarding muslin wrappers are true EXCEPT

    (A) muslin must be laundered, even if unused, in order to rehydrate it
    (B) a 140-thread count of unbleached muslin is used for wrappers
    (C) muslin is flexible and easy to handle
    (D) small holes can be repaired by stitching on a patch

310. Packages wrapped in muslin must have

    (A) one thickness
    (B) two thicknesses
    (C) three thicknesses
    (D) four thicknesses

311. The maximum storage life for a muslin-wrapped item in a closed cabinet is

    (A) 7 days
    (B) 14 days
    (C) 21 days
    (D) 30 days

312. An item dropped on the floor is considered safe only if

    (A) it is wrapped in woven material
    (B) it is enclosed in an impervious material
    (C) it is used right away
    (D) it is inspected carefully

313. When using a pour solution

    (A) a portion may be poured and the cap replaced
    (B) the contents must be used or discarded after the bottle is opened
    (C) the cap may be replaced if it has not been placed on an unsterile surface
    (D) the solution may be used on the same case if the cap is not replaced

314. What is the standard safety margin on package wrappers?

   (A) up to the edge
   (B) less than 1 inch
   (C) 1 inch or more
   (D) none of the above

315. When opening a wrapper, the circulator should open the top flap

   (A) toward self
   (B) away from self
   (C) after the sides
   (D) over sterile field

316. When the scrub nurse opens an inner sterile wrapper

   (A) the side nearest the body is opened first
   (B) the side nearest the body is opened last
   (C) the lateral areas are done first
   (D) A or B

317. When flipping a sterile item onto the field, the circulator may

   (A) lean over the sterile field to shake item out of package
   (B) project item without reaching over the sterile field
   (C) shake item into sterile basin stand
   (D) lean over sterile linen pack and drop item onto it

D. Operating Room Environment

318. The room temperature in an operating room (OR) should be

   (A) below 50°F
   (B) below 60°F
   (C) between 68 and 76°F
   (D) between 80 and 86°F

319. If an OR staff member wears eyeglasses

   (A) the glasses should be wiped with an antiseptic solution before each operation
   (B) the glasses should be soaked for 5 minutes in an antiseptic solution before the day begins

   (C) the glasses should be wiped with an antiseptic solution daily
   (D) no special care is necessary

320. Each statement regarding OR attire is true EXCEPT

   (A) lab coats worn out of the OR suite should be clean, closed, and knee length
   (B) scrub suits are always changed upon re-entry to the OR suite
   (C) scrub suits may be worn out of the OR uncovered, if they are changed upon OR re-entry
   (D) nonprofessional personnel and visitors must wear approved attire in the OR

321. The most effective protection from the radiation of x-rays is a

   (A) lead apron
   (B) double thick muslin apron
   (C) 3-foot distance from machine
   (D) 3-foot distance from patient

322. It is considered good technique to

   (A) change the mask only if it becomes moistened
   (B) hang the mask around the neck
   (C) criss-cross the strings over the head
   (D) handle the mask only by the strings

323. Sterile gloves

   (A) should be wiped off after donning to remove lubricant
   (B) need not be wiped off
   (C) should be wiped off only in septic cases
   (D) should be wiped off only in eye cases

324. Electrical cords should be

   (A) removed from outlets by the cord
   (B) wrapped tightly around equipment
   (C) removed from pathways so equipment is not rolled over them
   (D) disconnected from the unit before disconnection from the wall

325. Scatter radiation effects are directly related to

(A) amount of radiation
(B) length of exposure
(C) accumulation of radioactive substances in OR room
(D) amount of radiation and length of exposure time

III. CONCEPTS OF PATIENT CARE

A. Transportation

326. When using a patient roller, how many people are necessary to move the patient safely and efficiently?

(A) two
(B) three
(C) four
(D) five

327. When moving the patient from the OR table, who is responsible for guarding the head and neck from injury?

(A) circulating nurse
(B) scrub nurse
(C) anesthesiologist
(D) surgical technician

328. To move the patient from the transport stretcher to the OR table

(A) one person stands at the head, one at the foot, while the patient moves over
(B) one person stands next to the stretcher, one adjacent to the OR table, while the patient moves over
(C) one person stands next to the stretcher, stabilizing it against the OR table, while the patient moves over
(D) one person may stand next to the OR table and guide the patient toward him if stretcher wheels are locked

329. When moving a patient with a fracture in the OR, all of the following are true EXCEPT

(A) extra personnel are necessary
(B) support of the extremity should always be from below the site of fracture

(C) lifters on the affected side support the fracture
(D) the surgeon should be present

330. Which statement is false regarding the position on the OR table?

(A) elbow should not rest against the metal table
(B) feet should be uncrossed
(C) pillows provide support and comfort to prevent strain
(D) safety strap is 4 inches below the knee

331. To avoid compromising the venous circulation, the restraint or safety strap should be placed

(A) at knee level
(B) at the midthigh area
(C) 2 inches above the knee
(D) 2 inches below the knee

332. A patient with a fractured femur is being moved to the OR table. Who is responsible for supporting and protecting the fracture site?

(A) the nurse assistant
(B) the physician
(C) the circulating nurse
(D) the scrub nurse

B. Positioning

333. Crossing the patient's arms across his or her chest may cause

(A) pressure on the ulnar nerve
(B) interference with circulation
(C) postoperative discomfort
(D) interference with respiration

334. A precaution always taken when the patient is in the supine position is to

(A) place the pillows under the knees for support
(B) place the safety strap 3 to 4 inches below the knee
(C) place the head in a headrest
(D) protect the heels from pressure on the OR table

335. During lateral positioning, a

(A) pillow is placed between the legs
(B) sandbag is placed between the knees
(C) rolled towel is placed under the bottom leg
(D) sheet is folded flat between the legs

336. To prevent strain to the lumbosacral muscles and ligaments when the patient is in the lithotomy position

(A) the buttocks must not extend beyond the table edge
(B) the legs must be placed symmetrically
(C) the legs must be at equal height
(D) a pillow should be placed under the sacral area

337. The lithotomy position requires each of the following EXCEPT

(A) patient's buttocks rest along the break between the body and leg sections of the table
(B) stirrups are at equal height on both sides of the table
(C) stirrups are at the appropriate height for the length of the patient's legs to maintain symmetry
(D) each leg is raised slowly and gently as it is grasped by the toes

338. All of the following are requirements of the Kraske position EXCEPT

(A) patient is prone with hips over the break of the table
(B) a pillow is placed under lower legs and ankles
(C) a padded knee strap is applied 2 inches above knees
(D) arms are tucked in at sides

339. When using an armboard, the most important measure is to

(A) support the arm at the intravenous site
(B) strap the patient's hand to it securely
(C) avoid hyperextension of the arm
(D) avoid hypoextension of the arm

340. Anesthetized patients should be moved slowly to

(A) prevent fractures
(B) prevent circulatory overload
(C) allow the respiratory system to adjust
(D) allow the circulatory system to adjust

341. If the patient is in a supine position, the circulator must always

(A) place a pillow between the knees
(B) place a pillow under the knees
(C) see that the ankles and legs are not crossed
(D) see that the thoracic area is padded adequately

342. Extreme positions of the head and arm can cause injury to the

(A) cervical plexus
(B) radial nerve
(C) ulnar nerve
(D) brachial plexus

343. Ulnar nerve damage could result from

(A) poor placement of legs in stirrups
(B) hyperextension of the arm
(C) using mattress pads of varying thickness
(D) placing an arm on an unpadded table edge

344. In the prone position, the thorax must be elevated from the OR table to prevent

(A) compromised respiration
(B) pressure areas
(C) circulatory impairment
(D) brachial nerve damage

345. The anesthesiologist closes the eyelids of a general anesthetic patient for all of the following reasons EXCEPT

(A) prevent drying of the eye
(B) prevent the patient from seeing the procedure
(C) prevent eye trauma
(D) protect the eye from anesthetic agents

C. Observation and Monitoring

346. Diastolic blood pressure refers to

    (A) the force created by the contraction of the left ventricle of the heart
    (B) the relaxation phase between heartbeats
    (C) the first sound heard when taking the pressure on a manometer
    (D) the high point of the cycle

347. Systolic blood pressure represents

    (A) the pressure in the heart chambers, great vein, or close to the heart
    (B) the relaxation phase between heartbeats
    (C) the low point of the cycle
    (D) the greatest force caused by contraction of the left ventricle of the heart

348. Tachycardia is a(n)

    (A) heartbeat over 100 beats per minute
    (B) irregular heartbeat
    (C) thready, weak heartbeat
    (D) heartbeat less than 60 beats per minute

349. The most common artery used to feel the pulse is the

    (A) dorsalis pedis artery
    (B) femoral artery
    (C) radial artery
    (D) carotid artery

350. The body temperature taken orally is 98.6°F. What is it in Celsius?

    (A) 37°C
    (B) 52°C
    (C) 110°C
    (D) 212°C

351. Which term indicates low or decreased blood volume?

    (A) anoxemia
    (B) hypovolemia
    (C) hypoxia
    (D) hypocapnia

352. If the surgeon wants to assess the patient's ability to void voluntarily via the urethra, yet sees the need for urinary drainage, he could use a

    (A) Bonanno suprapubic catheter
    (B) Foley catheter
    (C) urethral stent
    (D) perineal urethrostomy

353. When catheterizing a patient

    (A) the patient must be shaved
    (B) the tip of the catheter must be kept sterile
    (C) sterile technique is not necessary
    (D) the bag must be maintained above table level

354. In which burn classification are the skin and subcutaneous tissue destroyed?

    (A) first
    (B) second
    (C) third
    (D) fourth

355. Uncontrolled increased positive pressure in one side of the thorax causes collapse of the opposite side, which is called

    (A) flail chest
    (B) Cheyne–Stokes syndrome
    (C) emphysema
    (D) mediastinal shift

356. Why is the obese patient at greater surgical risk than one of normal weight?

    (A) fat has poor vascularity
    (B) fluid and electrolyte balance is compromised
    (C) kidney function is altered
    (D) immune system lacks integrity

357. The patient has received preoperative medication. The action to be taken when this patient complains of dry mouth (thirst) and requests water would be to

    (A) provide the patient with unlimited water for thorough hydration
    (B) restrict water to 2 ounces

(C) restrict fluids completely and explain the reason for action of medication

(D) report to the surgeon immediately

358. When drawing a blood sample for arterial blood gases (ABGs), what is considered a safe time lapse between blood drawing and analysis?

(A) 10 minutes
(B) 20 minutes
(C) 30 minutes
(D) 1 hour

359. A patient is on anticoagulant drugs. Which of the following tests may be done to check the clotting time of his or her blood?

(A) serum amylase
(B) complete blood count
(C) bleeding time
(D) prothrombin time

D. Documentation and Records

360. The preoperative urinalysis test done on a patient indicates that the specific gravity is 1.050. This

(A) is within normal range
(B) is below normal range and he or she is dehydrated
(C) is above normal range and he or she is dehydrated
(D) is indicative of sugar in the urine

361. A type and crossmatch is done

(A) on all surgical patients
(B) if the surgeon anticipates in advance of the operation that blood loss replacement may be necessary
(C) on all hospital patients
(D) in the OR

362. A patient scheduled for surgery has a hematocrit reading of 40% of whole blood volume. This is

(A) within normal range
(B) below normal range
(C) above normal range
(D) inconclusive

363. Inherited deficiencies of coagulation in which bleeding occurs spontaneously after minor trauma is

(A) Tay–Sachs disease
(B) hemophilia
(C) pernicious anemia
(D) erythroblastosis fetalis

364. Preoperative chest x-rays

(A) are not necessary for the surgical patient
(B) are necessary only for the thoracic surgical patient
(C) are necessary only on the surgical patient with a chronic cough
(D) should be done on all surgical patients

365. An electrocardiogram is

(A) an electrical recording of heart activity
(B) an x-ray defining heart structures
(C) an x-ray of the cardiac portion of the stomach
(D) a stress test on the heart

366. After being scheduled in the OR for a routine tonsillectomy, the nurse checking the chart of a patient notes that the hemoglobin is 9.0 g. This reading is

(A) within normal range
(B) below normal range
(C) above normal range
(D) inconclusive

367. A microscopic blood exam that estimates the percentages of each type of white cell is called a

(A) red blood count
(B) white blood count
(C) differential blood count
(D) blood grouping

368. Which procedure is NOT absolutely necessary in patient identification?

    (A) identification by the anesthesiologist, who checks the wristband, chart, and operating schedule
    (B) identification by the surgeon before administration of an anesthetic
    (C) identification by the circulating nurse, who checks the wristband, chart, and operating schedule
    (D) identification by the scrub nurse before the procedure begins

369. Operative records documenting all aspects of perioperative care are required by

    (A) JCHO
    (B) OSHA
    (C) ASTM
    (D) CDC

E. Cardiopulmonary Resuscitation

370. Except for endotracheal tube installation, basic life support cannot be interrupted for more than

    (A) 1 minute
    (B) 2 to 3 minutes
    (C) 5 seconds
    (D) 30 seconds

371. External cardiac compression

    (A) restores and maintains oxygenation
    (B) provides pulmonary ventilation
    (C) provides oxygen to vital tissues
    (D) provides peripheral pulse

372. Which action is the responsibility of the scrub person during an intraoperative CPR effort?

    (A) remain sterile, keep track of counted items, and assist as necessary
    (B) document all medications given and draw up as necessary
    (C) start time clock, guard sterile field
    (D) bring defibrillator into the room and reposition the patient

F. Medical, Ethical, and Legal Responsibilities

373. A patient was burned on the lip with a hot mouth gag. Which of the following actions would have prevented this incident?

    (A) the circulator cooled the item in the sterilizer
    (B) the scrub nurse warned the surgeon that the item was hot
    (C) the scrub nurse cooled the item in a basin with sterile water
    (D) the surgeon had checked the item before using it

374. A patient signs a permission form for surgery, but because of a language barrier he or she does not fully understand what she or he has signed. This could constitute a liability case for

    (A) assault and battery
    (B) lack of accountability
    (C) improper documentation
    (D) invasion of privacy

375. If a patient falls because he or she was left unattended, the OR team member could be cited in a lawsuit for

    (A) misconduct
    (B) assault
    (C) doctrine of Respondeat Superior
    (D) abandonment

376. Which is not considered a safe procedure when caring for dentures inadvertently sent to the OR?

    (A) place in a properly labeled container
    (B) place in a properly labeled denture cup
    (C) return to the patient unit immediately and obtain a receipt, which is placed on the chart
    (D) wrap in a plastic bag and attach to the patient's chart

377. A lack of care or skill that any nurse or technician in the same situation would be expected to use is the legal definition of

(A) assault
(B) abandonment
(C) negligence
(D) default

378. The legal doctrine that mandates every professional nurse and technician to carry out their duties according to national standards of care practiced throughout the country is the

(A) doctrine of Res ipsa Loquitor
(B) doctrine of Respondeat Superior
(C) Nurse Practice Act
(D) doctrine of Reasonable Man

379. The doctrine of Respondeat Superior refers to

(A) the legal terms for assault and battery
(B) invasion of privacy
(C) employer liability for employee's negligent conduct
(D) professional misconduct

380. Liability is a legal rule that

(A) applies only in criminal actions
(B) holds the hospital responsible for its personnel
(C) holds each individual responsible for his or her own acts
(D) has no significance in malpractice suits

381. A criteria that identifies, measures, monitors, and evaluates patient care is

(A) audits
(B) automated information systems
(C) quality control circles
(D) quality assurance programs

382. Each of the following applies to an incident report EXCEPT

(A) notation is made on the patient's OR record
(B) statement should be factual and non-interpretive
(C) description includes action taken
(D) details are complete and accurate

7. Emotional Support

383. In which way could a patient's response to impending surgery exhibit itself?

(A) tension and anxiety
(B) fear and suspicion
(C) anger and hostility
(D) all of the above

IV. OCCUPATIONAL HAZARDS

384. Excessive exposure to radiation can affect the

(A) integumentary system
(B) brain
(C) reproductive organs
(D) stomach

385. Radiation exposure of the staff is monitored with

(A) a homing device
(B) a Holter monitor
(C) film badges
(D) a notation on each operative record

386. Ionizing radiation protection is afforded by the use of

(A) iron
(B) ebonized coating
(C) zinc
(D) lead

387. A potential safety hazard associated with laser surgery is

(A) eye injury
(B) electrical shock
(C) carcinogenic activity
(D) ionizing radiation exposure

388. An OR hazard that has been linked to increased risk of spontaneous abortion in female OR employees is exposure to

(A) x-ray control
(B) radium
(C) sterilization agents
(D) waste anesthetic gas

389. Which virus can be transmitted by a needle puncture or splash in the eye?

(A) hepatitis A
(B) hepatitis B
(C) non-A hepatitis
(D) non-B hepatitis

390. While using this mixture, a scavenging system is used to collect and exhaust or absorb its vapors. It is called

(A) glutaraldehyde
(B) polypropylene
(C) methyl methacrylate
(D) halon

391. The best measure for staff protection against HIV is

(A) handling all needles and sharps carefully
(B) using barriers to avoid direct contact with blood and body fluids
(C) immunization of all staff with vaccine
(D) A & B

392. Which body organ is most susceptible to laser injury?

(A) skin
(B) gonads
(C) eye
(D) thyroid

393. How is inhalation of the laser plume best prevented?

(A) double mask worn by scrub team
(B) filter on suction
(C) laser on standby whenever possible
(D) mechanical smoke evacuator on field

Fundamental Knowledge
Answers and Explanations

I. BASIC SCIENCES

A. Terminology

1. **(D)** Tissues or structures that are adjacent to or near another, related structure. The ovaries and the uterine tubes are adnexa to the uterus (*Mosby's Medical, Nursing, and Allied Health Dictionary*, 5th ed.).

2. **(A)** The abbreviation gt means a drop, derived from gutta, a Latin word (*Mosby's Medical, Nursing, and Allied Health Dictionary*, 5th ed.).

3. **(B)** Ung refers to ointment (*Mosby's Medical, Nursing, and Allied Health Dictionary*, 5th ed.).

4. **(A)** Proximal means nearer to a point of reference or attachment, usually the trunk of the body; proximal meaning closest (*Mosby's Medical, Nursing, and Allied Health Dictionary*, 5th ed.).

5. **(B)** Movement of a limb toward the axis of the body (*Mosby's Medical, Nursing, and Allied Health Dictionary*, 5th ed.).

6. **(A)** A condition in which there is decreased supply of oxygenated blood to a body part or organ (*Mosby's Medical, Nursing, and Allied Health Dictionary*, 5th ed.).

7. **(A)** A cystocele is a herniation or protrusion of the urinary bladder through the wall of the vagina (*Mosby's Medical, Nursing, and Allied Health Dictionary*, 5th ed.).

8. **(D)** Nulli means none. A woman who has never been pregnant is nulligravida. A woman who has not given birth to a viable infant is nullipara. The designation "para 0" indicates nulliparity (*Mosby's Medical, Nursing, and Allied Health Dictionary*, 5th ed.).

9. **(C)** The prefix pseudo means false, as in pseudoarthrosis (false joint) or pseudocyesis (false pregnancy) (*Mosby's Medical, Nursing, and Allied Health Dictionary*, 5th ed.).

10. **(A)** Petechiae are a result of tiny hemorrhages, and they range from pinpoint to pinhead size and are flush with the skin surface (*Mosby's Medical, Nursing, and Allied Health Dictionary*, 5th ed.).

11. **(C)** Kera, kerat, and kerato mean horn or also could refer to the cornea of the eye (*Mosby's Medical, Nursing, and Allied Health Dictionary*, 5th ed.).

12. **(C)** Lysis is a suffix meaning breaking down as in freeing adhesions from tissue, lysis of adhesions (*Mosby's Medical, Nursing, and Allied Health Dictionary*, 5th ed.).

13. **(C)** The letters OS mean left eye, oculus sinister (*Mosby's Medical, Nursing, and Allied Health Dictionary*, 5th ed.).

14. **(A)** Localized tissue death that occurs in groups of cells in response to disease or injury is necrosis (*Mosby's Medical, Nursing, and Allied Health Dictionary*, 5th ed.).

15. **(D)** Diaphoresis is the secretion of sweat, especially the profuse secretions associated with an elevated body temperature, physical exertion, exposure to heat and mental and emotional stress (*Mosby's Medical, Nursing, and Allied Health Dictionary,* 5th ed.).

B. Anatomy and Physiology

16. **(C)** The MRI, magnetic resonance imaging, uses radio frequency radiation as its source of energy. It affords superior soft tissue contrast, has the ability to image in multiple planes, and lacks ionizing radiation hazards. The CT scan produces a detailed cross section of tissue structure. A PET (positron emission tomography) scan examines the metabolic activity of various body structures in color-coded images. The ultrasound images deep structures by measuring and recording sound waves (*Mosby's Medical, Nursing, and Allied Health Dictionary,* 5th ed.).

17. **(D)** Atresia is the absence of a normal body opening, duct, or canal, such as the anus, vagina, external ear canal, or biliary structure (*Mosby's Medical, Nursing, and Allied Health Dictionary,* 5th ed.).

18. **(B)** Epistaxis is bleeding from the nose caused by local irritation of mucous membranes, violent sneezing, and a variety of other reasons. Also know as nose bleed (*Mosby's Medical, Nursing, and Allied Health Dictionary,* 5th ed.).

19. **(C)** Arterial blood gas (ABG) assesses the oxygen and carbon dioxide in arterial blood, measured by various methods to assess the adequacy of ventilation and oxygenation and the acid-base status (*Mosby's Medical, Nursing, and Allied Health Dictionary,* 5th ed.).

20. **(D)** A knot or knotlike mass; nerve cell bodies collected in groups (*Mosby's Medical, Nursing, and Allied Health Dictionary,* 5th ed.).

21. **(C)** Each lung is enveloped in a sac of serous membrane called the pleura. The chest cavity is lined with the parietal pleura. The lung covering is called the visceral pleura (Tortora and Grabowski).

22. **(D)** The muscular pharynx serves as a passageway for food and liquids into the digestive tract. It is also the path for air into the respiratory system. The throat runs from the nares and runs partway down the neck, where it opens into the esophagus (posterior) and the larynx (anterior) (Tortora and Grabowski).

23. **(A)** The vocal cords lie in the upper end of the larynx. They are responsible for voice production (Tortora and Grabowski).

24. **(D)** The windpipe, or trachea, conducts air to and from the lungs. It is a tubular passageway located anterior to the esophagus. It further divides into the right and left bronchi (Tortora and Grabowski).

25. **(B)** The nasal cavity is a hollow behind the nose. It is divided into right and left portions by the nasal septum. The anterior septum is made of cartilage (Tortora and Grabowski).

26. **(C)** The metacarpal bones form the palm of the hand. There are five on each side. The heads of the metacarpal are commonly called the knuckles (Tortora and Grabowski).

27. **(D)** The intercostal muscles are inserted in the spaces between the ribs. These are particularly important in respiration. They serve to enlarge the thoracic cavity upon inspiration (Tortora and Grabowski).

28. **(C)** The pectoralis major is a thick, fan-shaped muscle located in the upper chest. Its fibers extend from the center of the thorax through the armpits to the humerus (Tortora and Grabowski).

29. **(B)** The deltoid is a thick, triangular muscle that covers the shoulder joint. It is responsible for the roundness of the shoulder. It acts to abduct the arm (Tortora and Grabowski).

30. **(A)** On the anterior portion of the abdominal wall, the rectus abdominis forms a strap-like mass of muscle. It runs from the pubic bone at the floor of the abdominal cavity straight up to the xiphoid process of the sternum and the lower margins of the rib cage (Tortora and Grabowski).

31. **(B)** The pelvic floor, or perineum, has its own form of diaphragm, shaped somewhat like a shallow dish. One of the principal muscles of this pelvic diaphragm is the levator ani, which acts on the rectum and aids in defecation (Tortora and Grabowski).

32. **(A)** The gastrocnemius is the chief muscle of the calf of the leg. It is a large muscle on the posterior part of the leg. It extends the foot and helps to flex the knee upon the thigh (Tortora and Grabowski).

33. **(D)** A ligament is a band or sheet of strong fibrous tissue connecting the articular ends of bones. It serves to bind them together and facilitate or limit motion. It is a cord-like structure (*Mosby's Medical, Nursing, and Allied Health Dictionary*, 5th ed.).

34. **(A)** One parietal bone is located on each side of the skull just posterior to the frontal bone. They form the bulging sides and the roof of the cranium (Tortora and Grabowski).

35. **(A)** The sternocleidomastoid muscle extends along the side of the neck. It is sometimes referred to as the sternomastoid. It arises from the sternum and the inner part of the clavicle (*Mosby's Medical, Nursing, and Allied Health Dictionary*, 5th ed.).

36. **(A)** The forearm is the ulna. It is on the same side as the little finger. On the proximal end is the olecranon process, which forms the prominence of the elbow (Tortora and Grabowski).

37. **(B)** The sphenoid bone is a large wedge-shaped bone at the base of the skull. It lies between the occipital and ethmoid in the front, and between the parietal and temporal bones on the side (Tortora and Grabowski).

38. **(B)** The occipital bone forms the posterior part and a good portion of the base of the cranium. It is the bone in the lower part of the skull between the parietal and the temporal bones (Tortora and Grabowski).

39. **(B)** The mandible is the lower jawbone. It is the only movable bone in the skull. It is horseshoe shaped (Tortora and Grabowski).

40. **(D)** The hyoid bone is located in the neck between the mandible and the larynx. It supports the tongue and provides an attachment for its muscles. It does not articulate with any other bone (Tortora and Grabowski).

41. **(C)** In an infant there are 33 separate bones in the vertebral column. Five of these bones eventually fuse to form the sacrum, and four others join to become the coccyx. As a result, an adult vertebral column has 26 parts (Tortora and Grabowski).

42. **(A)** There are seven cervical vertebrae in the neck, 12 thoracic vertebrae, and five lumbar vertebrae (lower back) (Tortora and Grabowski).

43. **(D)** The single hyoid bone does not articulate with any other bone. It supports the tongue providing attachment sites for muscles of the tongue, neck and pharynx (Tortora and Grabowski).

44. **(A)** Regardless of age, each person usually has 12 pairs of ribs, one pair attached to each of the 12 thoracic vertebrae. Each rib articulates posteriorally with its corresponding thoracic vertebrae (Tortora and Grabowski).

45. **(C)** The clavicles are slender, rodlike bones with elongated "s" shapes. They are located at the base of the neck and run horizontally between the sternum and the shoulders. Another name is collarbone (Tortora and Grabowski).

46. **(A)** Each disk is composed of a tough outer layer of fibrocartilage (annulus fibrosus) and an elastic central mass (nucleus pulposus). This structure is soft and pulpy (Tortora and Grabowski).

47. **(C)** The upper, flaring portion or prominence of the hipbone is the ilium. Its superior border is the iliac crest. The internal surface is the iliac fossa (Tortora and Grabowski).

48. **(D)** The foramen magnum is a large hole in the inferior part of the bone (occipital) through which the medulla oblongata and its membranes, the accessory nerve (XI), and the vertebral and spinal arteries pass (Tortora and Grabowski).

49. **(D)** The tibia is the larger medial bone of the lower leg. It bears the major portion of the weight on the leg. Another name is shinbone (Tortora and Grabowski).

50. **(B)** The head of the femur fits into a lateral depression in the os coxae (the acetabulum), forming a joint. It is held in place by a ligament and by a tough fibrous capsule surrounding the joint (Tortora and Grabowski).

51. **(A)** The patella, or kneecap, is a small, triangular bone anterior to the knee joint. It is a lens-shaped sesamoid bone situated in front of the knee in the tendon of the quadriceps femoris muscle (Tortora and Grabowski).

52. **(B)** There are two categories of membranes: epithelial and connective tissue. The epithelial is further divided into the mucous membrane, which lines tubes and other spaces that open to the outside of the body, and the serous membrane, which lines closed cavities within the body (Tortora and Grabowski).

53. **(A)** Long bones consist of a rodlike shaft with knoblike ends. The longest bone in the body is the femur. Another name is the thighbone (Tortora and Grabowski).

54. **(D)** A condyle is a rounded protuberance found at the point of articulation with another bone. The distal end of the femur has large condyles. These condyles articulate with the tibia at the knee joint (Tortora and Grabowski).

55. **(B)** Osteomyelitis is an infection of bone caused by bacteria that may reach the bone from outside the body, from other sites of infection, and from adjacent structures (Tortora and Grabowski).

56. **(A)** The ends of long bones are called epiphyses. They have a somewhat bulbous shape, which provides roomy areas for muscle attachments and gives stability to the joints (Tortora and Grabowski).

57. **(C)** Several kinds of exocrine glands are associated with the skin: sebaceous (oil) glands, sudoriferous (sweat) glands, ceruminous glands and mammary glands (Tortora and Grabowski).

58. **(A)** The periosteum is a fibrous vascular membrane covering bones, except at the extremities (*Mosby's Medical, Nursing, and Allied Health Dictionary*, 5th ed.).

59. **(D)** The lens is a transparent, colorless structure in the eye that is biconvex in shape. It is enclosed in a capsule. It is capable of focusing rays so that they form a perfect image on the retina (Tortora and Grabowski).

60. **(A)** The purpose of the iris is to regulate the amount of light entering the eye. The pupil is the contractile opening in the center of the eye (Tortora and Grabowski).

61. **(D)** The iris is a thin, muscular diaphragm that is seen from the outside as the colored portion of the eye (Tortora and Grabowski).

62. **(B)** The optic nerve carries visual impulses received by the rods and cones in the retina to the brain. This is the second cranial nerve (Tortora and Grabowski).

63. **(B)** The eyeball has three separate coats or tunics. The outermost layer is called the sclera and is made of firm, tough connective tissue. It is known as the white of the eye (Tortora and Grabowski).

64. **(C)** Aqueous humor is a watery, transparent fluid found in the anterior and posterior chambers of the eye. It helps maintain the eye's conical shape and assists in focusing light rays. The posterior cavity lies between the lens and the retina and contains a jelly-like substance called vitreous humor, which helps prevent the eyeball from collapsing (Tortora and Grabowski).

65. **(C)** Normally the air pressure on the two sides of the eardrum is equalized by means of the eustachian tube. This connects the middle ear cavity and the throat. This allows the eardrum to vibrate freely with the incoming sound waves (Tortora and Grabowski).

66. **(B)** Conjunctiva is the mucous membrane that lines the eyelids and covers the anterior surface of the globe, except for the cornea. It is reflected onto the eyeball (Tortora and Grabowski).

67. **(D)** There are 31 pairs of spinal nerves. Each nerve is attached to the spinal cord by two roots, the dorsal root and the ventral root. By pairs there are eight cervical, twelve thoracic, five lumbar, five sacral, and one coccygeal (Tortora and Grabowski).

68. **(D)** The trigeminal nerve is the great sensory nerve of the face and head. It has three branches that carry general sense impulses. The third branch is joined by motor fibers to the muscles of chewing (mastication) (Tortora and Grabowski).

69. **(C)** The acoustic nerve, VIII, contains special sense fibers for hearing as well as balance from the semicircular canal of the internal ear. It is also called the vestibulocochlear (Tortora and Grabowski).

70. **(A)** The cerebellum aids in coordinating the voluntary muscles, helps maintain balance in standing, walking, and sitting, and aids in maintaining muscle tone (Tortora and Grabowski).

71. **(D)** The lobes of the cerebral hemispheres are named after the skull bones that they underlie. They are the frontal, parietal, temporal, and occipital lobes (Tortora and Grabowski).

72. **(D)** Within the medulla are three vital reflex centers of the reticular system. The cardiac center regulates heartbeat, the respiratory center adjusts the rate and depth of breathing, and the vasoconstrictor center regulates the diameter of the blood vessels (Tortora and Grabowski).

73. **(B)** The largest part of the brain is the cerebrum, which is divided into the two cerebral hemispheres (a right and a left side). It is supported by the brain stem (Tortora and Grabowski).

74. **(B)** The meninges are three layers of connective tissue that surround the brain and the spinal cord to form a complete enclosure. The outermost layer of these membranes is called the dura mater. The second layer around the brain and spinal cord is the arachnoid membrane. The third layer is the pia mater (Tortora and Grabowski).

75. **(A)** Between the arachnoid and the pia mater is the subarachnoid space. This is where the cerebral fluid circulates (Tortora and Grabowski).

76. **(B)** Within the brain are four fluid-filled spaces called the ventricles. They are cavities that communicate with each other, with the central canal of the spinal cord, and with the subarachnoid space (Tortora and Grabowski).

77. **(B)** The tympanic membrane (eardrum) transmits sound vibrations to the internal ear by means of the auditory ossicles (*Mosby's Medical, Nursing, and Allied Health Dictionary*, 5th ed.).

78. **(D)** The cochlea looks like a small spiral-shaped shell. It is a tube coiled for about two and a half turns into a spiral, around a central axis of the bone (Tortora and Grabowski).

79. **(A)** Expanding across the middle ear area are three exceedingly small bones called the auditory ossicles: the malleus, the incus, and the stapes (Tortora and Grabowski).

80. **(C)** In a cross-match of blood, the donor RBCs are mixed with the recipients serum. If agglutination does not occur, the recipient does not have antibodies that will attack the donor RBCs. If no agglutination (clumping) occurs, the donor's blood may be safely transfused to the recipient providing all the other criteria have been met (Tortora and Grabowski).

81. **(A)**   Red blood cells contain oxygen-carrying protein hemoglobin. They are called RBCs or erythrocytes (Tortora and Grabowski).

82. **(C)**   The differential white count (an estimate of the percentage of each type of white cell) is done using a stained blood slide. Some blood diseases and inflammatory conditions can be recognized this way (Tortora and Grabowski).

83. **(A)**   Incompatibility of blood transfusions may be attributable to either the plasma or red cells of the donor's blood. The red cells of the donor's blood may become clumped or held together in bunches. This process is called agglutination (Tortora and Grabowski).

84. **(A)**   Platelets are formed by the red bone marrow and are essential for the coagulation of blood and in maintenance of hemostasis (Tortora and Grabowski).

85. **(C)**   A normal adult has an average of 5,000 to 10,000 leukocytes per cubic millimeter of circulating blood, or about 1 leukocyte to 700 erythrocytes. A high white blood count is indicative of infection (Tortora and Grabowski).

86. **(B)**   The saphenous vein is the longest vein in the body. The greater saphenous vein, which is superficial, extends up the medial side of the leg, the knee, and the thigh. At the groin, it empties into the femoral vein (Tortora and Grabowski).

87. **(C)**   In the bend of the elbow, the median cubital vein ascends from the cephalic vein on the lateral side of the arm to the basilic vein on the medial side. It is the preferred vein for venipuncture (Tortora and Grabowski).

88. **(A)**   The external iliac artery changes to the femoral in the thigh. This vessel branches off in the thigh and then becomes the popliteal artery at the back of the knee joint. It subdivides below the knee. The popliteal vein is also behind the knee (Tortora and Grabowski).

89. **(B)**   The superior mesenteric artery, which is the largest branch of the abdominal aorta, carries blood to most of the small intestine as well as to the first half of the large intestine. The much smaller inferior mesenteric artery, which is located near the end of the abdominal aorta, supplies the major part of the large intestine and the rectum (Tortora and Grabowski).

90. **(A)**   The azygos vein drains the veins of the thorax and empties into the superior vena cava just before the latter empties into the heart. It also may serve as a bypass for the inferior vena cava that drains blood from the lower body (Tortora and Grabowski).

91. **(D)**   Blood from the face, scalp, and superficial regions of the neck is drained by the internal and external jugular vein. The internal jugulars flow into the superior vena cava. The external jugulars flow into the subclavian veins (Tortora and Grabowski).

92. **(C)**   Blood is supplied to the heart by the right and left coronary arteries. Branches of these two arteries encircle the heart and supply all the parts of the myocardium. Branches lead to the atrial and ventricular myocardium (Tortora and Grabowski).

93. **(B)**   Impulses that start at the sinoatrial node spread through the atrial muscle fibers, producing atrial contractions. When the impulses reach the A-V node they are relayed to the ventricles via the bundle of His and the Purkinje fibers, producing synchronized contraction of the ventricles (Tortora and Grabowski).

94. **(A)**   The right primary bronchus is more vertical, shorter, and wider than the left. As a result, foreign objects in the air passageways are more likely to enter it than the left and frequently lodge in it (Tortora and Grabowski).

95. **(D)**   The spleen is an organ containing lymphoid tissue designed to filter blood. It is frequently damaged in abdominal trauma, causing it to rupture. This causes severe hemorrhage, which requires prompt splenectomy (Tortora and Grabowski).

96. **(B)** Most parts of the body receive branches from more than one artery. The junction of two or more vessels supplying the same body region is an anastomosis. Anastomosis between arteries provides alternate routes for the blood. If a vessel becomes occluded, circulation is taken over by the alternate route; this is known as collateral circulation (Tortora and Grabowski).

97. **(B)** The left and right carotid arteries supply the head and neck. The external carotid supplies the right side of the thyroid, tongue, throat, face, ear, scalp, and the dura mater (Tortora and Grabowski).

98. **(A)** Pericardium forms the outermost layer of the heart wall. It also lines the pericardial sac. It is a loose-fitting membrane. Pericarditis is an inflammation of the lining (Tortora and Grabowski).

99. **(C)** The posterior cerebral arteries help to form an arterial circle at the base of the brain called the circle of Willis, which creates a connection between the vertebral artery and internal carotid artery systems. It equalizes blood pressure to the brain and provides alternate routes for blood to the brain (Tortora and Grabowski).

100. **(B)** The external iliac arteries continue into the thigh, where the name of these tubes is changed to femoral. Both femorals go to the genitals and abdominal wall. Other branches run to the thigh and become the popliteal (back of the knee) (Tortora and Grabowski).

101. **(D)** The descending aorta travels through the thorax, branching off to supply the thoracic organs and structure. It then passes through the diaphragm into the abdomen, supplying the abdominal organs via numerous branches. It terminates at the level of the fourth vertebra, dividing into the two common iliac arteries, which supply the pelvis and lower extremities (Tortora and Grabowski).

102. **(A)** The contractions of the heart are synchronized, and their rate is controlled by specially modified muscular tissue. The sinoatrial node, the pacemaker, is found in the right atrial wall near the opening of the superior vena cava (Tortora and Grabowski).

103. **(D)** The arterioles lead into a vast network of very fine blood vessels, the capillaries. These are the blood vessels that permeate the tissues and service the body cells directly. They play a key role in regulating blood flow from arteries to capillaries (Tortora and Grabowski).

104. **(D)** The human heart is a double pump. The two sides are completely separated from each other by a partition called the septum (Tortora and Grabowski).

105. **(D)** the tricuspid valve (right atrioventricular) closes at the time the right ventricle begins pumping in order to prevent blood from going back into the right atrium. It has three flaps or cusps and is between the right atrium and the right ventricle (Tortora and Grabowski).

106. **(B)** The endocardium, which lines the inner surface of the heart cavity, is a thin, delicate membrane composed of endothelial cells. It covers the valves, surrounds the chordae tendineae, and is continuous with the lining membrane of the large blood vessels (Tortora and Grabowski).

107. **(A)** The spleen is located in the upper left hypochondriac region of the abdomen and is normally protected by the rib cage. It is between the fundus of the stomach and the diaphragm (Tortora and Grabowski).

108. **(A)** Lymph, lymph vessels, lymph nodes, tonsils, the thymus, and the spleen make up the lymphatic system. Its function is to drain protein-containing fluid that escapes from the blood capillaries from the tissue spaces. It also transports fats from the digestive tract to the blood (Tortora and Grabowski).

109. **(D)** The s-shaped bend where the colon crosses the brim of the pelvis and enters the pelvic cavity (where it becomes the rectum) is the sigmoid colon. It begins at the left iliac crest, projects toward the midline, and terminates at the rectum (Tortora and Grabowski).

110. **(B)** The large intestine has little or no digestive function. It serves to absorb water and electrolytes. It also forms and stores feces until defecation occurs (Tortora and Grabowski).

111. **(D)** The narrow, distal part of the large intestine is called the anal canal. The rectum is the last 8 inches of the gastrointestinal tract. The terminal 2 inches is the anal canal (Tortora and Grabowski).

112. **(D)** Some organs lie on the posterior abdominal wall and are covered by peritoneum on the anterior surface only. Such organs, including the kidney and pancreas, are said to be retroperitoneal (Tortora and Grabowski).

113. **(B)** The beginning (proximal) portion of the large intestine is the cecum. It hangs below the ileocecal valve. It is a blind pouch 2.5 inches long (Tortora and Grabowski).

114. **(C)** To the cecum is attached a small blind tube known as the appendix. It is a twisted, coiled tube, 3 inches in length (Tortora and Grabowski).

115. **(A)** The gallbladder stores bile between meals and releases it when stimulated by gastric juice, fatty foods, and the hormone cholecystokinin. Bile is produced in the liver. The gallbladder stores and concentrates bile (Tortora and Grabowski).

116. **(B)** When the gallbladder contracts, it ejects concentrated bile into the duodenum. Bile is forced into the common bile duct when it is needed (Tortora and Grabowski).

117. **(B)** Pancreatic juice leaves the pancreas through the pancreatic duct, the duct of Wirsung. The pancreatic duct unites with the common bile duct from the liver and gallbladder and enters the duodenum in a small raised area called the ampulla of Vater (Tortora and Grabowski).

118. **(A)** The greater omentum is the largest peritoneal fold and hangs loosely like a "fatty apron" over the transverse colon and coils of the small intestine (Tortora and Grabowski).

119. **(B)** The hepatic duct joins the slender cystic duct from the gallbladder to form the common bile duct. The common bile duct and the pancreatic duct enter the duodenum in a common duct, the hepatopancreatic (Tortora and Grabowski).

120. **(D)** The bile pigments, bilirubin and biliverdin, are products of red blood cell breakdown and are normally excreted in bile. If their excretion is prevented, they accumulate in the blood and tissues, causing a yellowish tinge to the skin and other tissues. This condition is called obstructive jaundice (Tortora and Grabowski).

121. **(A)** The pancreas is an oblong, fish-shaped gland that consists of a head, tail, and body. The head rests in the curve of the duodenum, and its tail touches the spleen. It is linked to the small intestine by a series of ducts (Tortora and Grabowski).

122. **(B)** The ileocecal sphincter or valve joins the large intestine to the small intestine (Tortora and Grabowski).

123. **(C)** The duodenum receives secretions from the pancreas and the liver. The duodenum originates at the pyloric sphincter and extends 10 inches, where it merges with the jejunum (*Mosby's Medical, Nursing, and Allied Health Dictionary*, 5th ed.; Tortora and Grabowski).

124. **(C)** The pylorus is the region of the stomach that connects to the duodenum (Tortora and Grabowski).

125. **(A)** A broad fan-shaped fold of peritoneum suspending the jejunum and the ileum from the dorsal wall of the abdomen is the mesentery (*Mosby's Medical, Nursing, and Allied Health Dictionary*, 5th ed.).

126. **(B)** The stomach has four main regions: the cardia, fundus body, and pylorus. The large central portion is the body (Tortora and Grabowski).

127. **(D)** At the end of the pyloric canal, the muscular wall is thickened, forming a circular muscle called the pyloric sphincter. Pyloric stenosis is a narrowing of the pyloric sphincter, which prevents food from passing through (Tortora and Grabowski).

128. **(D)** The esophagus is a straight, collapsible tube about 10 inches long. It lies behind the trachea. It pierces the diaphragm at the esophageal hiatus (Tortora and Grabowski).

129. **(A)** The esophagus penetrates the diaphragm through an opening, the esophageal hiatus, which then empties into the stomach (Tortora and Grabowski).

130. **(B)** Adenoids are also known as pharyngeal tonsils. They have a glandular appearance, particularly lymphoidlike (*Mosby's Medical, Nursing, and Allied Health Dictionary*, 5th ed.).

131. **(B)** The molars job is to crush and grind food (Tortora and Grabowski).

132. **(C)** Mumps typically attack the parotid glands. It is an inflammation and enlargement (swelling) (Tortora and Grabowski).

133. **(B)** The sublingual glands are located under the tongue. They open into the floor of the mouth in the oral cavity (Tortora and Grabowski).

134. **(A)** The liver is the largest gland in the body. It is divided into left and right segments or lobes. It is located under the diaphragm. Bile is one of its chief products (Tortora and Grabowski).

135. **(D)** The glomerulus is a cluster of capillaries located on one end of the nephron. It is a rounded mass of nerves or blood vessels (Tortora and Grabowski).

136. **(D)** The ureter expands to form a collecting basin for urine in the renal pelvis. Tube-like extensions project from the renal pelvis into active kidney tissue to increase the area for collection. These are calyces (Tortora and Grabowski).

137. **(C)** Contractions of the muscular coat of the ureters produce peristaltic waves, which transport urine along the ureters. Peristalsis is the main function of the musculature (Tortora and Grabowski).

138. **(C)** The smooth, triangular area at the bottom of the bladder is the trigone. The two ureters enter the bladder at the upper corners of the trigone. Urine flows out of the urethra through the internal orifice located at the bottom of the trigone (Tortora and Grabowski).

139. **(B)** The kidneys are positioned retroperitoneally. This means that they are behind the parietal peritoneum and against the deep back muscles. Other retroperitoneal structures are the ureters and the suprarenal glands (Tortora and Grabowski).

140. **(A)** Nephrons are the functional unit of the kidney that filters blood, returns useful substances to the blood so they are not lost from the body, and removes substances from the blood that are not needed by the body (Tortora and Grabowski).

141. **(C)** Blood is supplied to the kidney through the renal artery, which arises from the abdominal aorta. The renal arteries transport about one-fourth of the total cardiac output to the kidney (Tortora and Grabowski).

142. **(A)** The hilus is a concave indentation of the medial surface of the kidney through which all structures that enter or leave the kidney pass. These structures are the renal artery, the renal vein, and the renal pelvis (Tortora and Grabowski).

143. **(D)**   The cortex is the outer part or layer of the kidney. The inner layer is the medulla (Tortora and Grabowski).

144. **(C)**   The male urethra passes through the prostate gland (prostatic portion), the pelvic floor (membranous portion), and along the length of the penis (cavernous portion) (Tortora and Grabowski).

145. **(C)**   A lack of voluntary control over micturition (urination); stress incontinence is a leakage of urine from the bladder as a result of a physical stress such as coughing or sneezing (Tortora and Grabowski).

146. **(A)**   Urine empties from the bladder through a tube called the urethra. It emerges at an opening on the exterior surface of the body called the urinary meatus (Tortora and Grabowski).

147. **(A)**   If an ovum is fertilized by a sperm cell, it most often occurs in the upper third of the uterine tubes. Fertilization may occur at any time up to 24 hours following ovulation. The ovum, whether fertilized or not, descends into the uterus within several days (Tortora and Grabowski).

148. **(D)**   In the female, the area located between the vagina and the anus is the perineum. It is cut during delivery (episiotomy) to prevent rectal tearing and subsequent damage (Tortora and Grabowski).

149. **(B)**   The small protuberance that contains specialized nerve endings sensitive to stimulation is the clitoris. It lies about 1 inch superior to the urethral orifice and is homologous to the male penis (Tortora and Grabowski).

150. **(B)**   There is no direct connection between the ovaries and the fallopian tubes. The ova are swept into the tubes by a current in the peritoneal fluid, produced by small, fringe-like projections from the abdominal openings of the tubes. These are known as fimbriae (Tortora and Grabowski).

151. **(A)**   The endometrium is the inner lining, serosa the outer layer, and the myometrium, the middle. Ovaries produce oocytes (incompletely developed ovum) (Tortora and Grabowski).

152. **(C)**   The ovaries are attached to the broad ligament of the uterus by a fold or peritoneum called the mesovarian, anchored to the uterus by the ovarian ligaments, and attached to the pelvic wall by the suspensory ligament (Tortora and Grabowski).

153. **(D)**   The spermatic cord is the supporting structure of the male reproductive system. It consists of veins, arteries, lymphatics, nerves, the vas deferens, and a small band of skeletal muscle called the cremaster muscle (Tortora and Grabowski).

154. **(B)**   A loose fold of skin called the prepuce, or foreskin, begins just behind the glans penis and extends forward as a sheath. In the female, it is formed where the labia minora unite and cover the entire body of the clitoris (Tortora and Grabowski).

155. **(A)**   The distal end of the penis is slightly enlarged and is called the glans, meaning shaped like an acorn. Covering the glans is the foreskin (Tortora and Grabowski).

156. **(B)**   The prostate gland surrounds the posterior urethra just below the urinary bladder. In older males, it often enlarges, causing interference with the excretion of urine. It is doughnut shaped and about the size of a chestnut (Tortora and Grabowski).

157. **(C)**   The urethra, in males is subdivided into three portions: the prostatic, the membranous, and the spongy (penile) urethra (Tortora and Grabowski).

158. **(A)**   The ductus (vas) deferens stores sperm and propels them toward the urethra during ejaculation (Tortora and Grabowski).

159. (B) Sperm mature in the epididymis, where they are stored and propelled toward the urethra during ejaculation (Tortora and Grabowski).

C. Microbiology

160. (D) In 1867, Lister began the age of chemical control of the atmosphere. He used aqueous phenol to disinfect instruments, soak dressings, and spray the air of surgical rooms (Bergquist and Pogosian).

161. (C) Osmosis allows the passage of a solvent, usually water, to pass through the membrane from the region of lower concentration of solute to the region of higher concentration. This tends to equalize the concentration of the two solutions (Tortora, Funke, and Case).

162. (D) The majority of microbes are aerobes. This means they grow and flourish in the presence of oxygen (Tortora, Funke, and Case).

163. (D) Leukocytes known as phagocytes rush to a wound to engulf and destroy the bacteria present. Phagocytosis means "cell eating" (Tortora, Funke, and Case).

164. (A) Agents that destroy or inactivate microorganisms are bacteriocidal. An agent that inhibits the growth of bacteria is known as a bacteriostatic agent (Bergquist and Pogosian).

165. (C) *Staphylococcus aureus* is commonly present on skin and mucous membranes, especially those of the nose and the mouth. It is Gram-positive and is the cause of such suppurative conditions as boils, carbuncles, and internal abscesses (*Mosby's Medical, Nursing, and Allied Health Dictionary*, 5th ed.).

166. (C) Microbial death occurs when an organism, or population of organisms, is no longer capable of reproduction (Bergquist and Pogosian).

167. (B) In passive natural immunity, maternal antibodies cross the placenta. Infants are immune to the same infectious diseases as their mothers for 6 to 12 months after birth. Breast fed babies receive additional protection from the breast milk (Bergquist and Pogosian).

168. (B) Microorganisms can multiply in the blood. Infection of bacterial origin carried through the bloodstream is referred to as bacteremia or septicemia. Microorganisms invade from a focus of infection in the tissue (Tortora, Funke, and Case).

169. (A) A toxoid is an inactivated toxin. Toxins are poisons produced by some infectious agents (Bergquist and Pogosian).

170. (A) When the exudate of the inflammatory process is thick and yellow with a large number of leukocytes, it is called purulent or suppurative. Suppurative is to form or generate pus (*Mosby's Medical, Nursing, and Allied Health Dictionary*, 5th ed., and Tortora, Funke, and Case).

171. (B) The unbroken skin acts as a mechanical barrier to pathogens. Only when it is cut, scratched, or burned can pathogens gain entrance. Mucous membranes entrap invaders (Tortora, Funke, and Case).

172. (A) Bacteria generally appear in one of several shapes: bacilli are rod-shaped, cocci are spherical, and spirilla and spirochetes are corkscrew-shaped (Tortora, Funke, and Case).

173. (D) In debridement damaged tissue that provides growth conditions for pathogens, is removed (Tortora, Funke, and Case).

174. (A) Herpes simplex, commonly called "cold sores" or fever blisters, is an example of a viral agent capable of latent periods where the virus is not multiplied. It remains intact until stress encourages growth. Its appearance is associated with trauma, sun, hormonal changes, and emotional upset (Tortora, Funke, and Case).

175. **(C)** Local irritation causes the small blood vessels to dilate and become more permeable. The tissue spaces become engorged with fluid, and edema results. In inflammation there is pain, redness, heat, swelling, vasodilation, and disturbance of function (Tortora, Funke, and Case).

176. **(C)** *Clostridium tetani* is the causative organism of tetany, or lockjaw. Commonly found in soil contaminated with animal fecal waste. Protection is provided by receiving tetanus toxoid to stimulate antibodies against tetanus toxins. A booster may be given when a dangerous wound is received (Tortora, Funke, and Case).

177. **(A)** The Gram stain is very useful because it classifies bacteria into two large groups: Gram-positive and Gram-negative. This provides valuable treatment options. Gram-positive bacteria tend to be killed easily by penicillins and cephalosporins. Gram-negative bacteria are generally more resistant (Tortora, Funke, and Case).

178. **(B)** When the organisms of gas gangrene are introduced into tissues where conditions permit anaerobic multiplication, they utilize amino acids and carbohydrates freed from dead or dying cells (Tortora, Funke, and Case).

179. **(A)** *Clostridium tetani* is found in soil contaminated with fecal animal waste. Improperly cleaned deep puncture wounds provide the anaerobic condition necessary for its growth. DPT immunization (which includes tetanus toxoid) is a standard immunization. A booster of toxoid may be given when a dangerous wound is received (Tortora, Funke, and Case).

180. **(B)** A beta-hemolytic streptococci, *Streptococcus pyogenes,* sometimes leads to the development of rheumatic fever. This disease usually is expressed as an arthritis. It frequently also takes the form of an inflammation of the heart, causing damage to the valves (Tortora, Funke, and Case).

181. **(C)** Anaphylactic shock is the state of collapse resulting from injection of a substance to which one has been sensitized. It is a severe allergic reaction. Death may occur if emergency treatment is not given (Tortora, Funke, and Case).

182. **(A)** *Staphylococcus aureus* is associated with skin infections such as boils, carbuncles, furuncles, and impetigo (Tortora, Funke, and Case).

183. **(B)** *Pseudomonas aeruginosa* most frequently found in burns, presents very difficult problems because the organism is generally resistant to many clinically useful antibiotics (Tortora, Funke, and Case).

184. **(A)** *S. aureus* produces furuncles, carbuncles, and impetigo. One of the most important skin invaders, it produces tissue destruction and abscesses if it escapes localization (Tortora, Funke, and Case).

185. **(B)** A wound with a poor blood supply (ischemia) can lead to necrosis (death of tissue). The death of soft tissue caused by loss of blood supply is gangrene. Gas gangrene caused by *Clostridium perfringens* develops with ischemia and necrosis (Tortora, Funke, and Case).

186. **(D)** Gas gangrene is caused by the microorganism *Clostridium perfringens* (Tortora, Funke, and Case).

187. **(A)** The most resistant form of microbial life is the endospore. Spores have a thick wall making them difficult to destroy. This enables them to withstand unfavorable conditions such as heat. They require a prolonged exposure time to high temperatures to destroy them (Tortora, Funke, and Case).

188. **(A)** *E. coli* is by far the best known enteric bacterium and is found in the intestinal tract of animals and humans (Bergquist and Pogosian).

189. **(C)**   A third-degree burn includes the skin with all its epithelial structures and subcutaneous tissue destroyed. It is characterized by a dry, pearly white, or charred-appearing surface void of sensation. The destroyed skin forms a parchmentlike eschar over the burned area (Fortunato).

190. **(B)**   In 1991, the Occupational Safety and Health Administration (OSHA) adopted requirements designed to prevent transmission of blood-borne pathogens in the work environment. It can fine health care facilities for noncompliance with regulations (Bergquist and Pogosian).

191. **(C)**   The inflammatory response is the body's attempt to neutralize and destroy toxic agents at the site of injury and prevent their spread. After injury, the metabolic rate increases, quickening heartbeat. More blood circulates to the area, causing dilation of vessels. The large amount of blood in the area is responsible for redness (Fortunato).

192. **(B)**   After debris and infected or contaminated tissue is removed by debridement, the wound is irrigated thoroughly. Devitalized tissue is removed because it acts as a culture medium. The third intention of healing requires debridement (Fortunato).

193. **(D)**   Serum or blood clots can form in this dead space and prevent healing by keeping the cut edges of the tissue separated. It is the space caused by separation of wound edges that have not been closely approximated (Fortunato).

194. **(A)**   Closure that is too tight or under tension causes ischemia, a decrease in blood supply to the tissues, and eventually tissue necrosis (Fortunato).

195. **(B)**   When the collagen in the tissue remains constant, the fiber pattern reforms crosslinks to increase tensile strength in the tissue. Tensile strength is the ability of the tissues to resist rupture (Fortunato).

196. **(A)**   Fibrinogen unites with thrombin (a product of prothrombin and thromboplastin) to form fibrin, which is the basic structural material of blood clots. It is essential for the clotting of blood (Fortunato).

197. **(B)**   A cicatrix or scar is formed by the intertwining of cells surrounding the capillaries and binding together in final closure of a wound. It is a scar left by a healing wound (Fortunato).

198. **(C)**   A keloid is a scar formation of the skin following trauma or surgical incision. The result is a raised, firm, thickened red scar. Black people are especially prone to keloids (Fortunato).

199. **(B)**   Healing by granulation (second intention) involves a wound that is either infected or one in which there is excessive loss of tissue. The skin edges cannot be adequately approximated. Generally, there is suppuration (pus formation), and abscess, or necrosis (Fortunato).

200. **(A)**   Precautions must be taken to prevent injuries. To prevent needle stick injuries, needles should not be recapped, purposely bent or broken by hand, removed from the disposable syringes, or otherwise manipulated by hand. Sharps should be place in a puncture-resistant container for disposal (Bergquist and Pogosian).

201. **(C)**   Healing by third intention implies that suturing is delayed for the purpose of walling off an area of gross infection involving much tissue removal, as in debridement of a burn when suturing is done later. Third intention of healing means that two opposing granulation surfaces are brought together. Granulation usually forms a wide, fibrous scar (Fortunato).

202. **(D)**   Loose sutures prevent the wound edges from meeting and create dead spaces, which discourage healing. Tight sutures or closure under tension causes ischemia (Fortunato).

203. **(C)** Second-intention healing is commonly referred to as granulation healing. This form of wound healing takes longer than first intention, but is equally as strong once healed. It heals from the inside to the outside surface (Fortunato).

204. **(C)** Hazardous body fluids include amniotic fluid, blood, pericardial fluid, peritoneal fluid, pleural fluid, semen, spinal fluid, synovial fluid, and vaginal secretions. Saliva has not been implicated in HIV transmission (Bergquist and Pogosian).

205. **(B)** A band of scar tissue that binds together two anatomical surfaces that are normally separate from each other is an adhesion. They are not commonly found in the abdomen, where they form after abdominal surgery, inflammation, or injury (*Mosby's Medical, Nursing, and Allied Health Dictionary*, 5th ed.).

D. Pharmacology and Anesthesia

206. **(C)** Heparin and warfarin are anticoagulant drugs that interfere with blood clotting mechanism (Association of Surgical Technologists).

207. **(B)** Kilograms, grams, milligrams, and micrograms are the metric weight designations (Association of Surgical Technologists).

208. **(D)** Dextran, artificial plasma, is used when plasma is not available (Association of Surgical Technologists).

209. **(B)** An inch is equal to 2.54 cm. To convert inches to centimeters, multiply by 2.54. To convert centimeters to inches, multiply by 0.3937 (*Mosby's Medical, Nursing, and Allied Health Dictionary*, 5th ed.).

210. **(B)** An ounce (fluid, apothecaries) is a measure for liquids. It is equal to 29.6 mL; thus, 30 mL (Tortora and Grabowski).

211. **(B)** One gram (g) is equal to 1000 mg (Association of Surgical Technologists).

212. **(B)** Epinephrine is an adrenergic which increases blood pressure (Association of Surgical Technologists).

213. **(D)** Anticholinergics block secretions, an example is atropine or scopolamine (Association of Surgical Technologists).

214. **(A)** One fluid ounce equals 29.573 mL. One milliliter equals 1 cc. Thus, 30 cc equals 1 ounce (Tortora and Grabowski).

215. **(A)** A narcotic antagonist is given to reverse the effects of a narcotic (Association of Surgical Technologists).

216. **(A)** Avitene is a microfibrillar collagen hemostatic agent. It is an adjunct to hemostasis when conventional methods are ineffective. It is an absorbable topical agent of purified bovine collagen, and it must be applied in its dry state. It is very expensive (Fortunato).

217. **(D)** Gelfoam is an absorbable hemostatic agent that aids in clot formation and absorbs 45 times its own weight in blood. Frequently it is soaked in thrombin or epinephrine solution and dipped in it before handing to the surgeon (Association of Surgical Technologists).

218. **(A)** Gelfoam can be used wet or dry. Each of the others must be applied dry (Fortunato).

219. **(C)** Heparin prolongs clotting time and may be given simultaneously, intravenously, or as a flush to keep IV lines open or to flush the lumen of a blood vessel (1 mL heparin in 100 mL normal injectable saline) (Fortunato).

220. **(A)** Warfarin sodium is a coumarin derivative that depresses blood prothrombin and decreases tendency of blood platelets to cling together, thus decreasing blood clotting. The others are either sedatives or help provide a calm, hypnotic state pre-operatively (Fortunato).

221. **(D)** An antibiotic used intraoperatively is Gentamicin (Association of Surgical Technologists).

222. **(A)** Bacitracin is a topical antibiotic (Meeker and Rothrock).

223. **(C)** Bone wax, made of refined and sterilized bee's wax is used on cut edges of bone to seal off oozing blood. Soften by kneading before use (Association of Surgical Technologists).

224. **(A)** Lasix (furosemide) increases the amount of urine secreted and is a common diuretic (Fortunato).

225. **(D)** Mannitol, an osmotic diuretic, is given prophylactically to prevent renal failure. It is also used to decrease intracranial and intraocular pressure (Fortunato).

226. **(B)** Pitocin is a trademark for an oxytocic (oxytocin), a hormone produced by the pituitary gland, which is prepared synthetically for therapeutic injection. In labor and delivery, it is given to contract the uterus after placenta delivery or systemically to control uterine hemorrhage (Fortunato; *Mosby's Medical, Nursing, and Allied Health Dictionary*, 5th ed.).

227. **(C)** Steroids reduce tissue inflammation and postoperative swelling. Examples are Decadron and Cortisporin ophthalmic ointment. In eye surgery, they are applied topically to reduce postoperative swelling. In plastic surgery, they are applied in and around the site in patients who tend to form keloids (Meeker and Rothrock).

228. **(D)** Methylprednisolone (Medrol) is an adrenal corticosteroid drug. Corticosteroids prevent the normal inflammatory response; thus, it is anti-inflammatory. In eye surgery, they reduce the resistance of the eye to invasion by bacterial viruses and fungi (Fortunato; *Mosby's Medical, Nursing, and Allied Health Dictionary*, 5th ed.).

229. **(C)** To test tubal patency, methylene blue or Indigo carmine in a saline solution are introduced into the uterine cavity. The tubes are viewed through a laparoscope. Dye seen coming from one or both tubes indicates patency (Fortunato).

230. **(B)** This dilates the pupil (Fortunato).

231. **(D)** A retrobulbar block results in a quiet eye and also immobility of the eye and lowered intraocular pressure (Fortunato).

232. **(C)** Miochol is a myotic (mytocic, miotic) used to constrict the pupil. It reduces intraocular pressure or in cataract surgery helps prevent the loss of the vitreous (Fortunato).

233. **(D)** Balanced salt solution is used to keep the cornea moist during surgery and also is an irrigant for the anterior or posterior segment (Meeker and Rothrock).

234. **(B)** Dextran is an artificial volume expander that acts by drawing the fluid from the tissues. It remains in the circulation for several hours. It is used in emergency situations to treat shock by increasing blood volume (Fortunato).

235. **(B)** Heparin is the most common drug used in vascular surgery to anticoagulate the patient. Protamine reverses heparin (Meeker and Rothrock).

236. **(C)** Heparin is reversed by protamine. It should be given slowly (Meeker and Rothrock).

237. **(C)** Type O blood is the universal donor blood. The four main types are A, B, O, and AB (Fortunato).

238. **(B)** Normal saline is used because it is isotonic (contains an amount of salt equal to that of intracellular and extracellular fluid), thus won't alter sodium, chloride, or fluid balance (Fortunato).

239. **(D)** Levophed (norepinephrine) restores and maintains blood pressure following peripheral vascular collapse or as a result of severe hypotensive or cardiogenic shock (Fortunato).

240. **(C)** Sodium bicarbonate treats acidosis. It should not be mixed in an IV line (Fortunato).

241. **(A)** During the induction phase, the patient retains an exaggerated sense of hearing until the last moment. Thus, it is essential that all personnel in the room remain as quiet as possible (Fortunato).

242. **(D)** Succinylcholine (Anectine) is an ultra-short acting agent with rapid onset and is useful to produce paralysis during intubation as well as continuing muscle relaxation when used in a dilute solution (Fortunato).

243. **(B)** The combination of a narcotic (potent analgesic) and a tranquilizer (neuroleptic) produce neuroleptoanalgesia. When these are reinforced with an inhalation anesthetic, it is call neuroleptoanesthesia (balanced anesthesia) (Association of Surgical Technologists).

244. **(A)** Benzodiazepines (sedative tranquilizers) are used in two ways to reduce the anxiety and apprehension of the patient and as an adjunct to general anesthesia to reduce the amount and concentration of other more potent agents; Valium and Versed are examples (Association of Surgical Technologists).

245. **(C)** Antimuscarinics (formerly known as anticholinergics) act as blockers of the cholinergic effects thus limit salivation and bradycardia; for example, Atropine sulfate and glycopyrrolate (Association of Surgical Technologists).

246. **(D)** Balanced anesthesia is a technique whereby the properties of anesthesia (hypnosis, analgesia, and muscle relaxation) are produced in varying degrees by a combination of agents (Fortunato).

247. **(D)** A bolus is a rapid medication dose injected all at once intravenously (Fortunato).

248. **(C)** Sedatives are drugs that soothe and relieve anxiety. The only difference between a hypnotic and a sedative is one of degree. A hypnotic produces sleep; whereas, a sedative provides mild relaxation. It is quieting and tranquilizing (*Mosby's Medical, Nursing, and Allied Health Dictionary,* 5th ed.).

249. **(A)** A Bier block provides anesthesia to the distal portion of the upper extremity by injecting an anesthetic agent into a vein at a level below a tourniquet (double cuffed). The limb is exsanguinated with Esmarch, and the cuff is inflated (Association of Surgical Technologists).

250. **(A)** Nitrous oxide has a rapid induction and recovery. It is used on short procedures, when muscle relaxation is unimportant (Fortunato).

251. **(D)** Pentothal (thiopental sodium) is potent; it has a cumulative effect and very rapid uptake from the blood. It is the most frequently used and it is short acting (Fortunato).

252. **(D)** A widely used halogenated hydrocarbon is Fluothane, also known as halothane. It is nonflammable and provides smooth induction (Fortunato).

253. **(D)** Spinal anesthesia is an extensive nerve block, sometimes called a subarachnoid block. It affects the lower spinal cord and nerve roots. It is used for lower abdominal or pelvic procedures (Fortunato).

254. **(A)** An epidural is used for anorectal, vaginal, perineal, and obstetrical procedures. Injection is made into the space surrounding the dura mater within the spinal canal (the epidural space) (Fortunato).

255. **(A)** Compazine is an antiemetic that minimizes nausea and vomiting (Fortunato).

256. **(B)** Pontocaine is tetracaine hydrochloride. It is commonly used for infiltration and nerve block (Fortunato).

257. **(C)** Nerve blocks may be used preoperatively, intraoperatively, and postoperatively to prevent pain or therapeutically to relieve chronic pain. In a field block, the surgical site is blocked off with a wall of anesthetic drug (Fortunato).

258. **(D)** Lidocaine hydrochloride (Xylocaine) is a most widely used agent. It is potent, has rapid onset and lacks local irritation effects. Allergic reactions are rare (Fortunato).

259. **(B)** Adrenalin is another name for epinephrine (Fortunato).

260. **(B)** Epinephrine is added to a local anesthetic when a highly vascular area is to be injected. It causes vasoconstriction at the operative site. This holds the anesthetic in the tissue, prolongs its effect, and minimizes local bleeding (Fortunato).

261. **(A)** LMA (laryngeal mask airway) is a device placed into the laryngopharynx through the mouth to form a low pressure seal (with an inflated balloon) around the laryngeal inlet. It is a simple, effective way of establishing a patent airway (Association of Surgical Technologists).

262. **(D)** Levophed is a potent peripheral vasoconstrictor. It is useful in peripheral vascular collapse, such as hypotension or cardiogenic shock. Some of its actions are similar to epinephrine (Fortunato).

263. **(A)** A rapid infusion pump aids in rapidly delivering blood or other fluids by means of a pressurized cuff around the administration bag to exert external force. It may also have a fluid warmer component (Association of Surgical Technologists).

264. **(C)** The pulse oximeter measures blood oxygenation. The finger tip is commonly used. It is a continuous, rapid, and easy means of assessment (Association of Surgical Technologists).

265. **(C)** Neostigmine, also known as Prostigmin, reverses the effect of muscle relaxants (Fortunato).

266. **(C)** Arterial blood gases (ABGs) involve invasive monitoring of pH, oxygen saturation, and CO_2 levels. A common site is the radial artery (arterial line or a-line). Direct blood pressure monitoring may also be performed this way (Association of Surgical Technologists).

267. **(D)** Suction must always be available and ready, along with assistance to the anesthesiologist, as induction begins for the safety of the patient (Association of Surgical Technologists).

II. INFECTION CONTROL

A. Aseptic Technique

268. **(B)** All unsterile persons should remain at least 1 foot from any sterile surface (Fortunato).

269. **(D)** Sterile tables should be set up just before the surgical procedure. Covering of tables is not recommended (Fortunato).

270. **(D)** A sterile draped table is considered sterile only on the top. The edges and sides extending below table level are considered unsterile (Fortunato).

271. **(D)** Check drapes for instruments. Roll drapes off the patient to prevent sparking and airborne contamination. Wet areas should be placed in the center to prevent soaking through the laundry bag (Fortunato).

272. **(B)** If a solution soaks through a sterile drape to an unsterile area, the wet area is covered with impervious sterile drapes or towels (Fortunato).

B. Sterilization and Disinfection

273. **(A)** Fifteen to seventeen pounds of pressure is necessary in the steam sterilizer set at 250°F It is 27 psi if set at 270°F (Fortunato).

274. **(A)** Positive assurance that sterile conditions have been achieved by either steam, ethylene oxide, or dry heat sterilization can be obtained only through a biologic control test. These should be done at least weekly. The most dependable is a preparation of living spores resistant to the sterilizing agent (Fortunato).

275. **(C)** Instruments wrapped as a set in double-thickness wrappers are autoclaved at a setting of 250°F for 30 minutes (Fortunato).

276. **(B)** In a flash (high-speed pressure) sterilizer set at 270°F, the minimum exposure time is 3 minutes for unwrapped items. With this cycle, the entire time for starting, sterilizing, etc., is 6–7 minutes (Fortunato).

277. **(D)** Rubber tubing should not be folded or kinked because steam cannot penetrate it nor displace air from folds. A residual of distilled water should be left in the lumen. Rubber bands must not be used around solid items because steam cannot penetrate through or under rubber (Fortunato).

278. **(A)** Linen packs must not weigh more than 12 pounds. Linen must be freshly laundered. Items must be fan-folded or loosely rolled (Fortunato).

279. **(D)** Gravity displacement utilizes steam under pressure to effect moist heat sterilization (Fortunato).

280. **(B)** The ultrasonic cleaner (which is not a sterilizer) utilizes ultrasonic energy and high-frequency sound waves. Instruments are cleaned by cavitation. In this process, tiny bubbles are generated by high-frequency sound waves. These bubbles generate minute vacuum areas that dislodge, dissolve, or disperse soil (Fortunato).

281. **(C)** Hinged instruments must be open with box locks unlocked to permit steam contact on all surfaces. All detachable parts should be disassembled (Fortunato).

282. **(D)** Solutions are sterilized alone on a slow exhaust cycle to prevent them from boiling over. The pressure gauge must read 0°F before opening the door. This is so the caps will not pop off (Fortunato).

283. **(D)** Wrapped basin sets are sterilized at 250°F for a minimum of 20 minutes. They are placed on their sides to allow air to flow out of them. This also helps water flow out (Fortunato).

284. **(A)** Basins and solid utensils must be separated by a porous material if they are nested, to permit permeation of steam around all surfaces, and condensation of steam from the inside during sterilization. Sponges or linen are not packaged in basins (Fortunato).

285. **(B)** EO gas is an effective substitute for most items that cannot be sterilized by heat or that would be damaged by repeated exposure to heat. It is noncorrosive and does not damage items. It completely penetrates porous materials (Fortunato).

286. **(D)** Ethylene oxide gas is used to sterilize items that are either heat or moisture sensitive. It kills microorganisms, including spores, by interfering with the normal metabolism of protein and reproductive processes (Fortunato).

287. **(B)** A proprietary (steris) chemical formulation of peracetic acid, hydrogen peroxide, and water causes cell death by inactivating the cell systems (Fortunato).

288. **(B)** Any tubing or other item with a lumen should be blown out with air to force dry before packaging, as water combines with EO gas to form a harmful acid, ethylene glycol (Fortunato).

289. (A) EO gas is highly flammable and explosive in air. By diluting it with a chlorofluorocarbon, a safe, nonflammable agent is provided. Chlorofluorocarbons destroy the ozone shield of the Earth and will be outlawed by the year 2000; thus, new alternatives are being explored (Fortunato).

290. (D) Glutaraldehyde, a high-level disinfectant is known commercially as Cidex (Association of Surgical Technologists).

291. (A) Peracitic acid is used in a machine (STERIS) that heats the sterilant and can be used for endoscopes. The cycle takes 30 minutes, and the sterilant can only be used for a single sterilization cycle, thus is more expensive than other methods (Association of Surgical Technologists).

292. (A) Items must be thoroughly rinsed before use. Solution is reusable for the time set by the manufacturer. Items must be clean and dry before submersion (Fortunato).

293. (A) Shelf life is defined as the period of time between activation, mixing, and disposal. For products without a surfactant it is 14 days, and with a surfactant it increases to 28 days. The concentration must be frequently tested during the 14- to 28-day period (using commercial test strips) (Association of Surgical Technologists).

294. (C) In cystoscopy, sterilization of instruments with steam or EO provides the greatest elimination of the risk of infection; however, it is not essential. High-level disinfection is recommended and provides reasonable assurance that items are safe to use (Meeker and Rothrock).

295. (B) The minimum exposure time at 270° with 27 psi is 3 minutes for unwrapped nonporous items only (Fortunato).

296. (C) Immersion in a 2% aqueous solution of activated, buffered alkaline glutaraldehyde is sporicidal (kills spores) within 10 hours. It is chosen for heat-sensitive items that cannot be steamed or if ethylene oxide gas (ETO) is unavailable or impractical (Fortunato).

297. (B) Lumens of instruments or tubing must be completely filled with solution. All items should be placed in a container deep enough to completely immerse them. All items should be dry before immersion so that the solution is not diluted (Fortunato).

298. (C) Moisture is essential in gas sterilization. Desiccated or highly dried bacterial spores are resistant to EO gas; therefore, they must be hydrated in order for the gas to be effective (Fortunato).

299. (B) Solutions are sterilized alone on slow exhaust so solutions will not boil over and so caps will not blow off (Fortunato).

300. (C) The most efficient dry heat sterilizer is the convection hot air oven. It is used for anhydrous oils, petroleum products and talc that steam cannot penetrate (Fortunato).

301. (B) Aeration following EO sterilization can be accomplished at room temperature; however, aeration of exposed items at an elevated temperature (in an aerator) enhances the dissipation rate of absorbed gases, resulting in faster removal. The aerator is a separate unit (Fortunato).

302. (A) EO or ETO is a chemical agent that kills microorganisms, including spores. It interferes with the normal metabolism of protein and reproductive processes, resulting in cell death (Fortunato).

303. (C) A minimum of 20 minutes is used to kill vegetative bacteria, fungi, hepatitis B, and HIV. It is 45 minutes for tuberculocidal activity (Fortunato).

304. (B) Scopes and all accessories that are soaked in activated glutaraldehyde are rinsed well in sterile distilled water to prevent tissue irritation from the solution (Fortunato).

305. **(D)** Peracetic acid or acetic acid mixed with a solution of salts (Bionox) kills microorganisms. It is used only in the STERIS system for heat-sensitive and immersible instruments. Processing is 20–30 minutes, temperature is controlled at 131°F, it is cost-effective, and environmentally friendly (Fortunato; Meeker and Rothrock).

306. **(B)** The Endoflush system is an economical, practical, and effective way to initially clean reusable, channeled instruments by removing organic debris by force flushing in a retrograde fashion (Meeker and Rothrock).

C. Packaging and Dispensing Supplies

307. **(A)** Nylon is not used for EO sterilization because of inadequate permeability; however, muslin, nonwoven fabric, paper, and plastic are safely used. Items wrapped for gas sterilization should be tagged to avoid inadvertent steam sterilization (Fortunato).

308. **(B)** Polypropylene film of 1- to 3-mm thickness is the only plastic acceptable for steam sterilization. It is used in the form of pouches presealed on two or three sides. The open sides are then heat sealed (Fortunato).

309. **(D)** Small holes can be heat sealed with double-vulcanized patches; they never can be stitched because this will leave needle holes in the muslin (Fortunato).

310. **(D)** Muslin wrappers must have two layers of double thickness (four thicknesses) to serve as a sufficient dust filter and microbial barrier. A 140-thread count muslin is used for wrappers (Fortunato).

311. **(D)** The storage life for muslin is 30 days maximum in closed cabinets. Muslin wets easily and dries quickly so water stains may not be obvious. On open shelving, the storage life is 21 days (Fortunato).

312. **(B)** If a sterile package is dropped, the item may be considered safe for immediate use only if it is enclosed in an impervious material and the integrity of the package is maintained. Dropped items wrapped in woven materials should not be used (Fortunato).

313. **(B)** After a sterile bottle is opened, the contents must be used or discarded. The cap cannot be replaced without contamination of the pouring edges. The edges of anything that encloses sterile contents are considered unsterile (Fortunato).

314. **(C)** A 1-inch safety margin is usually considered standard on package wrappers. After a package is open, the edges are unsterile (Fortunato).

315. **(B)** The top flap is opened away from self, the sides turned under, and secured. The last flap is pulled toward the person opening the package (Fortunato).

316. **(A)** When a scrub nurse opens a sterile wrapper, the side nearest the body is opened first. The portion of the drape then protects the gown, enabling the nurse to move closer to the table to open the opposite side (Fortunato).

317. **(B)** When flipping a sterile item onto a sterile field, the circulator may never reach over the sterile field and shake the item from the package (Fortunato).

D. Operating Room Environment

318. **(C)** Room temperature is maintained within a range of 68–76°F (Fortunato).

319. **(A)** Eyeglasses should be cleaned with an antiseptic solution before each operation to prevent cross contamination (Fortunato).

320. **(C)** Anyone entering the OR must wear approved, clean attire. Clean lab coats, buttoned and knee length, may be worn out of the department; however, scrub attire is changed upon OR re-entry. OR attire is not worn, uncovered, out of the OR. These policies protect the OR environment from "outside" as well as protect "outside" from OR contamination (Fortunato).

321. **(A)** Lead-lined aprons should be worn to protect the staff from radiation, especially during the use of an image intensifier. Thyroid collars are also particularly useful for protection (Fortunato).

322. **(D)** Masks should be handled only by the strings, thereby keeping the facial area of the mask clean. The mask should never be worn around the neck. Upper strings are tied at the top of the head; lower strings are tied behind the neck because criss-crossing distorts mask contours and makes the mask less efficient (Fortunato).

323. **(A)** Gloves are prelubricated with an absorbable dry powder before sterilization. This lubricant may at times cause serious complications (such as granulomas or peritonitis) if it is introduced to wounds. Therefore, gloves should be thoroughly wiped after donning (Fortunato).

324. **(C)** Electrical cords should not be kinked, curled, or tightly wrapped. They should be handled by the plug, not the cord, when disconnecting. Always remove cords from pathways before rolling in equipment because this can break the cord (Meeker and Rothrock).

325. **(D)** The effect of radiation is directly related to the amount and length of time of exposure. Exposure is cumulative (Fortunato).

III. CONCEPTS OF PATIENT CARE

A. Transportation

326. **(C)** Four people are needed to move the patient safely when using a roller. One lifts the head, one lifts the feet, one is beside the stretcher, and one is beside the OR table (Fortunato).

327. **(C)** It is the responsibility of the anesthesiologist to guard the neck and head. It also puts him or her in a better position to observe the patient. Four people are needed, and the action must be synchronized (Fortunato).

328. **(B)** There should be an adequate number of personnel to safely transfer the patient to the OR table. One person should stand next to the stretcher to stabilize it against the adjacent OR table. Another receives the patient from the opposite side of the table (Fortunato).

329. **(B)** Fractures should be handled gently. Support should be both above and below the fracture site when moving the patient. Adequate personnel should be available. The lifters on the affected side support the fracture site (Fortunato).

330. **(D)** The safety strap is 2 inches above the knee, not too tight but secure (Association of Surgical Technologists).

331. **(C)** The safety strap should be applied securely but loosely about 2 inches above the knee. This is to avoid compromise of venous circulation or pressure on bony prominences or nerves (Meeker and Rothrock).

332. **(B)** The physician is responsible for supporting and protecting the fracture site when moving the orthopedic patient. A fracture is handled gently with support above and below the fracture site (Fortunato).

B. Positioning

333. **(D)** Patient's arms should not be crossed on the chest in order to prevent hindrance of diaphragmatic movement and airway. This is essential to maintain respiratory function, to prevent hypoxia, and to facilitate inhalation anesthesia induction (Fortunato).

334. **(D)** In the supine position, heels must be protected from pressure on the table by a pillow, ankle roll, or doughnut. The feet must not be in prolonged flexion; the soles are supported to prevent footdrop (Fortunato).

335. **(A)** When a patient is positioned on his or her side, a pillow is placed lengthwise between the legs to prevent pressure on blood vessels and nerves (Fortunato).

336. **(A)** The buttocks should be even with the table edge but should not extend over the edge; otherwise, it could cause strain to the lumbosacral muscles and ligaments because the body weight rests on the sacrum (Fortunato).

337. **(D)** Legs are raised simultaneously by two people who grasp the sole of a foot in one hand and support the knee area with the other. Stirrups must be of equal height and appropriate for the size of the patient's leg (Fortunato).

338. **(D)** The requirements of the Kraske position are: patient is prone with hips over break of table, wide armboard is under head of mattress to support arms, pillow is under lower legs and ankles, padded knee strap is 2 inches above knees, table is flexed to acute angle, and small rolled towel is under each shoulder (Fortunato).

339. **(C)** When using an armboard, caution should be taken so that the arm is not hyperextended or the infusion needle dislodged. Hyperextension can cause nerve damage (Fortunato).

340. **(D)** The anesthetized patient and the elderly patient must be moved slowly and gently. This allows the circulatory system to adjust. This is for patient safety (Fortunato).

341. **(C)** The patient must not have ankles or legs crossed as this could create pressure on blood vessels and nerves. A normal reaction is for a supine patient to cross his or her legs before going to sleep (Fortunato).

342. **(D)** Injury to the brachial plexus can result from extreme positions of the head and arm. This can be avoided with proper care and careful observation (Fortunato).

343. **(D)** Ulnar nerve damage can occur from pressure from the OR table edge. The arm resting on an unpadded surface places pressure on the ulnar nerve as it transverses the elbow. This can be prevented by the use of padding, by fastening the arm securely with a lift sheet, or by placing the arms on armboards (Fortunato).

344. **(A)** The thorax is elevated when the patient is in the prone position in order to facilitate respiration. This is accomplished with supports, rolls, elevating pads, body rests, or braces (Fortunato).

345. **(B)** The patient's eyes may remain open even when the patient is under anesthesia. This exposes them to drying or trauma from drapes or instruments. They can be protected with ophthalmic ointment or taped closed (Fortunato).

C. Observation and Monitoring

346. **(B)** Diastolic blood pressure is that which exists during the relaxation phase between heartbeats. It is the point at which sound is no longer heard. Normal is about 80 (Fortunato).

347. **(D)** Systolic blood pressure occurs when a great force is caused by contraction of the left ventricle of the heart. The first sound heard is recorded as the systolic pressure (Fortunato).

348. **(A)** Tachycardia is excessive rapidity of heart action. The pulse rate is over 100 beats per minute. Some of the most common causes are exercise, anxiety, fever, and shock (Fortunato).

349. **(C)** The radial artery, at the wrist, is the most commonly used to feel the pulse (Tortora and Grabowski).

350. **(A)** To convert Fahrenheit to Celsius, subtract 32 from the number of Fahrenheit degrees and multiply the difference by 5/9, as 98.6°F − 32.0 = 66.6, times 5/9 = 37°C (*Mosby's Medical, Nursing and Allied Health Dictionary*, 5th ed.).

351. **(B)** Hypovolemia means low or decreased blood volume. Hypovolemic shock is caused by a decrease in circulating blood volume from loss of blood, plasma, or extracellular fluid. It is reversed by prompt restoration of blood volume via a transfusion of whole blood or other IV fluid or plasma expander (*Mosby's Medical, Nursing, and Allied Health Dictionary*, 5th ed.).

352. **(A)**   A suprapubic catheter (Bonanno) can be used if the bladder or urethra is injured, after some surgeries of the bladder, prostate or urethra, or when assessment is desirable regarding voluntary voiding and maintenance of urethral function and tone (Fortunato).

353. **(B)**   Urinary catheterization requires sterile technique because contamination can lead to urinary tract infection. The drainage bag is always maintained below the table level. This prevents contamination by retrograde or backward flow of urine (Fortunato).

354. **(C)**   In a third-degree burn, the skin with all its epithelial structures and subcutaneous tissue are destroyed. These burns require skin graft for healing to occur (Fortunato).

355. **(D)**   Referred to as mediastinal shift, this reaction attends entrance of either air or fluid to the pleural cavity, compressing the opposite lung and causing dyspnea (Fortunato).

356. **(A)**   Fat is the tissue most vulnerable to trauma and infection because of its poor vascularity. Good wound closure is difficult (Fortunato).

357. **(C)**   Oral intake is discontinued; usually the patient is NPO (nothing by mouth) for 8 hours preceding operation. This is done to prevent regurgitation or emesis and aspiration of contents. The preoperative medication contains an anticholinergic for inhibition of mucous secretions. The patient usually complains of dry mouth after their administration (Fortunato).

358. **(A)**   Blood samples should be sent to the lab immediately. If more than 10 minutes elapse between blood drawing and analysis, the analysis cannot be considered accurate. In the event of delay, the syringe with blood should be immediately immersed in ice and refrigerated at near-freezing temperature (Fortunato).

359. **(D)**   A prothrombin time is a clotting time test used to judge the effect of administration of anticoagulant drugs. It determines the time for clotting to occur after thromboplastin and calcium are added to decalcified plasma (*Mosby's Medical, Nursing, and Allied Health Dictionary,* 5th ed.).

D. Documentation and Records

360. **(C)**   Specific gravity measures the density of particles in the urine, thus showing the concentrating or diluting powers of the kidneys. The normal range is from 1.010 to 1.025. A low specific gravity (under 1.010) may indicate poor renal function, with the kidneys unable to concentrate urine. A high specific gravity (over 1.025) may indicate a dehydrated state (*Mosby's Medical, Nursing, and Allied Health Dictionary,* 5th ed.).

361. **(B)**   A type and cross match of blood is done if the surgeon anticipates that blood loss replacement may be necessary. In emergency situations, a sample of blood may be sent from the OR for immediate typing and cross matching (Fortunato).

362. **(A)**   The normal range hematocrit reading in males is between 43 and 49%; in females it is between 37 and 43% of whole blood volume. Hematocrit is the percentage of blood made up of RBCs (*Mosby's Medical, Nursing, and Allied Health Dictionary,* 5th ed.).

363. **(B)**   The effects of all types of hemophilia are so similar they are hardly distinguishable from one another, but each is a deficiency of a different blood-clotting factor. The most common type is hemophilia A (*Mosby's Medical, Nursing, and Allied Health Dictionary,* 5th ed.).

364. **(D)**   Even though chest disease is not related to the patient's surgery, most surgeons consider a chest x-ray an important part of a preoperative preparation. The x-ray rules out unsuspected pulmonary disease that could be communicable or would contraindicate the use of inhalation anesthetics (Fortunato).

365. **(A)** Electrocardiogram (ECG) is a graph of the electrical activity of the heart made with an ECG machine (Fortunato).

366. **(B)** The hemoglobin concentration in the blood establishes the presence or absence of anemia (if low) or of polycythemia (if high). Values less than 14 g/100 mL in an adult male or less than 12 g/100 mL in an adult female would indicate anemia. A count above 18 g in either sex would indicate polycythemia. Surgery would be delayed because bleeding is expected in tonsil surgery (Fortunato; Meeker and Rothrock).

367. **(C)** In a differential blood count, the varieties of leukocytes and their percentages are estimated. It is a microscopic exam of a very thin layer of blood on a glass slide that has been stained (*Mosby's Medical, Nursing, and Allied Health Dictionary*, 5th ed.).

368. **(D)** The circulating nurse and anesthesiologist always check the label identifying the patient and surgeon; they also check the patient's chart and the operating schedule. The surgeon sees the patient before anesthetic agents are administered (Fortunato).

369. **(A)** The Joint Commission on Accreditation of Healthcare Organizations requires that a record be kept of each operation (preoperative diagnosis, description, specimens, postoperative diagnosis, names of participants, and the intraoperative case record) (Meeker and Rothrock).

E. Cardiopulmonary Resuscitation

370. **(C)** Basic life support (BLS) should not be interrupted for more than 5 seconds at a time except for endotracheal intubation. If intubation is difficult, the patient must be ventilated between short attempts, and CPR should never be suspended for more than 30 seconds (Fortunato).

371. **(C)** External, cardiac compression maintains circulation, which provides oxygen to vital body tissues and keeps them viable. It also preserves cardiac tone and reflexes and prevents intravascular clotting. It is the rhythmic application of pressure that compresses the ventricles (Fortunato).

372. **(A)** The scrub person remains sterile, guards the sterile field, covers and packs incision, keeps counts, and gives attention to field and surgeon's needs. The other jobs are done by the circulator or additional personnel (Fortunato).

F. Medical, Ethical, and Legal Responsibilities

373. **(C)** It is the responsibility of the scrub nurse to cool an instrument in cool sterile water before handing it to the surgeon. Burns are one of the most frequent causes of lawsuits (Fortunato).

374. **(A)** Lack of consent is an aspect of assault and battery. Consent must be given voluntarily with full understanding of the implications. The procedure must be explained fully, in understandable language, so that the patient fully comprehends what will be done (Fortunato).

375. **(D)** Abandonment may be a cause for a lawsuit if an unattended patient falls from a stretcher or an OR table. It is the responsibility of a staff member to stay with the patient at all times (Fortunato).

376. **(D)** The nurse should place dentures in a properly labeled container and return them immediately to the unit. He or she will obtain a receipt, which is placed on the patient's chart. The transaction is recorded in the nurse's notes (Fortunato).

377. **(C)** Negligence is legally defined as "the omission to do something which a reasonable person, guided by those ordinary considerations which ordinarily regulate human affairs, would do, or doing something which a reasonable and prudent person would not do" (Fortunato).

378. **(D)** The Doctrine of Reasonable Man means that a patient has the right to expect all professional and technical nursing personnel to utilize knowledge, skill, and judgment in performing duties that meet the standards exercised by other reasonable, prudent persons involved in a similar circumstance (Fortunato).

379. **(C)** An employer may be liable for an employee's negligent conduct under the Respondeat Superior master–servant employment relationship. This implies that the master will answer for the acts of the servant (Fortunato).

380. **(C)** An unconditional general rule of law is that every person is liable for the wrongs he or she commits that cause injury, loss, or damage to any person's property. Liability means to be legally bound, answerable, and responsible. A patient or family member may institute a civil action against the person who caused the injury, loss, or damage (Fortunato).

381. **(D)** Quality Assurance (QA) establishes the criteria for measuring, monitoring, and evaluating patient care as well as setting standards for improvement (Fortunato).

382. **(A)** Details of an incident report must be complete and accurate. They should be written as a statement of facts without interpretation or opinion. Describe the action taken, care or treatment given, and complete according to hospital policy. The fact that an incident report was completed should *not* be mentioned in the patient's medical record, including the nurses' notes, or in the OR record (Fortunato).

7. Emotional Support

383. **(D)** Anxiety, tension, fear, questioning, suspicion, guilt, depression, withdrawal, anger, and hostility are some of the reactions a patient may experience (Fortunato).

IV. OCCUPATIONAL HAZARDS

384. **(C)** Exposure to radiation can cause genetic changes, cancer, cataracts, injury to bone marrow, burns, tissue necrosis, and spontaneous abortion and congenital anomalies (Fortunato).

385. **(C)** Film badges are the most widely used monitors measuring total rems of accumulated exposure. Data are reviewed (Fortunato).

386. **(D)** Shielding with lead is the most effective protection against gamma rays and x-rays in the form of lead-lined walls, portable lead screens, lead aprons, lead-impregnated rubber gloves, lead thyroid–sternal collars, and lead glasses (Fortunato).

387. **(A)** Eye and skin exposure must be avoided. Fire must be prevented. Avoid inhalation of laser plume. Ionizing radiation is from x-ray exposure (Fortunato).

388. **(D)** Waste anesthetic gas is gas and vapor that escape from the anesthesia machine and equipment, as well as gas released through the patient's expiration. The hazards to personnel include an increased risk of spontaneous abortion in females working in the OR, congenital abnormalities in their children as well as in the offspring of unexposed partners of exposed male personnel, cancer in females administering anesthesia, and hepatic and renal disease in both males and females. This problem can be reduced by a scavenging system that removes waste gases (Fortunato).

389. **(B)** Hepatitis B (HBV) is a major nosocomial problem. Carriers are a main source of infection. Immunization is recommended for high-risk providers because it is easily transmitted by direct contact with blood and body fluids via a needlestick or scalpel cut, a break in skin entry point, or a splash (Fortunato).

390. **(C)** Methyl methacrylate, bone cement, is mixed at the sterile field. Vapors are irritating to eyes and respiratory tract. It may be a mutagen, a carcinogen, or toxic to the liver. It can cause allergic dermatitis. A scavenging system is used to collect vapor during mixing and exhaust it to the outside or absorb it through activated charcoal (Fortunato).

391. **(D)** A patient may come to the OR infected but may not yet test positive. Careful handling of needles and sharps and using barriers to avoid direct contact with blood and body fluids are the best measures to prevent transmission. A vaccine has not been developed for immunization (Fortunato).

392. **(C)** The eye is the organ most susceptible to laser injury. Safety goggles should be worn at all times when the laser is in use. The patient's eyes must also be protected (Fortunato).

393. **(D)** A mechanical smoke evacuator or suction with a high-efficiency filter removes toxic substances including carcinogens and viruses from the air. Personnel should not inhale the fumes (Fortunato).

REFERENCES

Association of Surgical Technologists. *Surgical Technology for the Surgical Technologist: A Positive Care Approach.* Albany, NY: Delmar, 2001.

Bergquist L, Pogosian B. *Microbiology Principles and Health Science Applications.* Philadelphia: W.B. Saunders, 2000.

Fortunato N. *Berry and Kohn's Operating Room Technique,* 9th ed. St. Louis: Mosby, 2000.

Meeker M, Rothrock J. *Alexander's Care of the Patient in Surgery,* 11th ed. St. Louis: Mosby-Year Book, 1999.

Mosby's Medical, Nursing, and Allied Health Dictionary, 5th ed. St. Louis: Mosby-Year Book, 1998.

Tortora G, Funke B, Case C. *Microbiology, An Introduction,* 7th ed. Menlo Park, CA: Benjamin Cummings, 2001.

Tortora G, Grabowski S. *Principles of Anatomy and Physiology,* 9th ed. New York: John Wiley & Sons, 2000.

PART 2

Preoperative Preparation
Questions

DIRECTIONS (Questions 394 through 718): Each of the numbered items or incomplete statements in this section is followed by answers or completions of the statement. Select the ONE lettered answer or completion that is BEST in each case. Check your answers with the correct answers at the end of the chapter.

I. PHYSICAL ENVIRONMENT OF THE OPERATING ROOM

A. Preparation

394. Room temperature for infants and children should be maintained as warm as

    (A) 70°
    (B) 80°
    (C) 85°
    (D) 95°

395. Areas needing special cleaning attention on a weekly or monthly routine would include

    (A) furniture
    (B) air conditioning grills and walls
    (C) ceiling and wall mounted fixtures and tracks
    (D) kick buckets

B. Maintenance

396. A glass suction bottle should ideally be

    (A) rinsed with tap water between each case
    (B) cleaned with a disinfectant solution and autoclaved before reuse
    (C) rinsed with sterile distilled water between each case
    (D) autoclaved daily

397. Storage shelves must be cleaned with a germicide

    (A) each case
    (B) each day
    (C) each week
    (D) each month

398. While a surgical case is in progress

    (A) doors remain open so staff can easily move in or out
    (B) doors should remain closed
    (C) doors remain open to circulate air
    (D) doors may be opened or closed

399. When cleaning the floor between cases

    (A) a clean mop head must be used each time
    (B) a two-bucket system, one detergent and one clear water, is used
    (C) buckets must be emptied and cleaned between each case
    (D) all of the above

400. A dropped sterile item may only be used if the

    (A) wrapper is muslin
    (B) wrapper is impervious and contact area is dry
    (C) wrapper is impervious with contact area wet or dry
    (D) wrapper is dusted off thoroughly

II. PATIENT-RELATED PROCEDURES

A. Consents

401. In the event that a child needs emergency surgery, and the parents cannot be located to sign the permission

    (A)   no permission is necessary
    (B)   permission is signed by a court of law
    (C)   permission is signed by the physician
    (D)   a written consultation by two physicians other than the surgeon will suffice

402. The patient is scheduled for an appendectomy. After completing this procedure the surgeon decides to remove a mole from the shoulder while the patient is still under anesthesia. No permission was obtained for this. The circulating nurse should

    (A)   report it to the anesthesiologist
    (B)   report it to the chief of surgery
    (C)   report it to the supervisor or proper administrative authority
    (D)   let the surgeon proceed because it is his or her responsibility to obtain the consent

403. The surgical consent form can be witnessed by each of the following EXCEPT

    (A)   the surgeon
    (B)   a nurse
    (C)   an authorized hospital employee
    (D)   the patient's spouse

404. The patient is premedicated and brought to the operating room for a cystoscopy and an open reduction of the wrist. Upon arrival in the operating room, it is observed that the patient has only signed for the cystoscopy. The correct procedure would be to

    (A)   cancel surgery until a valid permission can be obtained
    (B)   have the patient sign for the additional procedure in the operating room
    (C)   ask the patient verbally for consent and have witnesses attest to it
    (D)   let the surgeon make the decision as to whether surgery could be done

405. A general consent form is

    (A)   a form authorizing all treatments or procedures
    (B)   a form for all patients having general anesthesia
    (C)   a form for all patients having hazardous therapy
    (D)   another name for an operative permit

406. The ultimate responsibility for obtaining consent lies with the

    (A)   operating room supervisor
    (B)   circulating nurse
    (C)   surgeon
    (D)   unit charge nurse

407. The surgical consent is signed

    (A)   before induction
    (B)   in the holding area
    (C)   the morning of surgery
    (D)   before administration of preoperative medications

408. An informed consent

    (A)   authorizes routine duties carried out at the hospital
    (B)   protects patient from unratified or unwanted procedures
    (C)   protects the surgeon and the hospital from claims of an unauthorized operation
    (D)   B and C

409. Implied consent

    (A)   is the preferred option for consents
    (B)   is allowed by law in emergencies when no other authorized person may be contacted.
    (C)   is never legally valid
    (D)   is the permission for surgical action.

410. Which statement regarding the withdrawal of a consent by a patient is NOT true?

(A) the surgeon informs the patient of the dangers if the procedure is not carried out

(B) the surgeon informs the hospital administration of the patient's refusal

(C) the surgeon obtains a written refusal from the patient

(D) the surgeon may do the procedure if he documents that it is necessary as a lifesaving measure

B. Positions for Operative Procedures

411. Which position would be the most desirable for a pilonidal cystectomy or a hemorrhoidectomy?

(A) lithotomy
(B) Kraske
(C) knee–chest
(D) modified prone

412. A position often used in cranial procedures is called

(A) Fowler's
(B) Kraske
(C) Trendelenburg
(D) lithotomy

413. In positioning for laminectomy, rolls or bolsters are placed

(A) horizontally, one under the chest and one under the thighs

(B) longitudinally to support the chest from axilla to hip

(C) longitudinally to support the chest from sternum to hip

(D) below the knees

414. The position used for a patient in hypovolemic shock is

(A) modified Trendelenburg
(B) reverse Trendelenburg
(C) supine
(D) dorsal recumbent

415. A Mayfield table would be used for which type of surgery?

(A) ophthalmic
(B) gynecologic
(C) neurologic
(D) urologic

416. Good exposure for thyroid surgery is ensured by all of the following EXCEPT

(A) modified dorsal recumbent with shoulder roll

(B) hyperextension of the neck

(C) utilization of skin-stay sutures

(D) firm retraction of the laryngeal nerve and surrounding structures

417. A procedure requiring the patient to be positioned supine in modified lithotomy is

(A) colonoscopy
(B) abdominoperineal resection (APR)
(C) marsupilization of pilonidal cyst
(D) ileostomy

418. In which procedure may the patient be placed in a supine position with the right side slightly elevated by a wedge to tilt the patient to the left?

(A) cerclage
(B) marsupilization of Bartholin's cyst
(C) Shirodkar
(D) cesarean section

419. The position for most open bladder surgery would be

(A) lithotomy
(B) supine, bolster under pelvis
(C) reverse Trendelenburg
(D) Fowler's, modified

420. In which circumstance could the patient sustain injury to the pudendal nerves?

(A) positioned on the fracture table
(B) positioned in lateral chest
(C) positioned in lithotomy
(D) positioned on the urological table

421. Which factor is important to consider when positioning the aging patient?

(A) skeletal changes
(B) limited range of motion of joints
(C) tissue fragility
(D) all of the above

422. When positioning the patient for a procedure, which of the following provides maximum patient safety and maximum surgical site exposure?

(A) patient's body does not touch metal on table
(B) equipment, Mayo stand, or personnel are not resting on the patient
(C) bony prominences are padded
(D) all of the above

C. Skin Preparation

423. When preparing a patient for a breast biopsy, a breast scrub is either eliminated or done very gently because of

(A) patient anxiety
(B) dispersal of cancer cells
(C) contamination
(D) infection

424. The ideal place to do the shave prep is in the

(A) patient's room
(B) operating room (OR) suite
(C) holding area of the OR
(D) room where the surgery will be performed

425. Any area that is considered contaminated

(A) should be scrubbed last or separately
(B) should not be scrubbed at all
(C) should be scrubbed first
(D) needs no special consideration

426. In preparation for surgery, skin should be washed and painted

(A) from the incision site to the periphery in a circular motion
(B) from the periphery to the incision site in a circular motion

(C) in a side-to-side motion
(D) in an up-and-down motion

427. Preliminary preparation of the patient's skin begins

(A) with a preoperative shower
(B) with the shave preparation
(C) in the OR
(D) in the holding area

D. Draping

428. Suction tubing is attached to the drapes with a(n)

(A) towel clip
(B) nonperforating clamp
(C) Kocher clamp
(D) Allis clamp

429. All of the following statements regarding sterility are true EXCEPT

(A) wrapper edges are unsterile
(B) instruments or sutures hanging over the table edge are discarded
(C) sterile persons pass each other back to back
(D) a sterile person faces a nonsterile person when passing

430. When draping a table, the scrub nurse should drape

(A) back to front
(B) front to back
(C) side to side
(D) either A or B

431. A seamless, stretchable material often used to cover extremities during draping is

(A) Esmarch
(B) ace bandage
(C) Kling
(D) stockinette

432. Drapes are

(A) adjusted after placement for correct position
(B) unfolded before being carried to OR table

(C)   passed across the table to surgeon along with towel clips

(D)   placed on a dry area

433.   Which statement demonstrates a break in technique during the draping process?

(A)   gloved hands may touch the skin of the patient

(B)   discard a drape that becomes contaminated

(C)   discard a sheet that falls below table level

(D)   cover or discard a drape that has a hole

434.   A head drape consists of

(A)   medium sheet, towel, towel clip

(B)   two medium sheets, towel clip

(C)   one small sheet, one medium sheet, towel clip

(D)   towel, fenestrated sheet

III. SCRUB TASKS

A. Scrub, Gown, and Glove

435.   Gowns are considered sterile only from

(A)   waist to neck level in front and back, and the sleeves

(B)   waist to shoulder, front and back, and the sleeves

(C)   neck to thighs in front, and the sleeves

(D)   only in front from chest to sterile field level, and sleeves from elbow to cuffs

436.   An acceptable action when drying the hands and arms after the surgical scrub is to

(A)   dry from elbow to fingertip

(B)   dry thoroughly, cleanest area first

(C)   keep the hands and arms close to the body, at waist level

(D)   dry one hand and arm thoroughly before proceeding to the next

437.   All of the following statements regarding gowning another person are true EXCEPT

(A)   open the hand towel and lay it on the person's hand

(B)   hand the folded gown to the person at the neckband

(C)   keep hands on the outside of the gown under a protective cuff

(D)   release the gown once the person touches it

438.   Which statement regarding the scrub procedure is *not* true?

(A)   reduces the microbial count

(B)   leaves an antimicrobial residue

(C)   renders the skin aseptic

(D)   removes skin oil

439.   If the scrub nurse needs to change a glove during an operation

(A)   the scrub must also regown

(B)   the circulator pulls the glove off

(C)   the scrub pulls the glove off

(D)   the scrub uses closed-glove technique to reapply gloves

440.   Which statement regarding the removal of gown and gloves does *not* meet safe criteria?

(A)   the gloves are removed before the gown

(B)   the gown is pulled off inside-out

(C)   the gown is untied by the circulator

(D)   the gloves are removed inside-out

441.   An effective surgical scrub procedure is

(A)   time method

(B)   brush-stroke method

(C)   3-minute anatomic method

(D)   A and B

442.   Regarding the surgical scrub, which statement would violate acceptable practice?

(A)   fingernails should not reach beyond fingertip

(B)   nail polish may be worn if freshly applied

(C)   anyone with a cut, abrasion, or hang-nail should not scrub

(D)   a non-oil-based hand lotion may be used to protect the skin

443. Eyewear, goggles, and/or faceshields should be worn

(A) on every case
(B) on orthopedic cases
(C) on vascular cases
(D) on positive HIV cases

444. The surgical scrub is

(A) sterilization of the skin
(B) mechanical cleansing of the skin
(C) chemical cleansing of the skin
(D) mechanical washing and chemical antisepsis of the skin

445. Scrub technique ends

(A) 2 inches below the elbow
(B) just below the elbow
(C) at the elbow
(D) 2 inches above the elbow

446. Which statement regarding the surgical scrub indicates INAPPROPRIATE preparation by the scrub?

(A) artificial nails/devices must not cover nails
(B) nail polish may be worn, if not chipped
(C) finger nails should not reach beyond fingertips
(D) skin should be protected with a non-oil-based product

447. Which statement best describes an effective surgical hand scrub?

(A) time, no anatomical sequence
(B) number of strokes, no anatomical sequence
(C) time or number of strokes, hand to elbow sequence
(D) number of strokes, elbow to hand sequence

448. The brush-stroke method of scrubbing prescribes the number of strokes required. Indicate the number for each: nails, fingers, hand (back and palm) and arms.

(A) 40, 30, 30, 30
(B) 40, 40, 20, 20

(C) 30, 20, 20, 20
(D) 30, 20, 10, 10

B. Basic Setups

a. Instrumentation

449. A surgical treatment for scoliosis could employ the use of

(A) skeletal traction
(B) external fixation
(C) compression plate and screws
(D) Harrington rods

450. What is a Lebsche used for?

(A) to open the sternum
(B) to retract spinal nerves
(C) to elevate the periosteum
(D) to separate the ribs

451. A rongeur used extensively in surgery of the spine and in neurosurgery is the

(A) Adson
(B) Cobb
(C) Kerrison
(D) Cloward

452. Bakes are

(A) retractors
(B) common duct dilators
(C) uterine dilators
(D) elevators

453. A rib retractor is a

(A) Weitlaner
(B) Finochietto
(C) Harrington
(D) Beckman

454. A Doyen is a

(A) rib shears
(B) rib cutter
(C) rib spreader
(D) rib raspatory

455. The instrument used to enlarge the burr hole made during a craniotomy is a

(A) rongeur
(B) periosteal elevator
(C) Gigli saw
(D) Cloward punch

456. Wescott scissors are used in

(A) plastic surgery
(B) ophthalmic surgery
(C) vascular surgery
(D) orthopedic surgery

457. The instrument used in a splenectomy is a

(A) Doyen
(B) Allen
(C) Jacobs
(D) pedicle clamp

458. Bowman probes are used in

(A) common bile duct surgery
(B) lacrimal surgery
(C) kidney surgery
(D) bladder surgery

459. A Hurd dissector and pillar retractor is used for

(A) appendectomy
(B) plastic surgery
(C) nasal surgery
(D) tonsillectomy

460. The Lempert elevator is used in surgery of the

(A) eye
(B) nose
(C) ear
(D) bones

461. A Scoville retractor is used in a

(A) total knee replacement
(B) meniscectomy
(C) laminectomy
(D) carpal tunnel release

462. A Bailey is a

(A) clamp
(B) rongeur

(C) dissecting forceps
(D) rib approximator

463. A Sauerbruch is a(n)

(A) elevator
(B) raspatory
(C) retractor
(D) rongeur

464. An Auvard is a

(A) forceps
(B) dissector
(C) speculum
(D) sound

465. A Babcock is used to

(A) grasp bone
(B) grasp delicate structures
(C) clamp vessels
(D) retract soft tissue

466. Nasal cartilage is incised with a

(A) Ballenger swivel knife
(B) Freer elevator
(C) Duckbill rongeur
(D) Hurd dissector

467. A self-retaining retractor is a

(A) Weitlaner
(B) Lincoln
(C) Hibbs
(D) Deaver

468. A rectal speculum is a

(A) Percy
(B) Hirshmann
(C) Pennington
(D) Hill

469. A small fine needle holder used in plastic surgery is a

(A) Ryder
(B) Heaney
(C) Webster
(D) Castroviejo

470. A kidney pedicle clamp is a

(A) Lincoln
(B) Herrick
(C) Love
(D) Little

471. Uterine dilators are

(A) Hanks
(B) Van Buren
(C) Bakes
(D) Graves

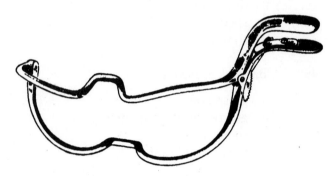

472. On which set would this instrument shown above be found?

(A) thyroidectomy set
(B) perineorrhaphy set
(C) tonsillectomy set
(D) orthopedic bone set

Illustrations above reprinted, with permission, courtesy of Pilling Surgical.

For Questions 474–481 refer to figures on page 67.

473. The instrument shown above used to retrieve a needle biopsy from either thyroid, liver, kidney, or prostate is

(A) Dorsey
(B) Chiba
(C) Bernardino–Sones
(D) Silverman

474. The instrument(s) used for a corrective rhinoplasty is/are

(A) 5
(B) 3 and 8

(C) 1 and 3
(D) 3 and 5

475. The instrument(s) found on a cholecystostomy setup is/are

(A) 4 and 5
(B) 4
(C) 1
(D) 3

476. Which instrument is an O'Sullivan–O'Connor?

(A) 2
(B) 3
(C) 4
(D) 5

477. The instrument(s) found on an intestinal setup is/are

(A) 1
(B) 2
(C) 4 and 5
(D) 1 and 5

478. The retractor in a thorocotomy set to separate the ribs is

(A) 1
(B) 3
(C) 6
(D) 2

479. The retractor known as a Green is

(A) 2
(B) 3
(C) 5
(D) 7

480. An instrument found in a major bone set is a

(A) 8
(B) 6
(C) 3
(D) 7

481. Which instrument is a Davidson?

(A) 1
(B) 2
(C) 3
(D) 7

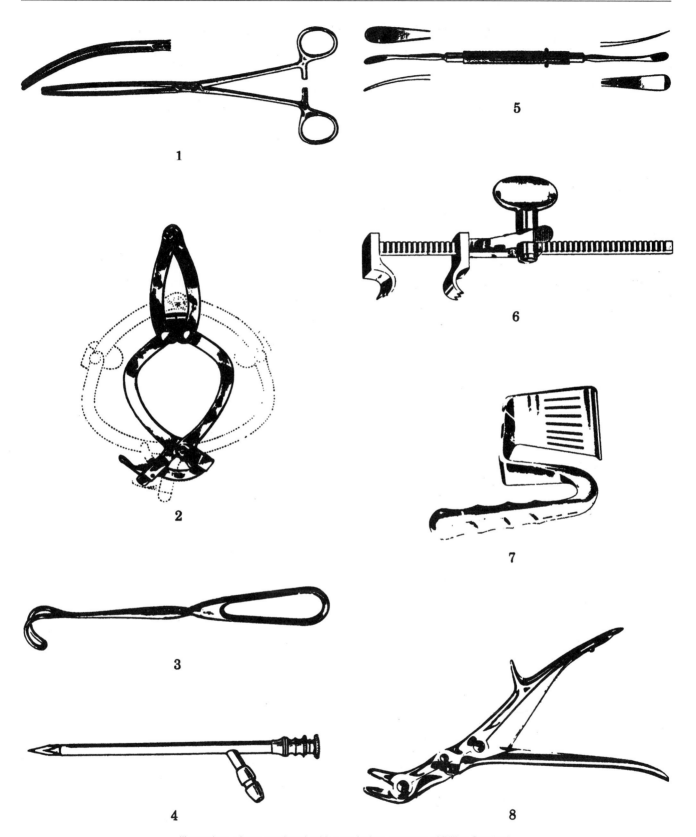

Illustrations above reprinted, with permission, courtesy of Pilling Surgical.

For Questions 482–487 refer to figures on page 69.

482. The instrument used to grasp lung tissue is

    (A) 1
    (B) 2
    (C) 3
    (D) 4

483. The instrument(s) found on a vascular setup is/are

    (A) 2, 3, 5, and 6
    (B) 1, 3, and 5
    (C) 3 and 5
    (D) 2 and 3

484. The instrument known as a bulldog is

    (A) 1
    (B) 2
    (C) 3
    (D) 6

485. Which instrument is a Heaney?

    (A) 1
    (B) 2
    (C) 3
    (D) 4

486. Which instrument is a Potts–Smith?

    (A) 1
    (B) 3
    (C) 5
    (D) 6

487. The instrument(s) used to clamp the aorta is/are

    (A) 1
    (B) 3
    (C) 6
    (D) 1 and 3

488. This needle holder is called

    (A) Jameson
    (B) Castroviejo
    (C) Wescott
    (D) Webster

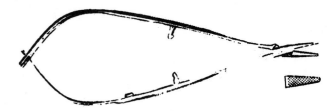

489. This kidney instrument is called

    (A) Mayo pedicle clamp
    (B) Herrick pedicle clamp
    (C) Randall stone forceps
    (D) Lewkowitz lithotomy forceps

490. The retractor pictured is called

    (A) Deaver
    (B) Oschner malleable
    (C) Harrington
    (D) Richardson

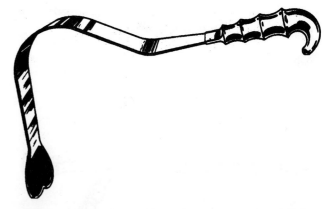

Illustrations above reprinted, with permission, courtesy of Pilling Surgical.

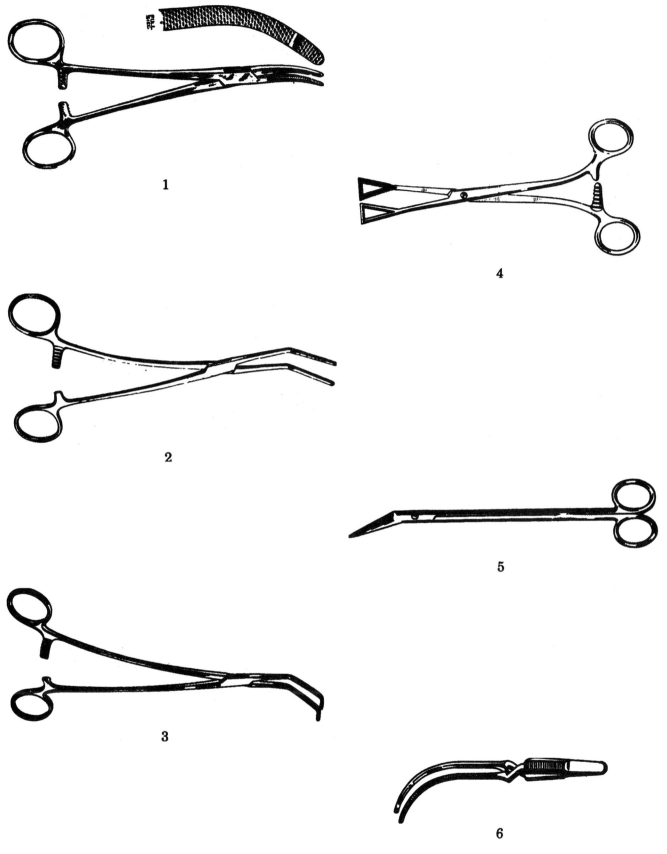

Illustrations above reprinted, with permission, courtesy of Pilling Surgical.

491. This forceps is called

    (A) Ferris–Smith
    (B) alligator
    (C) Adair
    (D) bayonet

Illustration above reprinted, with permission, courtesy of Pilling Surgical.

492. A technique utilizing the insertion of a needle or wire through a needle in order to identify suspicious breast tissue is a(n)

    (A) incisional biopsy
    (B) wire localization
    (C) Silverman needle biopsy
    (D) magnetic resonance imaging (MRI)

493. A forceps used to remove stones in biliary surgery is a

    (A) mixter
    (B) Lahey gall duct
    (C) Potts–Smith
    (D) Randall

494. Which procedure may require the preparation of a skin graft setup?

    (A) total radical mastectomy
    (B) modified radical mastectomy
    (C) adenomammectomy
    (D) lumpectomy

495. Right-angled pedicle clamps would be found on a setup for

    (A) splenectomy
    (B) cholecystectomy
    (C) hemorrhoidectomy
    (D) thyroidectomy

496. Blunt nerve hooks are selected for a _____ setup.

    (A) vagotomy
    (B) colostomy
    (C) gastrojejunostomy
    (D) abdominal–perineal resection

497. In which procedural setup would a T-tube be found?

    (A) exploration of the common bile duct
    (B) cholecystectomy
    (C) cholelithotripsy
    (D) choledochoscopy

498. Stapedectomy requires all of the following items EXCEPT

    (A) small microsuction
    (B) speculum
    (C) prosthesis
    (D) autograft

499. Cochlear implants utilize an electrode device

    (A) to restore hearing
    (B) to aerate the mastoid
    (C) to allow drainage
    (D) to relieve vertigo

500. All of the following are required for repair of a nasal fracture EXCEPT

    (A) bayonet forceps
    (B) Ballenger swivel knife
    (C) splint
    (D) Asch forceps

501. A forceps used in nasal surgery is a(n)

    (A) bayonet
    (B) Russian
    (C) rat–tooth
    (D) alligator

502. All of the following instruments can be found on a nasal setup EXCEPT

    (A) Freer elevator
    (B) bayonet forceps
    (C) Potts forceps
    (D) Frazier suction tube

503. On which setup would bougies be found?

    (A) tonsillectomy
    (B) esophagoscopy
    (C) radical neck
    (D) parotidectomy

504. All of the following can be found on a tonsillectomy setup EXCEPT

(A) Yankauer suction
(B) Hurd dissector and pillar retractor
(C) tongue depressor
(D) Jameson hook

505. Tissue expanders are used in

(A) augmentation mammoplasty
(B) reduction for gynecomastia
(C) transrectus myocutaneous flap
(D) breast reconstruction

506. The fracture treated with arch bars is

(A) nasal
(B) mandibular
(C) zygomatic
(D) orbital

507. Rib removal for surgical exposure of the kidney requires all of the following EXCEPT a(n)

(A) Alexander periosteotome
(B) Doyen raspatory
(C) Heaney clamp
(D) Stille shears

508. Stone forceps on a kidney set are

(A) Lewkowitz
(B) Randall
(C) Satinsky
(D) Mayo

509. A Sarot is a

(A) bronchus clamp
(B) scapula retractor
(C) lung retractor
(D) lung grasping clamp

510. Which item would not be included on a setup for a transvenous (endocardial) pacemaker?

(A) tunneling instrument
(B) intra-aortic balloon pump
(C) fluoroscopy
(D) defibrillator

511. The most frequent conditions requiring the use of a permanent pacemaker are

(A) coronary or mitral insufficiency
(B) pulmonary artery or vein stenosis
(C) heart block, bradyarrhythmia
(D) pulmonary stenosis, ventricular septal defect

512. Which setup would include distraction and compression components?

(A) Harrington rods
(B) intramedullary nail
(C) arthrodesis
(D) tibial shaft fracture

513. Traction applied directly on bone via pins, wires, or tongs is

(A) internal
(B) closed
(C) skeletal
(D) counter pressure

514. Skeletal traction of a lower leg is accomplished with the use of a(n)

(A) Kirschner wire
(B) Knowles pin
(C) Eggers plate
(D) Smith–Peterson nail

515. In orthopedic surgery, the viewing of the progression of a procedure on a television screen is known as

(A) image intensification
(B) radiography
(C) portable filming
(D) x-ray

516. A neurologic study in which a radiopaque substance is injected into the subarachnoid space through a lumbar puncture is called a(n)

(A) cerebral angiography
(B) myelogram
(C) encephalogram
(D) diskogram

517. A neuro headrest skull clamp is called a(n)

(A) Sachs
(B) Frazier
(C) Adson
(D) Mayfield

518. Maintenance of acceptable blood pressure and prevention of the development of air emboli in the neurosurgical patient can be effected by preoperative utilization of

(A) an antigravity suit
(B) Ace bandages
(C) thrombo-embolic device (TED) stockings
(D) adequate body support

519. A _____ is a mouth gag.

(A) Burlisher
(B) Blair
(C) Dingman
(D) Forman

520. Specialized instruments for a cleft lip repair would include

(A) Cupid's bow
(B) Logan's bow
(C) arch bar
(D) wire scissors

521. Cloward instrumentation would be included for surgery of the

(A) hip
(B) femur
(C) cervical spine
(D) lumbar spine

522. On which setup would a Beaver knife handle be found?

(A) orthopedic
(B) pediatric
(C) gynecologic
(D) eye

523. Which procedure requires a sterile setup?

(A) manual skin traction
(B) skin traction
(C) skeletal traction
(D) closed reduction

524. A craniotomy may employ the use of a(n) _____ for exposure.

(A) Mayfield
(B) Sugita
(C) Heifetz
(D) Leyla–Yasargil

525. On which setup would either a Pereyra or a Stamey needle be found?

(A) urologic
(B) eye
(C) orthopedic
(D) thoracic

526. Disintegration of kidney stones through a liquid medium is accomplished with a(n)

(A) nephroscope
(B) extracorporeal shock wave lithotriptor
(C) laser
(D) cystoscope

527. A urology perineal retractor system is called

(A) Bookwalter
(B) O'Sullivan–O'Conner
(C) Omni–Tract
(D) Lowsley

528. Which procedure would utilize a Mason–Judd retractor?

(A) bladder
(B) uterus
(C) hip
(D) nose

529. A Furlow inserter is used in

(A) penile implantation
(B) femoral–popliteal bypass
(C) total hip replacement
(D) intraocular lens (IOL) implant

530. On which case would a boomerang be found?

(A) prostate
(B) ovary
(C) eye
(D) nose

531. A Millin is a(n)

(A) prostatic enucleator
(B) urological needle holder
(C) stone forceps
(D) retropubic bladder retractor

532. Which setup would include a Gomco clamp?

(A) colostomy
(B) breast augmentation
(C) circumcision
(D) femoral popliteal bypass

533. In which surgical specialty would a Humi Cannula be used?

(A) gynecologic
(B) ophthalmic
(C) orthopedic
(D) vascular

534. An instrument used in laparoscopy to manipulate the uterus for increased structure visibility is the

(A) Verres
(B) Pratt
(C) Mayo–Hegar
(D) Hulka

535. A central venous pressure (CVP) catheter insertion requires

(A) a sterile setup
(B) a crash cart
(C) an IV technician
(D) none of the above

536. The purpose of a set of Bakes would be

(A) anal dilation
(B) esophageal dilation
(C) common duct dilation
(D) cervical dilation

537. A Steffee plate is a

(A) shoulder replacement
(B) knee joint replacement
(C) femoral implant
(D) spinal implant

538. Skeletal traction is accomplished with

(A) Sayre sling
(B) Minerva jacket
(C) Crutchfield tongs
(D) Steffee system

539. The Bookwalter is a _____ instrument.

(A) clamping
(B) holding
(C) suturing
(D) retracting

540. Which instrument is a retractor?

(A) Harrington
(B) Doyen
(C) Crile
(D) Allen

541. A long thoracic forceps is a

(A) Semb
(B) Schnidt
(C) Sauerbruch
(D) Doyen

542. A bougie is a

(A) clamp
(B) dilator
(C) retractor
(D) grasper

b. Equipment

543. Which graft must be obtained with a dermatome?

(A) split-thickness mesh graft
(B) full-thickness Wolfe graft
(C) free myocutaneous graft
(D) full-thickness pinch graft

544. A Cavitron unit is used for

(A) cyclodialysis
(B) photocoagulation
(C) phacoemulsification
(D) cryotherapy

545. The power source for Hall power equipment is

(A) carbon dioxide
(B) nitrous oxide
(C) nitrogen
(D) electricity

546. A neurosurgical drill used for precision cutting, shaping, and repair of bone is the

(A) Bermann
(B) Air Drill 100
(C) Mayfield
(D) Gardner

547. In what surgery would a small fragment compression set be used?

(A) hip fracture
(B) femoral fracture
(C) pelvic fracture
(D) olecranon fracture

548. A permanent pacemaker operates on a pulse generator powered by

(A) nitrogen
(B) titanium
(C) electricity
(D) lithium

549. Which item is an air drill?

(A) Reese
(B) Padgett–Hood
(C) Hall
(D) Brown

550. Hypothermia is employed in cardiac surgery

(A) to reduce oxygen consumption
(B) to reduce elevated temperature
(C) to slow metabolism
(D) to induce ventricular fibrillation

551. Which item is *not* a component of a cardiopulmonary bypass system?

(A) oxygenator
(B) heat exchanger
(C) ventricular fibrillator
(D) pump

552. Which movement in a power instrument drills holes or inserts screws, wires, or pins?

(A) rotary movement
(B) reciprocating movement
(C) oscillating movement
(D) alternating movement

553. The power instrument that is small, lightweight, free of vibration, and easy to handle for pinpoint accuracy at high speed is

(A) electrically powered
(B) battery-powered
(C) sonic energy-powered
(D) air-powered

554. The power source for the Air Drill 100 is

(A) electricity
(B) fiberoptic bundles
(C) ultrasonic power
(D) compressed nitrogen

555. The power source for air-powered dermatomes is

(A) compressed nitrogen
(B) nitrous oxide
(C) air
(D) A or C

556. Suction tubing should be processed in the following way

(A) residual of distilled water in lumen, steam sterilize, tubing coiled
(B) residual of saline in lumen, ethylene oxide sterilization (ETO), tubing coiled
(C) lumen dried thoroughly, ETO, tubing banded
(D) A or B

557. The suction tip that is right angled and is used for small amounts of fluid such as in brain surgery is

(A) Poole
(B) Ferguson–Frazier
(C) Yankauer
(D) Tungsten

558. Which suction tip has an angle and is used in the mouth or throat?

- (A) Ferguson
- (B) Ferguson–Frazier
- (C) Poole
- (D) Yankauer

559. Each of the following steps can assist in the immediate determination of intraoperative blood loss EXCEPT

- (A) visual inspection of blood in sponges
- (B) measurement of blood in sponges by weighing
- (C) estimation of blood in suction container
- (D) complete blood count

560. When using a cellsaver for autologous blood transfusion, the blood is suctioned through a double lumen tubing and is

- (A) heparinized
- (B) homogenized
- (C) sterilized
- (D) water-bathed

561. During orthopedic surgery the suction tubing should be

- (A) clamped off or kinked until needed
- (B) cleared frequently
- (C) sterilized with instrument sets
- (D) attached to a scavenging system

562. Which type of surgery would require several patent suction cannulas and suction often controlled by a foot pedal?

- (A) gynecologic
- (B) thoracic
- (C) urologic
- (D) ear, nose, throat (ENT)

563. When suctioning in neurosurgery a precaution taken is to

- (A) prepare one reserve canister
- (B) separate cells for study
- (C) avoid applying vacuum directly on brain or neural tissue
- (D) avoid evacuating cerebrospinal fluid

564. A tourniquet is utilized

- (A) only in lower extremity bleeding
- (B) only when hemorrhage is not controlled by other methods
- (C) in all venous bleeding
- (D) in all arterial bleeding

565. The proper setting for a tourniquet applied to an arm is

- (A) 100–200 mm Hg
- (B) 250–300 mm Hg
- (C) 350–450 mm Hg
- (D) 400–500 mm Hg

566. Exsanguination of a limb before tourniquet inflation is accomplished with wrapping the elevated extremity with

- (A) Kling
- (B) Esmarch
- (C) Stockingette
- (D) Webril

567. The amount of pressure used to inflate a tourniquet depends on all of the following EXCEPT

- (A) patient's age
- (B) size of extremity
- (C) depth of surgical incision
- (D) systolic blood pressure

568. A regional block that uses the tourniquet is a(n)

- (A) Bier block
- (B) intrathecal block
- (C) peridural block
- (D) field block

569. The tourniquet is contraindicated if

- (A) patient's circulation to distal part of extremity is poor
- (B) patient is elderly
- (C) patient is obese
- (D) patient has epidural anesthesia

570. Which action drains venous blood during tourniquet application?

(A)   elevate extremity after tightening tourniquet

(B)   ascertain extremity remains at body level as tourniquet is tightened

(C)   elevate extremity before tightening tourniquet

(D)   lower the extremity to below body level as tourniquet is tightened

571. At what point should the surgeon be informed of the time of tourniquet application?

(A)   after 15 minutes, then every 5 minutes

(B)   after 1 hour, then every 15 minutes

(C)   after 2 hours, then every hour

(D)   after 3 hours, then every 15 minutes

572. When would the use of Esmarch be contra-indicated?

(A)   patient has had previous anesthesia

(B)   patient has had recent injury

(C)   patient has had recent cast

(D)   B and C

573. Which agent is NOT used to inflate a pneumatic tourniquet?

(A)   nitrous oxide

(B)   air

(C)   oxygen

(D)   freon

574. A precaution necessary when using a pneumatic tourniquet is

(A)   limb must be continually elevated

(B)   tourniquet time must not exceed 20 minutes

(C)   solutions must be prevented from pooling under tourniquet

(D)   inflation is done before prep and draping

575. In which procedure would a tourniquet be contraindicated?

(A)   tendon repair, child

(B)   arthroscopy, adult

(C)   bunionectomy

(D)   gangrenous toe amputation

576. The following statements regarding a grounding plate for electrosurgery are true EXCEPT

(A)   the plate must have good contact with the patient's skin

(B)   the plate must be lubricated with electrosurgical gel

(C)   the plate must be placed directly over a bony prominence

(D)   the grounded pathway returns the electrical current to the unit after the surgeon delivers it to the operative site

577. A grounding pad is not required for the electrocautery in

(A)   a cutting current setting

(B)   a coagulation current setting

(C)   a monopolar unit

(D)   a bipolar unit

578. The inactive electrode of the cautery is the

(A)   ground pad

(B)   electrocautery pencil

(C)   cable connecting pad to pencil

(D)   blade tip pencil

579. The electrical circuit of the electrocautery when

(A)   current flows from generator to inactive electrode, through tissue and back to generator

(B)   current flows from active electrode to generator, to tissue and return

(C)   current flows to and from the generator to patient via the active electrode

(D)   current flows to generator to active electrode, through tissue, and back to generator via the inactive electrode

580. Why must the electrocautery tip be kept clean?

(A)   to ensure electrical contract effectiveness

(B)   to avoid fire via accidental drape ignition

(C)   to prevent burn injuries to staff

(D)   to prevent circuit overload

581. In electrosurgery, "buzzing" refers to

    (A) coagulation of vessel via a metal instrument touching the active electrode
    (B) coagulation of tissue via a metal instrument touching the inactive electrode
    (C) cutting current
    (D) blended current (cutting and coagulating simultaneously)

582. Which electrosurgical unit provides precise control of the coagulated area?

    (A) monopolar
    (B) blended
    (C) bipolar
    (D) Bovie

583. Which condition is MOST acceptable when using electrocautery?

    (A) ground pad placed on scar or hairy area
    (B) ground pad placed on patient's forearm
    (C) ground pad placed on skin over metal implant
    (D) ground pad placed close to operative site

584. The active electrode on the electrocautery is the

    (A) dispersive electrode
    (B) power unit
    (C) grounding pad
    (D) tip

585. A cautery would not be used

    (A) when Betadine skin prep is used
    (B) in cases requiring irrigation
    (C) in neck or nasopharynx surgery if nitrous oxide is used
    (D) in hernia repair if an epidural is used

586. Why are only moist sponges utilized during electrocautery use?

    (A) to prevent snagging of sponges on a cautery tip
    (B) to prevent fire
    (C) to reflect beam
    (D) none of the above

587. If the electrocautery is used through the colonoscope, carbon dioxide should be available to flush out the colon because

    (A) gases normally in colon could cause explosion
    (B) there is a need for good visability
    (C) a reduction of heat buildup may be necessary
    (D) there is a need for carbon dioxide replacement

588. Fulguration is utilized primarily in _____ surgery.

    (A) ENT
    (B) gynecologic
    (C) thoracic
    (D) transurethral resection (TUR) and prostate operations

589. When working in the bladder why is more or higher electrical current necessary during cautery use?

    (A) more current is needed when working in solution
    (B) bladder tissue is tougher
    (C) high voltage arcing requires it
    (D) eschar formation is to be avoided

590. Fulguration via the resectoscope is accomplished by the use of a(n) _____ tip.

    (A) electrode
    (B) ball
    (C) blade
    (D) needle

591. A direct visualization of the common bile duct is done by means of a(n)

    (A) cholangiocath
    (B) Fogarty catheter
    (C) choledochoscope
    (D) operative microscope

592. Fiberoptic lighting is

    (A) a cool light
    (B) made of plastic fibers
    (C) of low intensity
    (D) powered by battery

593. Complications can occur during endoscopy, such as

   (A) infection
   (B) bleeding
   (C) perforation
   (D) B and C

594. An endoscopy procedure that does not require a sterile set up is

   (A) laparoscopy
   (B) bronchoscopy
   (C) arthroscopy
   (D) mediastinoscopy

595. All are precautions when handling fiberoptic cables EXCEPT

   (A) light cables should be dropped or swing free when carried
   (B) cables are coiled loosely, no kinking
   (C) heavy items are not laid on cables
   (D) cables are only gas sterilized

596. Fiberoptic cable integrity is questionable when

   (A) illumination is bright
   (B) dark spots are evident
   (C) tubing has been coiled
   (D) tubing is scratched

597. When using a fiberoptic, burns and fires are prevented by

   (A) cable is kept away from drapes when disconnected from endoscope
   (B) personnel should not lean on cable end that is disconnected but is still on
   (C) cable end is kept on a moist towel when disconnected from endoscope
   (D) all of the above

598. An economical, practical, and effective way to clean reusable channeled endoscopic instruments initially is with the

   (A) Endoflush
   (B) ultrasonic washer
   (C) washer–sterilizer
   (D) STERIS system

599. A sterilant that is used on endoscopes that is bactericidal, fungicidal, and sporicidal in 20–30 minutes processing time is

   (A) Metaphen
   (B) aspartic acid
   (C) peracetic acid
   (D) ammonium chloride

600. Which statement is true regarding a STERIS system for endoscope sterilization?

   (A) only one scope or a few instruments can be processed in a cycle
   (B) it is not sporicidal
   (C) the processing time is lengthy
   (D) it is very costly

601. The endoscope that provides a view of the middle of the thorax, between the two pleural sacs is

   (A) bronchoscope
   (B) laryngoscope
   (C) thoracoscope
   (D) mediastinoscope

602. Loupes are used for

   (A) tissue retraction
   (B) magnification
   (C) hemostasis
   (D) patient transfer

603. Resolving power of an operating microscope means

   (A) the ability to discern detail
   (B) the ability to enlarge the image
   (C) the adaptation of operative procedure to individual patient requirements
   (D) the ratio of image size on viewer's retina with and without magnification

604. Which item in the optical lens system is responsible for magnification?

   (A) oculars
   (B) paraxial illuminators
   (C) objective lens
   (D) A and C

605. The range of focal lengths of the objective lenses in the operating microscope is

(A) 0–100 mm
(B) 100–200 mm
(C) 100–400 mm
(D) 5–25 mm

606. A continuously variable magnification system is afforded to the eye surgeon by the

(A) broadview viewing lens
(B) microadapter
(C) zoom lens with foot control
(D) couplings

607. The purpose of the "slit" lamp in eye surgery is

(A) defining depth perception
(B) focusing ability
(C) magnifying power
(D) discerning detail

608. The operating microscope that visually employs fiberoptics for its light source is

(A) halogen
(B) tungsten
(C) coaxial illuminators
(D) paraxial illuminators

609. Care of the microscope would include all of the following EXCEPT

(A) damp dust external surfaces with detergent–disinfectant before use
(B) damp dust lenses with detergent–disinfectant before use
(C) enclose in an antistatic plastic cover when not in use
(D) clean casters before each use

610. The purpose of the beam splitter in an operating microscope is to

(A) coincide the assistant's field of view with the surgeon's
(B) increase light intensity
(C) decrease vibration
(D) narrow the beam of light

611. The colpomicroscope affords a view of the

(A) fallopian tube
(B) intraperitoneal structures
(C) cervix
(D) uterine endometrium

612. The procedure employing the use of a self-retaining laryngoscope and microscope is called a _____.

(A) indirect laryngoscopy
(B) direct laryngoscopy
(C) suspension microlaryngoscopy
(D) laser microlaryngoscopy

613. The binocular microscope provides stereoscopic vision. This refers to

(A) the view afforded by double eyepieces
(B) the color projected on the field
(C) the magnification capability
(D) the illumination process

614. Which magnifying powers are available for the microscope eye pieces?

(A) 1×, 2×, 3×, and 4×
(B) 10×, 20×, 30×, and 40×
(C) 10×, 12.5×, 16×, and 20×
(D) 300 mm, 400 mm, 500 mm, 600 mm

615. Which procedure is inappropriate when caring for optic lenses?

(A) blood, water, and irrigating solutions are removed with cotton tipped applicators and distilled water
(B) lens is always cleaned in a circular motion, beginning at the center
(C) oil or fingerprints are removed by soaking in solvent for 10 minutes and drying with a cotton ball
(D) lint or dust are removed with a lens brush or rubber bulb syringe

616. The OR bed may have a metal crossbar between the two upper sections which may be raised to elevate the

(A) kidney
(B) breast
(C) gallbladder
(D) A and C

617. Which item is also known as an "airplane support"?

    (A) shoulder braces
    (B) arch bar
    (C) cranial headrest
    (D) double arm board

618. Operative accessibility in thyroid surgery may be aided by the use of a(n)

    (A) headrest
    (B) shoulder braces
    (C) arch bar
    (D) shoulder bridge

619. In which position would shoulder braces be indicted?

    (A) reverse Trendelenburg
    (B) extreme Trendelenburg
    (C) Fowler's
    (D) Kraske

620. A precaution necessary when using the kidney rests is

    (A) to press firmly but not too tightly against body
    (B) to pad well
    (C) to place the longer rest beneath iliac crest
    (D) all of the above

621. Chest rolls (bolsters)

    (A) secure position
    (B) minimize pressure on abdominal organs
    (C) facilitate respiration
    (D) minimize pressure on bony prominences

622. Bakelite orthopedic table attachments are sometimes used because

    (A) they clean very easily
    (B) the do not interfere with radiographic studies
    (C) they are unaffected by irrigation fluids
    (D) they can be sterilized

623. Sponges and towels used near the laser tissue impact site are kept wet in order to

    (A) prevent drying of tissue
    (B) prevent ignition of these materials by reflected beam
    (C) protect the instruments
    (D) absorb the gas produced

624. A laser plume is composed of

    (A) methane gas
    (B) carbonized particles, water, and odor
    (C) dry combustibles
    (D) gas vapor

625. When using lasers, nonreflective instrumentation

    (A) decreases accidental direct reflection of the laser beam to another area
    (B) decreases potential for infection
    (C) decreases explosibility
    (D) decreases short-circuiting of the laser

626. Which laser emission is primarily absorbed in tissue by hemoglobin or melanin?

    (A) CO_2
    (B) argon
    (C) Nd–YAG
    (D) helium–neon

627. The fire extinguisher of choice for a laser fire is a(n)

    (A) water pressurized
    (B) CO_2
    (C) Halon
    (D) dry chemical

628. In a surgical procedure employing the use of the laser, prep solution on the patient's skin should be pat-dried because

    (A) pooled fluids can retain laser heat and subsequently burn tissue
    (B) instrumentation cannot be exposed to prep solutions
    (C) vapors can cause damage to the laser beam impact point
    (D) laser retardant draping material must be placed on a thoroughly dry surface

629. Laser surgery performed in the rectal area should be preceded by

    (A) suctioning of lower bowel to remove methane gas
    (B) suctioning out of lower bowel contents
    (C) packing the rectum with dry, counted sponges
    (D) A and C

630. Ebonization refers to

    (A) escharing of tissue from thermal or chemical burn
    (B) coating of instruments to decrease reflectivity
    (C) removing of a growth or harmful substance
    (D) clumping together of cells as a result of interaction with antibodies

631. The use of each of the following items are measures employed to reduce laser-induced injuries EXCEPT

    (A) ebonized instruments
    (B) anodized instruments
    (C) plastic vaginal and rectal speculums
    (D) reflective drapes

632. When utilizing the laser, occupational exposure to surgical smoke via the skin, eye, and mucous membranes is best minimized by the use of

    (A) charcoal filters
    (B) copper shield
    (C) universal precautions
    (D) standard suction

633. Which specialty would employ the use of a slit lamp and the laser?

    (A) orthopedic
    (B) urologic
    (C) ophthalmic
    (D) ENT

634. The laser used primarily for port-wine stain lessons of the skin is the

    (A) argon
    (B) krypton

    (C) yttrium aluminum garnet (YAG)
    (D) ruby

635. People who are near the CO_2 laser impact area can guard against corneal injuries by

    (A) wearing amber-tinted lenses
    (B) wearing clear glass or plastic glasses with side guards
    (C) wearing green-tinted lenses
    (D) looking away from the energy source

636. Each of the following are measures used to control the effects of the laser plume EXCEPT

    (A) smoke evacuators
    (B) suctions
    (C) high filtration masks
    (D) moistened drapes

637. Which endotracheal tube is contraindicated during laser surgery?

    (A) flexible metal tube with external cuff attached
    (B) polyvinyl chloride (PVC) tube
    (C) red rubber tube wrapped with reflecting tape
    (D) commercial laser endotracheal (ET) tube

638. What item should be on the scrub person's instrument table while the laser is in use?

    (A) basin of sterile water or saline
    (B) basin of sterile baking soda
    (C) flame retardant sheets
    (D) cotton blanket

639. The following statements regarding lasers are true EXCEPT

    (A) laser unit is protected from bumping against walls during movement
    (B) flammable materials should not be used near laser impact site
    (C) water or other solutions should not be placed on laser unit
    (D) laser unit is in "on" position during entire case

640. The laser used most commonly for retinal detachment, tear, or hole is

(A) krypton
(B) Nd–YAG
(C) argon
(D) CO_2

641. The tunable dye laser used to disintegrate kidney stones is the

(A) ESWL
(B) candela
(C) CO_2
(D) Nd:–AG

c. Supplies

642. A device used to correct and counteract internal bleeding conditions and hypovolemia is a(n)

(A) CT
(B) IPB
(C) CVP
(D) MAST

643. Placement of a Levin tube would be in the

(A) ear
(B) large intestine
(C) stomach
(D) bladder

644. A sponge used in brain surgery is a(n)

(A) cottonoid patty
(B) Kitner
(C) impregnated gauze
(D) porcine

645. The dressing used after nasal surgery is

(A) collodion
(B) moustache
(C) pressure
(D) telfa

646. Seamless tubular cotton that stretches to fit a contour and is used for padding is called a(n)

(A) Ace bandage
(B) Webril
(C) sheet wadding
(D) stockinette

647. Which case would require the use of cottonoid strips?

(A) laminectomy
(B) tonsillectomy
(C) thorocotomy
(D) aortic aneurysmectomy

648. An item used for padding that has smooth and clingy layers is called

(A) Webril
(B) stockinette
(C) telfa
(D) gypsum

649. Rectal packing is made of

(A) petroleum-treated gauze
(B) heparin-treated gauze
(C) antibiotic-treated gauze
(D) telfa-treated gauze

650. An elastic adhesive bandage is

(A) flexible collodion
(B) Ace bandage
(C) elastoplast
(D) Scultetus binder

651. A dissecting sponge that is a small roll of heavy cotton tape is a

(A) Kitner
(B) peanut
(C) tonsil
(D) tape

652. A dissecting sponge made of gauze that is used to dissect or absorb fluid is called a

   (A) patty
   (B) tonsil
   (C) cottonoid
   (D) peanut

653. A temporary biologic dressing is

   (A) porcine
   (B) telfa
   (C) collagen
   (D) mesh

654. Which procedure would not require a pressure dressing?

   (A) plastic surgery
   (B) knee surgery
   (C) radical mastectomy
   (D) hysterectomy

655. A sponge that is cotton-filled gauze with a cotton thread attached is a

   (A) patty
   (B) tonsil
   (C) Kitner
   (D) peanut

656. Patties are

   (A) used dry
   (B) moistened with saline
   (C) moistened with water
   (D) moistened with silver nitrate solution

657. Which of the following can be a supplement to a subcuticular closure?

   (A) skin staples
   (B) swaged sutures
   (C) stent fixation
   (D) skin closure tapes

658. A protective skin coating is accomplished with

   (A) tincture of benzoin
   (B) merthiolate
   (C) iodoform
   (D) Lugol's solution

659. A dressing that is held in place by long suture ends crisscrossed and tied is called a

   (A) passive
   (B) strip closure
   (C) proxi-strip
   (D) stent

660. The smallest diameter on a French scale is a

   (A) 3
   (B) 5
   (C) 7
   (D) 9

661. A stab wound is a separate small incision

   (A) close to operative site
   (B) medial to operative site
   (C) always above operative site
   (D) superior to operative site

662. A tube placed into the tympanic membrane to facilitate aeration is the

   (A) myringotomy tube
   (B) stent tube
   (C) Robinson tube
   (D) plastipore tube

663. A common size chest tube is a

   (A) 3 Fr.
   (B) 10 Fr.
   (C) 30 Fr.
   (D) 60 Fr.

664. What type of catheter would facilitate the removal of small gallstones?

   (A) T-tube
   (B) Robinson
   (C) Fogarty
   (D) Rehfus

665. A catheter commonly used in a gastrostomy is a

   (A) mushroom
   (B) Rehfus
   (C) Cantor
   (D) Sengstaken–Blakemore

666. Which of the following is NOT a type of ureteral catheter tip?

(A) whistle
(B) olive
(C) Braasch bulb
(D) Pezzar

667. The drain that has a reservoir creating negative pressure to facilitate drainage is a

(A) Penrose
(B) hemovac
(C) Levin
(D) stent

668. All of the following statements are true of ureteral catheters EXCEPT that they

(A) are made of flexible woven nylon or plastic
(B) range in caliber from size 3 to 14 French
(C) have graduated markings in centimeters
(D) provide direct visualization of the bladder

669. Long-term or temporary ureteral drainage can be accomplished with a

(A) Braasch bulb
(B) Blassuchi
(C) stent
(D) Garceau

670. A central venous catheter is usually inserted into the

(A) brachial vein
(B) cephalic vein
(C) femoral vein
(D) external jugular vein

671. An indwelling catheter used for chemotherapy administration is a

(A) Fogarty
(B) Tenckhoff
(C) Palmaz
(D) Gruntzig

672. Which of the following is not used for urethral dilation?

(A) McCarthy dilator
(B) VanBuren sound
(C) Hegar dilator
(D) Phillips filliform and followers

673. A closed-wound suction system works by

(A) positive pressure
(B) negative-pressure vacuum
(C) air displacement
(D) constant gravity drainage

674. Why is a 30-cc bag Foley used after a transurethral resection (TUR) of the prostate?

(A) hemostasis
(B) decompression
(C) creation of negative pressure
(D) aspiration

675. The tube that collects bronchial washings is

(A) Broyles
(B) Lukens
(C) Ellik
(D) Toomey

676. Balloon angioplasty is accomplished with the use of a _____ catheter.

(A) Gruntzig
(B) Gibbons
(C) Garceau
(D) Harris

677. A Pezzer is a

(A) Foley catheter
(B) bat-wing catheter
(C) ureteral catheter
(D) mushroom catheter

678. The three lumens of a Foley are used for inflation, drainage, and

(A) prevention of urine reflux
(B) access for sterile urine specimens
(C) continuous irrigation
(D) additional hemostasis

679. An image intensifier

(A) is an x-ray machine
(B) is a microscope
(C) converts the x-ray beam into a fluoro-scopic optical image
(D) converts an x-ray image into film

680. Extracorporeal circulation refers to circulation

(A) of blood outside of the body
(B) through the muscular tissue of the heart
(C) established through an anastomosis between two vessels
(D) of blood through the whole body EXCEPT the lungs

681. The scoring system that assesses an infant's condition after birth is called a(n)

(A) Roentgen
(B) Romberg
(C) Apgar
(D) colostrum

682. Which procedure records the electrical activity of the brain?

(A) electrocardiogram
(B) brain scan
(C) electromyogram
(D) electroencephalogram

683. An x-ray's photographic image is called a(n)

(A) ultrasound wave
(B) magnetic image
(C) roentgenogram
(D) computerized tomography

684. Immobilization of the hip joints after surgery is accomplished by the use of

(A) traction
(B) abduction pillow
(C) cast
(D) compression device

685. All of the following are true of disposable chest drainage units EXCEPT

(A) provides drainage collection from intrapleural space

(B) maintains a seal to prevent air from entering the pleural cavity
(C) provides suction control determined by water level
(D) aids in re-establishing positive pressure in the intrapleural space

686. Which factor is not accomplished by chest drainage?

(A) drains fluid and air from pleural cavity
(B) provides water seal for gravity drainage
(C) suction controlled by level of water
(D) positive pressure re-establishment

687. A cast applied from the hips to the head, which is used to immobilize cervical fractures is a

(A) Minerva jacket
(B) body jacket
(C) shoulder spica
(D) cylinder

688. A motorized device whose action prevents venous stasis and reduces risk of deep-vein clotting in high risk patients is

(A) pneumatic antishock garment
(B) military antishock trousers (MAST)
(C) TED stockings
(D) sequential pneumatic compression boots

689. Which synthetic mesh may be used in the presence of infection?

(A) Prolene
(B) Gore-tex
(C) Mersilene
(D) none of the above

690. Mersilene mesh

(A) cannot be resterilized
(B) can be steam sterilized once, if unused but not soiled
(C) can be resterilized, if soil is carefully washed off
(D) can be cold soaked for 10 minutes

691. A common donor site for an autogenous bone graft is

   (A) femur
   (B) pelvis
   (C) ilium
   (D) ischium

692. The patient coming to the OR with rupture of esophageal varices may have a(n) _____ in place to control bleeding.

   (A) Miller–Abbott
   (B) Franklin
   (C) Swan–Ganz
   (D) Sengstaken–Blakemore

693. Either a Foley, Mallecot, Pezzer, or Mushroom catheter can be inserted for

   (A) gastroscopy
   (B) gastrostomy
   (C) vagotomy
   (D) gastric bypass

694. The risks of cone biopsy are minimized by using the

   (A) cervitome
   (B) cold knife
   (C) scalpel
   (D) CO_2 laser

695. Stereotactic surgery takes place in the

   (A) ear
   (B) eye
   (C) brain
   (D) nose

696. A blood flow detector is a

   (A) Doppler
   (B) Gruntzig
   (C) Moretz
   (D) Warren

697. A secondary video monitor is referred to as a(n)

   (A) MAC
   (B) SMA
   (C) CAM-2
   (D) "slave"

698. Which catheter facilitates the infusion of chemotherapeutic drugs?

   (A) Hickman
   (B) Dorsey
   (C) Silverman
   (D) Huber

699. TPN

   (A) maintains patient's nutrition
   (B) provides withdrawal site for blood samples
   (C) provides access route for chemo installation
   (D) records vital signs

700. An Ambu bag is a

   (A) container for specimens
   (B) bag for blood pressure apparatus
   (C) bag for blood transfusion
   (D) breathing bag

701. A blood warmer is used

   (A) to induce hypothermia
   (B) to aid in hemolysis
   (C) to maintain 89–105°F temperature
   (D) to eliminate microorganisms

702. Which is the most necessary item for a blood transfusion?

   (A) blood warmer
   (B) blood filter
   (C) blood pressure cuff
   (D) refrigerator

703. Each are measures to prevent heat loss in newborn, infant, or children in the OR EXCEPT

   (A) hypothermia blanket is prepared
   (B) water mattress is warmed
   (C) webril is wrapped on extremities
   (D) solutions for skin prep and intraoperative use are warmed

704. A setup that would include a 1000-cc bag of normal saline, sterile IV tubing, an IV pole, and a pressure bag is

(A) splenectomy
(B) choledochoscopy
(C) thyroideotomy
(D) ovarian cystectomy

705. A laminaria tent is used to

(A) suction uterine contents
(B) close cervix
(C) dilate cervix
(D) visualize uterus

706. In which procedure would be a radiant warmer be found?

(A) sterilization
(B) cesarean section
(C) blood transfusion
(D) Ramstedt operation

707. The C-arm employs the use of

(A) fluoroscope
(B) carbon dioxide
(C) cesium
(D) creatine

708. Equate the radiation exposure in fluoroscopy as compared to that of a single x-ray.

(A) the same exposure
(B) 2:1
(C) 5:1
(D) 10:1

709. A PCA pump affords

(A) patient-controlled pain relief
(B) vital sign monitoring
(C) infusion of antibiotics intravenously
(D) heparinized solution intravenously

C. Counts

710. The initial count requires

(A) a count of both plain and radiopaque sponges
(B) that counts be done in the right-hand corner on the back table

(C) that the count be done aloud by circulator and scrub
(D) the scrub to count each item and report to the circulator for recording

711. If a sponge pack contains an incorrect number of sponges, the circulating nurse should

(A) isolate the pack, do not use it
(B) document it on the count record
(C) use if after adding or subtracting the correct number
(D) return it to the original outer package and set it aside

712. In an instrument count

(A) all instruments and parts must be counted
(B) precounted sets eliminate the need for pre-case count
(C) large bulky instruments need not be counted
(D) count only instruments that will be used

713. Which of the following statements concerning sponges are true EXCEPT

(A) only radiopaque sponges should be used on the sterile field
(B) sponges should be counted from the folded edge
(C) a pack containing an incorrect number of sponges is discarded
(D) a count is unnecessary in a vaginal procedure

714. The following statements regarding counts are true EXCEPT

(A) the relief scrub or circulator does not need to repeat count if only one of them is relieved
(B) all counts are verified before person being relieved leaves room
(C) persons taking final count are held accountable
(D) persons taking final count must sign the count record

715. During the closure count a discrepancy

    (A)   is noted on patient's chart
    (B)   is reported to surgeon
    (C)   is reported to supervisor
    (D)   is reported to anesthesiologist

716. If a sponge is intentionally left in the patient

    (A)   a report is made to the supervisor
    (B)   an incident report is completed
    (C)   a notation is placed on the operative record
    (D)   none of the above

717. The following statements regarding counting sponges are true EXCEPT

    (A)   sponges are counted at folded edge
    (B)   shake pack to separate sponges
    (C)   separate each sponge and number aloud while placing it in a pile on table
    (D)   an incorrect number of sponges in a pack should be compensated for on count sheet with a notation

718. During the sponge count procedures, which action would constitute an UNACCEPTABLE technique?

    (A)   soiled sponges are separated, stacked, and counted in multiples
    (B)   soiled sponges used for prep remain in kick bucket and are not part of count
    (C)   sponges are not added or removed from operative field during count
    (D)   sponges are counted before being moistened or used

Preoperative Preparation
Answers and Explanations

I. PHYSICAL ENVIRONMENT OF THE OPERATING ROOM

A. Preparation

394. **(C)** Infants and children are kept warm to minimize heat loss and prevent hypothermia, 85°F should be maintained (Fortunato).

395. **(B)** Ceiling- and wall-mounted fixtures are cleaned daily. Walls are spot cleaned as necessary but should be regularly cleaned along with air conditioning grills. All furniture, room equipment, floors, and waste receptacles are cleaned between cases and at the end of the day (Fortunato).

B. Maintenance

396. **(B)** Glass suction bottles should be thoroughly cleaned with a disinfectant solution and autoclaved before reuse (Fortunato).

397. **(C)** Storage areas should be cleaned at least weekly to control dust (Fortunato).

398. **(B)** Doors should be closed during and in between cases to reduce the microbial count (Fortunato).

399. **(D)** A wet vacuum system is the best. However, if mopping is to be utilized, a clean mop is used. Each time the mop is used, a two-bucket system is recommended (one a detergent–germicide and the other clear water), and the buckets must be emptied and cleaned between uses (Fortunato).

400. **(B)** If a sterile package wrapped in a pervious muslin or other woven material drops to the floor or unclean area, do not use it. If the wrapper is impervious and contact area is dry, the item may be used. Dropped packages should not be put back into sterile storage (Fortunato).

II. PATIENT-RELATED PROCEDURES

A. Consents

401. **(D)** In a dire emergency, the patient's condition takes precedence over the permit. Permits may be accepted from a legal guardian or responsible relative. Two nurses should monitor a telephone consent and sign the form; it is then signed by the parent, guardian, or spouse upon arrival. A written consultation by two physicians, not including the surgeon, will suffice until the proper signature can be obtained (Fortunato).

402. **(C)** If the surgeon intends or wants to perform a procedure not specified on the permission or consent form, the OR nurse assumes the responsibility of informing the surgeon and/or the proper administrative authority of the discrepancy (Fortunato).

403. **(D)** The patient's (or suitable substitute's) signature must be witnessed by one or more authorized persons. They may be physicians, nurses, or other hospital employees authorized to do so. The witness is attesting to the proper identification of the patient and the fact that the signing was voluntary (Fortunato).

404.   **(A)**   The patient giving his or her consent must be of legal age, mentally alert, and competent. The patient must sign before premedication is given and before going to the OR. This protects the patient from unratified procedures as well as protecting the surgeon and the hospital (Fortunato).

405.   **(A)**   The general consent form authorizes the physician in charge and hospital staff to render such treatments or perform such procedures as the physician deems advisable. It applies only to routine hospital procedures. The consent document for any procedure possibly injurious to the patient should be signed before the procedure is performed (Fortunato).

406.   **(C)**   The ultimate responsibility for obtaining permission is the surgeon's. The circulating nurse (RN or charge nurse) and the anesthesiologist are responsible for checking that the consent is on the chart, properly signed, and that the information on the form is correct (Fortunato).

407.   **(D)**   All consent forms must be signed before the administration of preoperative medications. This is to ensure that the patient fully understands what the procedure is. If the permission is signed incorrectly, it may not be revised until the preoperative medication has worn off (Fortunato).

408.   **(D)**   An informed consent (operative permit) protects the patient from unratified procedures and protects the surgeon and the hospital claims of an unauthorized operation. A general consent authorizes the physician and staff to render treatment and perform procedures which are routine duties normally carried out at the hospital (Fortunato).

409.   **(B)**   Implied consent is never the preferred action. Law allows it in emergency situations when no other authorized person can be contacted or when conditions are discovered during a surgical procedure (Association of Surgical Technologists).

410.   **(D)**   The patient has a right to withdraw written consent if it is voluntary and if he or she is in a rationale state. The surgeon explains consequences, obtains a written refusal and informs hospital and administration. The surgery is postponed (Fortunato).

B. Positions for Operative Procedures

411.   **(B)**   The Kraske (jackknife) position is used for procedures in the rectal area such as pilonidal sinus or hemorrhoidectomy. Feet and toes are protected by a pillow. The head is to the side and the arms are on armboards (Fortunato).

412.   **(A)**   In the Fowler's position the patient lies on his or her back with knees over the lower break in the table. A footboard is raised and padded. The foot of the table is lowered slightly, flexing the knees. The body section is raised. Arms rest on a pillow on the lap. This position is used in some cranial procedures with the head supported by a headrest (Fortunato).

413.   **(B)**   The patient is in prone position with lumbar spine over the center break of the table; two laminectomy rolls (or other firm padding) are placed longitudinally to support the chest from axilla to hip. Additional padding protects bony prominences (Fortunato).

414.   **(A)**   A modified Trendelenburg position is used for patients in hypovolemic shock. This may aid in venous return and cardiac output (Fortunato).

415.   **(C)**   A Mayfield is a special neurosurgical overhead instrument table (Meeker and Rothrock).

416.   **(D)**   The patient is in modified dorsal recumbent position with a rolled sheet to extend the neck and raise the shoulders. Skin flaps may be held away with stay sutures. The laryngeal nerve is identified and carefully preserved (Meeker and Rothrock).

417. (B) For an abdominoperineal resection, the patient is initially positioned supine in modified lithotomy providing simultaneous exposure of both abdominal and perineal fields (Fortunato).

418. (D) In a C-section, uterine displacement to the left in order to shift the uterus away from the pelvic vessels is done to avoid maternal hypotension and maintain fetal well-being (Fortunato).

419. (B) For most open bladder surgery the patient is placed in the supine position with a bolster under the pelvis. Trendelenburg may be desired to allow viscera to fall toward the head, allowing excellent pelvic organ exposure (Meeker and Rothrock).

420. (A) On the orthopedic fracture table, the patient is positioned supine with the pelvis stabilized against a well-padded vertical post. Pressure on the genitalia from the perineal post can injure the pudendal nerves (Meeker and Rothrock).

421. (D) The aging patient's skin integrity is very important. Aging decreases range of motion of joints. Elderly people cannot fully extend the spine, neck, or upper and lower extremities. Pillows, padding, and support devices compensate for the skeletal changes to ensure patient comfort and ensure against postoperative pain or injury (Meeker and Rothrock).

422. (D) Maximum patient safety is accomplished by padding all bony prominences, protecting the brachial plexus in the axillary region from strain or pressure, ensuring that the legs are not crossed to prevent pressure on nerves and blood vessels, supporting and securing extremities to prevent them from falling off the bed, ensuring that no part of the patient's body touches metal on the OR bed, and making certain no equipment, Mayo, or personnel rests on the patient (Meeker and Rothrock).

C. Skin Preparation

423. (B) When a breast is prepped for suspected malignancy, it is done gently or not at all. Scrubbing the breast with the usual amount of pressure could cause cancer cells to break loose from the lesion and spread the disease (Fortunato).

424. (C) The patient should be shaved immediately before surgery, preferably in a holding area of the OR. This is thought to reduce the infection rate. The amount of time between the preoperative shave and the operation has a direct effect on wound infection rate (Fortunato).

425. (A) Contaminated areas (which can include draining sinuses, skin ulcers, vagina, or anus) should be scrubbed last or with separate sponges. This prevents dragging pathogens into the incisional area and, thus, reduces the possibility of infection (Fortunato).

426. (A) Skin should be washed from the incision site to the periphery in a circular motion. This keeps the incision site cleaner and prevents wound contamination (Fortunato).

427. (A) Patients may be advised to begin bathing with a 3% hexachlorophene solution before admission for an elective procedure. Patients should shower or be bathed before coming to the OR suite. This action is bacteriostatic and reduces microbial contamination (Fortunato).

D. Draping

428. (B) Suction tubing is attached to the drapes with a nonperforating clamp (Fortunato).

429. (D) A sterile person turns his or her back to a nonsterile person or area when passing (Fortunato).

430. (B) When draping a table, open the drape toward the front of the table first. This establishes a sterile area close to the scrub (Fortunato).

431. (D) Stockinette may be used to cover an extremity. It is a seamless, stretchable tubing material which contours snugly to skin. It may be covered with plastic. Some has vinyl on outside layer (Fortunato).

432. (D) Drapes are placed on a dry area. The scrub nurse takes towel clips and skin towels to the side of the OR table from which the surgeon will apply them. Folded drapes are carried to the OR table. Drapes are held high enough to avoid touching nonsterile areas. Once a drape is placed, it may not be adjusted (Fortunato).

433. (A) B, C, and D are acceptable techniques. Gloved hands should not touch the skin of the patient. Protect gloved hands by cuffing end of sheet over them (Fortunato).

434. (A) The surgeon places a drape under the head while the circulator holds up the head. This drape consists of a towel placed on a medium sheet. Center of towel edge is 2 inches in from center of sheet edge. Towel is drawn up on each side of face, over forehead or at hairline and fastened with a clip. Additional towels surround operative site (Fortunato).

III. SCRUB TASKS

A. Scrub, Gown, and Glove

435. (D) Gowns are considered sterile only in front from chest to level of sterile field, and the sleeves from elbow to cuffs (Fortunato).

436. (B) Dry both hands thoroughly but independently. Dry each arm using a rotating motion while moving up the arm to the elbow; do not retrace the area. Bend forward slightly from the waist, holding hands and elbows above the waist and away from the body. The towel should be opened full length and reversed for each arm (Meeker and Rothrock).

437. (B) Before handing a gown, unfold it carefully, holding it at the neckband (Fortunato).

438. (C) The surgical scrub removes skin oil, reduces the microbial count, and leaves an antimicrobial residue on the skin. The skin can never be rendered sterile (aseptic). It is considered surgically clean (Fortunato).

439. (B) To change a glove during an operation, the scrub nurse must turn away from the sterile field. The circulator pulls the glove off inside-out, and the open-glove technique is used to don a new pair of gloves (Fortunato).

440. (A) The gown is always removed before the gloves. It is pulled downward from the shoulders, turning the sleeves inside out as it is pulled off the arms. Gloves are turned inside out, using the glove-to-glove then skin-to-skin technique as they are removed. The circulating nurse unfastens the gown at the neck and waist (Fortunato).

441. (D) Either the time method or brush–stroke method is effective if properly executed. Studies have shown that a vigorous 5-minute scrub with a reliable agent is as effective as the 10-minute scrub with less mechanical action (Fortunato).

442. (B) Chipped nail polish harbors microorganisms. No polish is preferred (Fortunato).

443. (A) Using barriers to avoid direct contact with blood and body fluid are the best measures to prevent work-related HIV (Fortunato).

444. (D) The surgical scrub is the process of removing as many microorganisms from the hands and arms by mechanical washing and chemical antisepsis (Fortunato).

445. (D) The arm is scrubbed, including the elbow and the antecubital space to 2 inches above the elbow (Fortunato).

446. (B) Skin and nails should be clean and in good condition. A non-oil-based hand cream should be used. Fingernails should not reach beyond fingertips. No polish should be worn and artificial nails/devices must not cover nails (Fortunato).

447. **(C)** Time varies with the frequency of the scrub, the agent used, and the method used. The procedure may be time method or counted brush stroke, each of which follows an anatomical pattern of scrub ending 2 inches above the elbow. All steps begin with hands and end with elbow, with the hands having most direct contact (Fortunato).

448. **(C)** The nails are scrubbed 30 strokes; all sides of each finger, 20 strokes; the back of the hand and palm, 20 strokes; and the arms, 20 strokes to 2 inches above the elbow (Fortunato).

449. **(D)** Scoliosis is a lateral deviation of the spine. Harrington rods are internal splints that help maintain the spine as straight as possible (Meeker and Rothrock).

B. Basic Setups

a. Instrumentation

450. **(A)** A Lebsche sternum knife is used in chest surgery to open the sternum (Meeker and Rothrock).

451. **(C)** Kerrison refers to a rongeur. It is available in many angles and is used extensively in surgery of the spine and neurosurgery (Meeker and Rothrock).

452. **(B)** Bakes common duct dilators have malleable shafts in sizes 3–11 mm. They are used to explore the common bile duct (Meeker and Rothrock).

453. **(B)** A Finochietto is a rib retractor (Meeker and Rothrock).

454. **(D)** A Doyen is a rib raspatory (Meeker and Rothrock).

455. **(A)** An electric drill or a hand perforator is used to make the burr holes. A rongeur is used to enlarge the burr holes and increase exposure (Meeker and Rothrock).

456. **(B)** Wescott tenotomy scissors are fine scissors with a spring action used in eye surgery (Meeker and Rothrock).

457. **(D)** For splenectomy, prepare a basic laparotomy set plus two large right-angled pedicle clamps and long instruments and hemostatic materials (Meeker and Rothrock).

458. **(B)** Bowman probes are used to probe the lacrimal duct in a dacrocystorhinostomy and in lacrimal probing to open a closed lacrimal drainage system (Meeker and Rothrock).

459. **(D)** The tonsil lobe is freed from its attachments to the pillars with a Hurd dissector and pillar retractor (Meeker and Rothrock).

460. **(C)** The Lempert elevator is used in delicate ear surgery (Meeker and Rothrock).

461. **(C)** The Scoville is a retractor used in a laminectomy (Meeker and Rothrock).

462. **(D)** The Bailey rib approximator is used to approximate the ribs for closure of a thoracic incision before closure of the chest with interrupted suture (Meeker and Rothrock).

463. **(D)** A Sauerbruch is a rib rongeur used to resect a rib and is found in a thorocotomy rib instrument bone set (Meeker and Rothrock).

464. **(C)** An Auvard is a speculum that is weighted for use in the vagina. It is placed in the posterior vagina (Meeker and Rothrock).

465. **(B)** A Babcock forceps is a curved fenestrated blade clamp without teeth that grasps or encloses delicate structures such as the ureter, appendix, or fallopian tube (Meeker and Rothrock).

466. **(A)** A Ballenger swivel knife is used in rhinologic surgery. The nasal cartilage is incised with a Ballenger knife (Meeker and Rothrock).

467. **(A)** A Weitlaner is a self-retaining retractor (Meeker and Rothrock).

468. **(D)** A Hill is a rectal retractor (Meeker and Rothrock).

469. **(C)** A Webster needle holder is found in a basic plastic surgery instrument set (Meeker and Rothrock).

470. **(B)** The kidney pedicle containing the major blood vessels is isolated and doubly clamped with a Herrick, Satinsky, or Mayo pedicle clamp (Meeker and Rothrock).

471. **(A)** Uterine dilators are Hank uterine dilators (Meeker and Rothrock).

472. **(C)** In a tonsillectomy, the mouth is retracted open with a self-retaining retractor such as a Jenning's mouth gag (Meeker and Rothrock).

473. **(D)** A Silverman biopsy needle is used for obtaining biopsy specimens of thyroid, liver, kidney, prostate, or other organs. It has a 14-gauge thin-wall outer cannula with a beveled obturator. An inner-split needle fits into the outer cannula and protrudes beyond the end of it. The distal tips of this instrument are grooved inside. They enter tissue, close on the specimen, and trap it as the needle is withdrawn (Fortunato).

474. **(A)** A Freer elevator is used in corrective rhinoplasty to undermine the skin of the nose and free the periosteum and perichondrium (Meeker and Rothrock).

475. **(B)** A cholecystostomy is establishment of an opening into the gallbladder to permit drainage of the organ and removal of stones. It is selected for high-risk patients. A purse-string suture encircles the gallbladder fundus and a trocar is placed in it. Suction tubing is attached to the trocar sheath and the gallbladder contents are aspirated. The contaminated trocar and sheath are discarded. Stone removal may then take place (Meeker and Rothrock).

476. **(A)** The O'Sullivan–O'Connor is an adjustable ring-shaped abdominal retractor with two lateral blades permanently attached. There are three detachable blades as well. It is self retaining (Meeker and Rothrock).

477. **(A)** The Doyen is an intestinal clamping forceps that comes straight or curved (Meeker and Rothrock).

478. **(C)** A Bailey rib spreader is found in a thorocotomy set. After the incision is effected, the ribs and tissue are protected with moist sponges. The rib retractor (Bailey rib spreader) is placed and opened slowly to expose the lung (Meeker and Rothrock).

479. **(B)** The Green goiter retractor is also known as a loop retractor. It is used to retract the sternocleidomastoid muscle during thyroidectomy (Meeker and Rothrock).

480. **(A)** A Stille–Luer Duckbill rongeur is part of a major bone setup. It is used to bite off sharp, irregular bone edges (Meeker and Rothrock).

481. **(D)** A Davidson is a scapula retractor. It is found in a thorocotomy set (Meeker and Rothrock).

482. **(D)** The Duval is a lung-grasping forcep and is included in the instrumentation for lobectomy and pneumonectomy (Meeker and Rothrock).

483. **(A)** The Satinsky (3) and DeBakey (2) are vascular clamping instruments. The Potts–Smith (5) is an angled or straight vascular scissor. The DeBakey cross action bulldog (6) is a clamping instrument (Meeker and Rothrock).

484. **(D)** A DeBakey bulldog is a cross action clamp, straight or curved. It is used for occlusion of major peripheral arteries. They come in several sizes (Meeker and Rothrock).

485. **(A)** A Heaney is a hysterectomy forceps. It has double serrated jaws with cross grooves (Meeker and Rothrock).

486. **(C)** A Potts–Smith is a vascular scissor that is angled to the side (Meeker and Rothrock).

487. **(B)** The Satinsky, an aortic clamp, is used during abdominal aortic aneurysmectomy (Meeker and Rothrock).

488. **(B)** The Castroviejo needle holder is used in both eye and plastic surgery as well as other surgeries requiring fine, delicate sutures (Meeker and Rothrock).

489. **(C)** Randall stone forceps come in various sizes and are used to remove stones from urinary structures (Meeker and Rothrock).

490. **(C)** The Harrington retractor is an exposing instrument frequently used for gallbladder surgery. Its tip is heart-shaped, thus, it is sometimes called a sweetheart (Meeker and Rothrock).

491. **(D)** The instrument pictured is a bayonet, a tissue forceps. It is angled and fine-tipped (Meeker and Rothrock).

492. **(B)** A lesion detected by a mammogram can be localized by the insertion of a needle(s) or a wire that is inserted through a needle. Once the suspected area is identified, the patient is sent to the OR for a biopsy. After biopsy, the specimen can be sent back for mammography validation before pathological examination (Meeker and Rothrock).

493. **(D)** Randall stone forceps are available in various angles and are used to remove stones from inaccessible areas (Meeker and Rothrock).

494. **(A)** In a radical mastectomy, the surgeon may prepare the anterior surface of the thigh in the event a skin graft is needed. This requires a separate setup for taking the graft (Fortunato).

495. **(A)** Instrumentation for splenectomy is a basic laparotomy plus two, large right-angled pedicle clamps, long instruments, and hemostatic materials or devices (Meeker and Rothrock).

496. **(A)** Two blunt nerve hooks are required on a vagotomy setup (Meeker and Rothrock).

497. **(A)** In an exploration of the common bile duct, a drainage T-tube is placed into the common bile duct. It is used to confirm successful evacuation and patency of the ducts and stays in place as a drain (Fortunato).

498. **(D)** Prosthetic devices are of stainless steel and Teflon. Microsuctions are used. A speculum provides view (Meeker and Rothrock).

499. **(A)** Cochlear implantation is the placement of an electrode device in the cochlea in deaf people. Candidates should have a history of lingual skills before becoming deaf. The device receives sound and emits electrical impulses into the cochlea and along the acoustic nerve. Sound interpretations are taught to the patient postoperatively (Meeker and Rothrock).

500. **(B)** A Ballenger swivel knife is used in nasal surgery. An anesthesia setup, bayonet forceps, an Asch septum-straightening forceps, a straight hemostat, impregnated gauze, packing, a splint, and adhesive tape are prepared for a nasal fracture, closed reduction (Meeker and Rothrock).

501. **(A)** A bayonet forceps is used to introduce sponges into the nose (Meeker and Rothrock).

502. **(C)** The Potts tissue forceps is a fine forceps associated with vascular and fine intestinal surgery. Nasal surgery requires, intranasally, an angled forceps such as the bayonet forceps, a Freer elevator, and a fine Frazier suction tube (Meeker and Rothrock).

503. **(B)** Esophageal dilators (Bougies) may be on an esophagoscopy setup (Meeker and Rothrock).

504. **(D)** A Jameson hook is used in eye surgery. The Yankauer suction, Hurd dissector and pillar retractor, and tongue depressor are all found in a tonsil set (Meeker and Rothrock).

505. **(D)** A tissue expander stretches normal tissue to accommodate a breast prosthesis, used postmastectomy. The expander is placed in a created pocket and exchanged for a permanent prosthesis after desired expansion has occurred (Meeker and Rothrock).

506. **(B)** Mandibular and maxillary fracture reduction is most often accomplished by applying Arch bars to the maxillary and mandibular teeth for immobilization in order to restore the patient's preinjury dental occlusion (Meeker and Rothrock).

507. **(C)** The Alexander periosteotome, Doyen raspatory, and Stille shears are all instruments required to remove a rib. A Heaney clamp is a hemostatic clamp used in gynecologic surgery (Meeker and Rothrock).

508. **(B)** Randall stone forceps are part of a kidney instrument set (Meeker and Rothrock).

509. **(A)** A Sarot is a bronchus clamp (Association of Surgical Technologists).

510. **(B)** An IPB is not necessary. Fluoroscopy and a defibrillator are required plus vascular dissecting instruments, tunneling instrument, pacemaker and electrodes, introducer set, and an external pacemaker (Meeker and Rothrock).

511. **(C)** A permanent pacemaker initiates atrial or ventricular contraction or both. The most common indications are complete heart block bradyarrhythmias (Meeker and Rothrock).

512. **(A)** Harrington rods are internal splints—the distraction rods placed concave to the curve and the compression rods on the convex side (Meeker and Rothrock).

513. **(C)** Skeletal traction is the pulling force exerted to maintain proper alignment or position. It is applied directly on the bone following insertion of pins, wires, or tongs placed through or into the bone. Traction is applied by pulleys and weights to establish and maintain direction until fracture reunites (Fortunato).

514. **(A)** For a forearm or lower leg, a Kirschner wire or a Steinmann pin is drilled through the bone distal to the fracture site. Traction is applied (Fortunato).

515. **(A)** During orthopedic surgery, the mobile image intensification, also referred to as fluoroscopy or x-ray image, allows viewing of the case progression (Meeker and Rothrock).

516. **(B)** The myelogram outlines the spinal subarachnoid space and shows distortions of the spinal cord or dura sac by means of an injection of contrast media (Meeker and Rothrock).

517. **(D)** Sachs, Frazier, and Adson are metal suction tips that suck and also conduct coagulation. Gardner and Mayfield are skull clamps and part of a neuro headrest setup (Meeker and Rothrock).

518. **(A)** An antigravity suit applied before positioning may help prevent air embolism and assist in maintaining blood pressure (Meeker and Rothrock).

519. **(C)** A, B, and D are instruments found in a cleft palate repair set, which would also include a Dingman mouth gag with assorted blades (Meeker and Rothrock).

520. **(B)** After wound closure, a Logan's bow is applied to the cheeks with tape strips to relieve tension on the incision and to splint the lip. It is a curved metal frame (Fortunato, Meeker and Rothrock).

521. **(C)** A Cloward is the removal of anterior cervical disk with fusion using Cloward instruments. It entails removal of disk fusion of the vertebral bodies and the use of bone dowels for the fusion obtained from the patient's iliac crest (Meeker and Rothrock).

522. **(D)** A Beaver knife handle is found on the instrumentation for lens procedures in the eye (Meeker and Rothrock).

523. **(C)** Skeletal traction requires the use of sterile supplies (traction bow, pins and drills) (Meeker and Rothrock).

524. (D) A Leyla–Yasargil is a self-retaining retractor. The others are aneurysm clips (Meeker and Rothrock).

525. (A) A Pereyra or a Stamey are used for bladder neck suspensions to correct urinary stress incontinence. It is a ligature carrier and is inserted through a suprapubic incision (Meeker and Rothrock).

526. (B) ESWL, a noninvasive procedure, utilizes the lithotriptor, which introduces shock waves through a liquid medium to disintegrate stones. Fluoroscopy and the image intensifier are used for visualization (Meeker and Rothrock).

527. (C) The Omni–Tract is an adjustable urology perineal retractor system (Meeker and Rothrock).

528. (A) A Mason–Judd is a bladder retractor (Meeker and Rothrock).

529. (A) The Furlow inserter is used to place a penile implant (Meeker and Rothrock).

530. (A) A boomerang is a prostate instrument (Meeker and Rothrock).

531. (D) A Millin is a retropubic bladder retractor (Meeker and Rothrock).

532. (C) The Gomco is a circumcision clamp used for infants. For adults, a plastic instrument set is used (Meeker and Rothrock).

533. (A) A Humi cannula is used in gynecologic surgery for placement into the uterine cavity via the cervix for intraoperative chromotubation with diluted methylene blue or indigo carmine solution (Meeker and Rothrock).

534. (D) The Hulka forceps may be introduced into the cervix to manipulate the uterus for better visibility (Meeker and Rothrock).

535. (A) A central venous pressure catheter insertion is a minor operative procedure requiring sterile gloves, drapes, and instruments (Fortunato).

536. (C) Bakes are a set of common duct dilators (Meeker and Rothrock).

537. (D) A Steffee plate is an internal spinal implant fixation system used for treatment of fractures, spondylolisthesis, and idiopathic scoliosis of the thoraco–lumbar spine (Fortunato).

538. (C) Crutchfield tongs are for skeletal traction (Fortunato).

539. (D) The Bookwalter is a self-retaining retractor system (Meeker and Rothrock).

540. (A) A Harrington is a large retractor (Meeker and Rothrock).

541. (B) The Schnidt is a long thoracic forceps (Meeker and Rothrock).

542. (B) Bougie dilators are available in graduated sizes for esophageal dilation (Meeker and Rothrock).

b. Equipment

543. (A) After removal of the split-thickness mesh graft with dermatome, the graft is placed on a plastic dermacarrier, upside down. The mesher then cuts small parallel slits in the graft. This permits expansion to three times its original size (Meeker and Rothrock).

544. (C) Phacoemulsification (the fragmentation of a lens by use of ultrasonic energy and its subsequent aspiration from the capsule) is accomplished by the use of a Cavitron unit (Meeker and Rothrock).

545. (C) The power source is inert, nonflammable, and explosion-free gas. Compressed nitrogen is the power source for all air-powered equipment (Meeker and Rothrock).

546. (B) Air Drill 100 has replaced the Surgairtome or Hall II Air Drill for precision cutting, shaping, and bone repair. Compressed nitrogen is its power source (Meeker and Rothrock).

547. **(D)** To correct an olecranon fracture, small fracture compression screws and set, Kirschner wires, Steinmann pins, and figure-of-eight wire may be used along with small bone and tissue sets. The others require large bone sets (Meeker and Rothrock).

548. **(D)** A permanent pacemaker has a pulse generator and electrode–pulse generators are typically powered by lithium, which lasts 5 to 10 years. They are classified as fixed ventricular, demand, and physiologic (Meeker and Rothrock).

549. **(C)** Hall is an air drill. Reese, Padgett–Hood, and Brown are all dermatomes (Meeker and Rothrock).

550. **(A)** Hypothermia deliberately reduces body temperature to permit reduction of oxygen consumption by about 50% (Meeker and Rothrock).

551. **(C)** The oxygenator, heat exchanger, and pump are the three components of a cardiopulmonary bypass system. To restart the heart after surgery, the need for a ventricular fibrillator would be additional (Meeker and Rothrock).

552. **(A)** A powdered surgical instrument utilizing rotary movement to drill holes or insert screws, wires, or pins. Reciprocating movement cuts front to back, and oscillating cuts side-to-side. They can have a combination changed by adjusting controls (Fortunato).

553. **(D)** Air-powered instruments are small, lightweight, free of vibration, and easy to handle for pinpoint accuracy at high speed. Minimal heating of the bone is generated (Fortunato).

554. **(D)** The power source for Air Drill 100 is compressed nitrogen. This drill is known for its precision cutting, shaping, and repair of bone (Meeker and Rothrock).

555. **(D)** Dermatomes may be electric or air-powered with compressed nitrogen or air (Fortunato).

556. **(A)** A residual of distilled water should be left in the lumen of any tubing to be sterilized by steam. Tubing should be coiled without kinks and disassembled from suction tips. Rubber bands prevent steam penetration (Fortunato).

557. **(B)** A right-angled tube with a small diameter used for small amounts of fluid such as in brain, spinal, plastic, or orthopedic surgery is Ferguson–Frazier (Fortunato).

558. **(D)** The Yankauer tonsil tip is a hollow tube, with an angle, used in the mouth and throat (Fortunato).

559. **(D)** A blood count may take some time. However, visual inspection of blood in sponges, measurement of blood in the sponges by weighing them, and estimation of blood in the suction containers are immediate methods. When measuring the suction container, allowance must be made for the presence of other body fluids and irrigants. The scrub nurse estimates the amount of irrigant used by keeping track of amounts given on field (Fortunato).

560. **(A)** In the cellsaver, blood is suctioned, and an anticoagulant solution of heparinized saline or citrated dextrose mixes with blood at the tip of the tubing. It is filtered and separated, and red blood cells (RBCs) are washed, infused with saline, and go into a reinfusion bag (about 250 cc) (Fortunato).

561. **(B)** Suction tubing must be kept open and collection containers changed as necessary to maintain suction for irrigation during operation (Fortunato).

562. **(D)** In ENT surgery, wall suction must be available, including several patent cannulas. The degree of suction is variable and often is controlled by a foot pedal so that the surgeon has control of it for grasping and releasing an object (Fortunato).

563. **(C)** Suction is necessary to evacuate blood, cerebrospinal fluid, and irrigating fluid for better visualization. A Ferguson–Frazier tip is used. Avoid applying vacuum directly on brain or normal neural tissue (Fortunato).

564. **(B)** Apply a tourniquet only as a last resort when hemorrhage cannot be controlled by any other means. Tourniquets can cause irreparable vascular or neurologic damage (Fortunato).

565. **(B)** The average arm is 300 mm Hg. The average leg is 500 mm Hg (Fortunato).

566. **(B)** While elevated, the extremity is wrapped distally to proximally with an Esmarch rubber bandage to exsanguinate the limb. The tourniquet is then inflated (Meeker and Rothrock).

567. **(C)** The patient's age, the size of extremity, and the patient's systolic pressure are all factors to be considered when applying a tourniquet. The depth of the incision is of no consequence (Meeker and Rothrock).

568. **(A)** A Bier is a regional intravenous injection of a local to an extremity below level of the tourniquet. The extremity remains painless as long as the tourniquet is in place (Fortunato).

569. **(A)** A tourniquet should never be used when direct circulation in the distal part of an extremity is impaired. It could cause tissue injury, shutting off of blood supply to the part below causing gangrene and loss of the extremity (Fortunato).

570. **(C)** Elevate an arm or leg to encourage venous drainage before tightening a tourniquet (Fortunato).

571. **(B)** Tourniquet application and removal time is recorded. The surgeon is informed when it has been on for 1 hour and then every 15 minutes (Fortunato).

572. **(D)** If the patient has had a traumatic injury or casting, danger exists that thrombi might be in vessels because of injury or stasis of blood. These could become dislodged and result in emboli (Fortunato).

573. **(A)** Air, oxygen, freon, or ambient air are used. Nitrous oxide is an anesthetic gas (Fortunato).

574. **(C)** Caution must be taken to prevent solution from pooling under a tourniquet. Apply tourniquet and drape position before tourniquet is inflated (Fortunato).

575. **(D)** Tourniquets are not used if circulation is compromised. Arthroscopy, bunionectomy, and tendon repair on a child would be indications for use (Fortunato).

576. **(C)** The ground plate or inactive electrode is lubricated with an electrosurgical gel and is placed in good contact with a fleshy, non-hairy body surface. It should not be placed over a bony prominence. The grounded pathway returns the electrical current to the unit after the surgeon delivers it to the operative site (Fortunato).

577. **(D)** Bipolar units provide a completely isolated output with negligible leakage of current between the tips of the forceps. The need for a dispersive pad is eliminated (Meeker and Rothrock).

578. **(A)** The dispersive pad is the inactive electrode. It is placed as close to the operative site as possible, on the same side of the body as the operative site and over a large muscle if possible. Bony prominences and scar tissue should be avoided. Good contact is essential (Meeker and Rothrock).

579. **(D)** To complete the electric circuit to coagulate or cut tissue, current must flow from a generator (power unit) to an active electrode, through tissue, and back to generator via the inactive electrode (Fortunato).

580. **(A)** The tip is kept clean, dry, and visible. Charred or coagulated tissue is removed by wiping with a tip cleaner or scraping with the back of a knife blade. Charred tissue on the electrode absorbs heat and decreases effectiveness of current (Fortunato).

581. **(A)** Vessels are coagulated when any part of the metal instrument is touched with the active electrode. It is known as buzzing (Fortunato).

582. **(C)** The bipolar cautery provides extremely precise control of the coagulated area (Fortunato).

583. **(D)** The ground plate should be as close as possible to the site where the active electrode will be used to minimize current through body (Fortunato).

584. **(D)** The sterile active electrode directs the flow of current to the operative site. Style of the electrode tip may be blade, loop, ball, or needle. It may be attached to a pencil-shaped handle or incorporated into either a tissue-forceps or suction tube (Fortunato).

585. **(C)** Electrosurgery is not used in the mouth, around the head, or in the pleural cavity when high concentrations or oxygen or nitrous oxide are used because of fire and explosion hazards (Fortunato).

586. **(B)** Only moist sponges should be permitted on a sterile field while the electrosurgical unit is in use, to prevent fire (Fortunato).

587. **(A)** Hydrogen methane gases are normally present in the colon. These gases must be flushed out with carbon dioxide before laser or electrosurgery through the colonoscope to avoid possibility of explosion within the colon (Fortunato).

588. **(D)** In fulguration, sparks of high voltage current char the tissue producing eschar. It uses a high-frequency cutting current and is used primarily for transurethral resection (TUR) and prostate surgery (Fortunato).

589. **(A)** More electric current is needed when working in solution, as in the bladder, than in the air. During bladder surgery, continuous irrigation is necessary to distend bladder for visualization and wash out debris (Fortunato).

590. **(A)** Fulguration of a tumor is accomplished by use of a cutting electrode to destroy tissue. It both cuts and coagulates (Fortunato).

591. **(C)** Choledochoscopy is direct visualization of the common bile duct by means of a choledocoscope introduced into the common bile duct. This takes the place of operative cholangiography and provides a means for stones difficult to remove (Meeker and Rothrock).

592. **(A)** Fiberoptic lighting is an intense cool light that illuminates body cavities via a bundle of thousands of coated glass fibers. It is non-glaring (Fortunato; Meeker and Rothrock).

593. **(D)** Two major complications of endoscopy are perforation and bleeding (Fortunato).

594. **(B)** A bronchoscopy is considered surgically clean. The rest require a sterile setup (Fortunato).

595. **(D)** Most cables are autoclaved but according to manufacturers directions only (Meeker and Rothrock).

596. **(B)** A simple test for the integrity of the cable is to hold one end of the cable to a bright light and inspect the opposite end. Dark spots are an indication that some of the fibers are broken (Fortunato; Meeker and Rothrock).

597. **(D)** Light is cold, meaning that the heat is not transmitted throughout scope and tissue is not damaged. The ends, however, can get hot and should be kept out of contact with patient and personnel skin. Keep cable away from drapes or place on moist towel to prevent burns and fires (Meeker and Rothrock).

598. **(A)** The Endoflush system is an economical, practical, and effective way to clean channeled instruments. It removes organic debris and flushes out ports (Meeker and Rothrock).

599. **(C)** Peracetic acid is bactericidal, fungicidal, and sporicidal. It is used for heat-sensitive items that can be cleaned and completely immersed. The process cycle is less than 30 minutes and especially good for endoscopes (Meeker and Rothrock).

600. **(A)** Only one scope or a few instruments can be done in a cycle. It is sporicidal, the process is only 20–30 minutes, and it is cost-effective (Meeker and Rothrock).

601. **(D)** The mediastinoscope is used to view lymph nodes or masses in the superior mediastinum. The mediastinum contains all the thoracic viscera except the lungs (Meeker and Rothrock; *Mosby's Medical, Nursing, and Allied Health Dictionary*, 5th ed.).

602. **(B)** Loupes are glasses with telescopic lenses used for magnification in microvascular surgery and nerve repair (Meeker and Rothrock).

603. **(A)** The ability to discern detail is known as resolving power or resolution (Fortunato).

604. **(D)** The optical combination of the objective lens and the oculars determine the magnification of the microscope (Fortunato).

605. **(C)** Objective lenses are available in various focal lengths ranging from 100 to 400 mm with intervening increases by 25-mm increments. The 400 mm provides the greatest magnification (Fortunato).

606. **(C)** A continuously variable system of magnification for increasing or decreasing images is possible with zoom lens, usually operated with a foot control to free surgeons' hands from the task (Fortunato).

607. **(A)** The slit aperture permits a narrow beam of light to be brought into focus on the field. This slit image assists the surgeon in defining depth perception (relative distance of objects within the field) (Fortunato).

608. **(C)** Usually fiberoptic, coaxial illumination provides intense, cool light. Paraxial illuminators contain tungsten or halogen bulbs (Fortunato).

609. **(B)** Microscopes should be damp dusted before use. All external surfaces, except the lenses, are wiped with detergent–disinfectant solution. Casters are also cleaned. It is kept dust free with an antistatic cover (Fortunato).

610. **(A)** A beam splitter takes the image from one of the surgeon's oculars and transmits it through an observer tube; thereby, providing the assistant with an identical image of the surgeon's view (Fortunato).

611. **(C)** The culpomicroscope illuminates and permits identification of abnormal cervical (ectocervical, lower cervical canal, and vaginal wall) epithelium to target for biopsies (Fortunato).

612. **(C)** The laryngoscope becomes self-retaining by suspension in a special appliance placed over the patient's chest, thus enabling the surgeon freedom of his or her hands to use a microscope and perform procedures (Fortunato).

613. **(A)** A microscope is a monocular or binocular. The binocular has two telescopes mounted side-by-side that gives stereoscopic vision (Meeker and Rothrock).

614. **(C)** Eye pieces are interchangeable and are available in four magnifying powers: 10×, 12.5×, 16×, and 20× (Meeker and Rothrock).

615. **(C)** A, B, and D are appropriate techniques. Oil or fingerprints are removed with a solvent or lens-cleaning solution or 50% denatured alcohol; however, solvents should be used sparingly so that cemented surfaces are not destroyed (Meeker and Rothrock).

616. **(D)** Some tables have a metal crossbar or body elevator between the two upper sections that can be raised to elevate a gallbladder or kidney (Fortunato).

617. **(D)** A double arm board is sometimes called an "airplane support." Both levels must be padded. It is used in lateral positioning (Fortunato).

618. **(D)** The shoulder bridge (thyroid elevator) is a metal bar slipped under the mattress between the head (removed during placement) and body sections. This hyperextends the shoulder or thyroid area for accessibility (Fortunato).

619. **(B)** Concave metal supports or shoulder braces are used to prevent the patient from slipping when the head of the table is tilted down, as in the Trendelenburg position (Fortunato).

620. **(D)** The kidney rests provide position stability in kidney position. They should not press too tightly against body, should be well padded, and the longer rest is beneath the iliac crest to minimize pressure on abdominal organs (Fortunato).

621. **(C)** Chest rolls (bolsters) elevate the chest to facilitate respiration (Fortunato).

622. **(B)** Bakelite or other material that does not interfere with radiologic studies is used for attachments that might otherwise obscure findings (Fortunato).

623. **(B)** During surgery, such dry combustibles as sponges or towels, near the laser tissue impact site should be kept wet to prevent ignition (Meeker and Rothrock).

624. **(B)** Laser plume contains carbonized particles, water, and odor, thus adequate smoke evacuation is necessary to remove the potentially viable contaminants from the air (Meeker and Rothrock).

625. **(A)** Instrumentation used in the immediate vicinity of the laser tissue impact site should be nonreflective to decrease the chance of the laser beam bouncing off the surface and accidentally impacting another area (Meeker and Rothrock).

626. **(B)** The argon laser operates in the visible light region in the blue–green spectrum. It is easily delivered to the tissue through flexible fiber optics and can be coupled to a microscope or hand piece. Argon laser energy is primarily absorbed in tissue by melanin and hemoglobin (Meeker and Rothrock).

627. **(C)** A Halon fire extinguisher consisting of hydrogenated halocarbons is recommended for laser unit fires because it does not produce a residue and has low toxicity (Ball).

628. **(A)** Prep solutions should be pat-dried, because pooled fluids can retain the laser heat and subsequently burn the tissue (Ball).

629. **(A)** The patient should be instructed to self-administer a preoperative enema to clean the lower bowel. The surgeon uses suction to evacuate any methane gas which could cause a large bowel explosion fire. The lower rectal area is packed with wet, counted sponges to decrease methane gas from escaping into the surgical area and creating a fire hazard (Ball).

630. **(B)** Laser instruments can be ebonized to decrease the chance of laser beam reflection when used near impact site. Instruments are coated with a substance to decrease reflectivity, often producing a black surface (Ball).

631. **(C)** Plastic vaginal and rectal speculae should not be used because they can burn or melt when struck by the laser beam. Ebonized or anodized (dull) instruments decrease risk of injury. Reflective drapes are less flammable (Ball).

632. **(C)** Universal precautions should be used when one is exposed to surgical smoke in order to reduce occupational exposure through the skin, eye, and mucous membrane (Ball).

633. **(C)** The slit lamp is a stereoscopic biomicroscope that magnifies in three dimensions. It is used for the delivery of the laser beam especially in the treatment of glaucoma (Fortunato; Meeker and Rothrock).

634. **(D)** Ruby lasers are primarily used to eradicate port-wine stain lesions of the skin (Fortunato).

635. **(B)** Eye protection with lenses that filter specific wave lengths is needed. Argon and YAG lasers will be absorbed by the retina and the CO_2 laser by the cornea. Argon requires an amber-tinted lens filter, CO_2 requires clear glass or plastic with side shields, and YAG requires a green-tinted lens filter (Fortunato; Ball).

636. **(D)** Special high filtration masks should be worn (double masking is inadequate). A smoke evacuator or suction are also effective (Fortunato; Ball).

637. **(B)** A PVC can easily be ignited by a laser beam and support combustion. The others are less likely to ignite (Fortunato; Ball).

638. **(A)** The scrub person should have a basin of sterile water or saline on the instrument table when laser is in use in the event of fire (Fortunato).

639. **(D)** The unit is placed in the standby mode when not actually in use to prevent accidental and uncontrolled laser firing (Ball; Meeker and Rothrock).

640. **(C)** The blue–green argon is used for retinal detachment, tear, or hole (Fortunato).

641. **(B)** The Candela laser is a tunable pulse-dyed system that has the ability to disintegrate stones without damaging soft tissue. Gas lasers are CO_2 or Argon, a solid is Nd:YAG; or a semiconductor crystal is a dioxide (Meeker and Rothrock).

c. Supplies

642. **(D)** The medical antishock trouser (MAST) is a garment designed to correct and counteract internal bleeding conditions and hypovolemia. It creates an encircling pressure around both legs and abdomen. It slows or stops arterial bleeding, forces any available blood from the lower body to the heart, brain, and other vital organs, and it prevents the return of available circulating blood volume to the lower extremities (Fortunato).

643. **(C)** A Levin tube is a #16 French, plastic catheter used in gastric intubation that has a closed weighted tip and an opening on the side (*Mosby's Medical, Nursing, and Allied Health Dictionary*, 5th ed.).

644. **(A)** Cottonoid patties are compressed rayon or cotton sponges that are used moist on delicate structures such as nerves, brain, and spinal cord (Fortunato).

645. **(B)** A moustache dressing may be applied under the nose (nares) to absorb any bleeding (Meeker and Rothrock).

646. **(D)** Stockinette is a knitted, seamless tubing of cotton 1 to 12 inches wide. It stretches to fit any contour snugly (Fortunato).

647. **(A)** In a laminectomy, cottonoid strips or patties are placed in the extremes of the field for hemostasis (Meeker and Rothrock).

648. **(A)** Webril is a soft, lint-free cotton bandage. The surface is smooth but not glazed, so that each layer clings to the preceding one and the padding lies smoothly in place (Fortunato).

649. **(A)** Petroleum gauze packing is inserted into the anal canal following hemorrhoidectomy (Fortunato).

650. **(C)** This bandage is preferable for holding dressings in place over mobile areas such as the neck or extremities, or where pressure is required (Fortunato).

651. **(A)** Kitner dissecting sponges are small rolls of heavy cotton tape that are held in forceps (Fortunato).

652. **(D)** Peanut sponges are very small gauze sponges used to dissect or absorb fluid in delicate procedures (Fortunato).

653. **(A)** Pigskin (porcine) is used as a temporary biologic dressing to cover large body surfaces denuded of skin (Fortunato).

654. **(D)** Pressure dressings are used frequently following extensive operations, especially in plastic surgery, knee operations, and radical mastectomies (Fortunato).

655. **(B)** Tonsil sponges are cotton-filled gauze with a cotton thread attached (Fortunato).

656. **(B)** Patties are moistened with saline and pressed out flat on a metal surface. They could pick up lint if placed on a towel (Fortunato).

657. **(D)** Skin closure tapes may be used instead of or supplementary to closure if very close approximation of skin is required for good cosmetic results (Fortunato).

658. **(A)** Tincture of benzoin is a protective coating substance frequently applied to the skin before adhesive dressings are used (Fortunato).

659. **(D)** A stent dressing or fixation is a method of applying pressure and stabilizing tissues when it is impossible to dress an area. In the case of the nose, for example, long suture ends are criss-crossed over a small dressing and tied (Fortunato).

660. **(A)** Instruments and catheters are measured on a French scale; the diameter (in millimeters) is multiplied by 3. The smallest is 1 mm in diameter times 3, or 3 French (Fortunato).

661. **(A)** Drains may be inserted directly from the incision or through a separate small incision, known as a stab wound, close to the operative site (Meeker and Rothrock).

662. **(A)** A myringotomy is the incision of the tympanic membrane to treat acute otitis media. Frequently tubes are inserted into the tympanic membrane to allow ventilation of the middle ear. Once the tube falls out, the tympanic membrane incision usually heals (Meeker and Rothrock).

663. **(C)** Chest tubes (28–30 Fr.) are used to effect chest drainage via the pleural opening (Meeker and Rothrock).

664. **(C)** A Fogarty-type biliary catheter is a balloon-tipped catheter used to facilitate the removal of small stones and debris in the duct of the gallbladder. It also demonstrates patency of the common bile duct to the duodenum (Meeker and Rothrock).

665. **(A)** Mushroom, Malecot, or Foley catheters are frequently used in the anterior gastric wall and are held in place by a purse-string suture (Meeker and Rothrock).

666. **(D)** A Pezzar or mushroom catheter is for drainage of body cavities. The others are commonly used ureteral catheter tips (Meeker and Rothrock).

667. **(B)** A hemovac is a closed-wound suction system that creates negative pressure in a reservoir attached to the drain (fluid collects here) (Meeker and Rothrock).

668. **(D)** Ureteral catheters are made of flexible woven nylon or other plastic materials, range in size from 3 to 14 French, and have graduated markings in centimeters (Fortunato).

669. **(C)** Ureteral stent is an indwelling stent. It is inserted for long-term or temporary drainage for ureteral obstruction (Fortunato).

670. **(D)** The preferred site of placement is the external jugular vein. Its insertion is indicated for infants and children who require TPN (total parenteral nutrition) because feeding through the GI tract is impossible, inadequate, or hazardous (Meeker and Rothrock).

671. **(B)** A Tenckhoff catheter is an indwelling infusion catheter that is placed percutaneously or directly into a vein or artery or into a body cavity for the administration of chemotherapy (Fortunato).

672. **(C)** Hegar dilators are cervical dilators. The others are all used for urethral dilatation (Meeker and Rothrock).

673. **(B)** This portable system is used to apply suction to a large closed-wound site post-operatively. A constant, negative vacuum evacuates tissue fluid and blood to promote healing by reducing edema and media for microbial growth (Meeker and Rothrock).

674. **(A)** Pressure from a 30-cc catheter balloon inserted after closure of the urethra helps obtain hemostasis by controlling venous bleeding (Meeker and Rothrock).

675. **(B)** Suction tubing with a Lukens tube collects washing specimens during a bronchoscopy (Meeker and Rothrock).

676. **(A)** A Gruntzig balloon dilation catheter is used for balloon angioplasty to dilate occluded vessels (Fortunato).

677. **(D)** A Pezzar or mushroom is a self-retaining catheter and is straight or angulated with a large single channel with the tip in the shape of a mushroom. This catheter is used primarily to drain the bladder suprapubically (Meeker and Rothrock).

678. **(C)** The third lumen provides a means for continuous irrigation of the bladder for a time postoperatively to prevent formation of clots in the bladder (Meeker and Rothrock).

679. **(C)** The image intensifier converts the x-ray beam through the body into a fluoroscopic optic image projected onto a television screen (Fortunato).

680. **(A)** Extracorporeal refers to the outside of the body. Many cardiac surgical procedures are done while the patient is placed on partial or complete cardiopulmonary bypass (CPB) (extracorporeal circulation). A pump removes blood from the systemic circulation, filters it, passes it through an oxygenator, and returns it to the patient via a cannula in the ascending aorta or the femoral artery. The oxygenated blood is used by the organs and tissues of the body and then returned to the pump or heart–lung machine, where the process is once again repeated (*Mosby's Medical, Nursing, and Allied Health Dictionary*, 5th ed.).

681. **(C)** The Apgar score is a system that scores an infant's physical condition 1 minute after birth. The heart rate, respiration, muscle tone, color, and stimuli response are scored. The maximum total score for a normal baby is 10. Those with low scores require immediate attention if they are to survive (*Mosby's Medical, Nursing, and Allied Health Dictionary*, 5th ed.).

682. **(D)** An electroencephalogram (EEG) records electrical activity of the brain via electrodes applied to the scalp (*Mosby's Medical, Nursing, and Allied Health Dictionary*, 5th ed.).

683. **(C)** A roentgenogram is a photographic image produced as x-rays pass through the body and expose the x-ray film (*Mosby's Medical, Nursing, and Allied Health Dictionary*, 5th ed.).

684. **(B)** An abduction pillow is placed between the patient's legs postoperatively to aid in immobilization of the hip joints after surgery (Meeker and Rothrock).

685. **(D)** Disposable chest drainage collects drainage, maintains a water seal, and provides suction control. It is aimed at providing a conduit for air, blood, and other fluids as well as the re-establishment of negative pressure in the intrapleural space (Meeker and Rothrock).

686. **(D)** Drainage systems consist of drainage collection, water seal, and suction. Air, blood, and other fluid from the interpleural space are drained to re-establish negative pressure in the interpleural space that has resulted from a collapsed lung (Meeker and Rothrock).

687. **(A)** A Minerva jacket is applied from the hips to the head. If the head is to be completely immobilized, it is included in the jacket. It is used for fractures of the cervical or upper thoracic vertebra (Fortunato).

688. **(D)** Inflatable, double-walled vinyl boots use alternating compression and relaxation to reduce risk of deep-vein clotting in legs of high-risk patients undergoing general anesthesia (Fortunato).

689. **(A)** Prolene mesh is inert. It can be used in the presence of infection. Mersilene and Gore-tex cannot (Fortunato).

690. **(B)** Mersilene mesh comes in sterile sheets. Unused, but *not* soiled or blood stained, mesh may be steam sterilized only *once*. It is important that it to be marked so it is not reused more than once (Fortunato).

691. **(C)** Autogenous bone, from the patient is taken from the ilium, tibia, or rib cage (Fortunato).

692. **(D)** The patient may come to the OR with this in place to control bleeding by pressure from the inflated balloon in the tube (Fortunato).

693. **(B)** A temporary or permanent opening in the stomach for decompression or alimentation is accomplished with either a Foley, Mallecot, Pezzer, or Mushroom catheter (Fortunato).

694. **(D)** Complications such as hemorrhage, infection, cervical stenosis, incompetent cervix, and infertility are minimized by obtaining the biopsy with a carbon dioxide laser cutting beam (Fortunato).

695. **(C)** Stereotaxis is the accurate location of a definite area within the brain from external points or landmarks on the skull via the computer. The stereotactic surgery can be performed through a burr hole, endoscope, or open craniotomy. Various intracranial procedures are performed with computer-assisted stereotaxis (Fortunato).

696. **(A)** The Doppler is a blood flow detector. Ultrasonic imaging records flowing blood (Fortunato).

697. **(D)** A secondary monitor is called a "slave" (Meeker and Rothrock).

698. **(A)** The Hickman catheter is used for long-term intermittent chemo or antibiotic infusion. It is introduced via the jugular, cephalic, or subclavian vein into the superior vena cava or the right atrium (Fortunato).

699. **(A)** Any patient who cannot be nutritionally maintained by other means is a candidate for total parenteral hyperalimentation nutrients provided via long-term indwelling catheter (Fortunato).

700. **(D)** An Ambu, or breathing bag, controls flow of respiratory gases entering the lungs (*Mosby's Medical, Nursing, and Allied Health Dictionary*, 5th ed.).

701. **(C)** A blood warmer is used to maintain 89°–105°F temperature. Cold blood may induce hypothermia; whereas, blood too warm may cause hemolysis (Fortunato).

702. **(B)** A blood filter is used for all transfusions to filter out microaggregates (Fortunato).

703. **(A)** A hyperthermia blanket is warmed and maintained at 95°–100°F and is double thickness covered. The other statements are all true (Fortunato).

704. **(B)** Choledochoscopy is direct visualization of the common bile duct requiring distention of the common bile duct (CBD) for better visualization. This is done by irrigating the ducts with saline via a pressure bag (300 Hg) around an IV (saline) bag. Sterile tubing is passed off-field and attached to saline. Scrub nurses attach the distal end of IV tubing to irrigating stopcock on choledochoscope (Meeker and Rothrock).

705. **(C)** A laminaria tent is a cone composed of dried seaweed that swells as it absorbs water and, therefore, is used to dilate the cervix nontraumatically in preparation for induced abortion (Meeker and Rothrock; *Mosby's Medical, Nursing, and Allied Health Dictionary,* 5th ed.).

706. **(B)** A radiant warmer provides immediate postdelivery care of the infant delivered by C-section. These infants are at risk until there is evidence of physiologic stability (Meeker and Rothrock).

707. **(A)** In fluoroscopy, a fluorescent light reproduces optical images of body structures identified by x-rays onto a luminescent screen. These images can be amplified with an image intensifier and can be projected onto a TV monitor (Fortunato).

708. **(D)** Radiation exposure can be as much as 10 times greater during 1 minute of fluoroscopy that than of a single x-ray (Meeker and Rothrock).

709. **(A)** A patient controlled analgesia (PCA) is a pain management device which administers a predetermined intravenous dose of narcotic substitute for pain relief. It allows a continuous and bolus administration when the patient believes it is necessary (Meeker and Rothrock).

C. Counts

710. **(C)** The scrub nurse and the circulator count each item aloud and together. The nurse then records the number. Count additional items away from already counted items. Counting should be uninterrupted (Fortunato).

711. **(A)** If a pack contains an incorrect number of sponges, it is the responsibility of the circulator to isolate it, and it is not used. The danger of error is great if attempts are made to correct or compensate for discrepancies (Fortunato).

712. **(A)** Each item used must be considered a foreign object that can cause unnecessary harm should it be left inside the patient. Detachable parts of instruments must be counted. This ensures that part of an instrument does not remain in the wound (Fortunato).

713. **(D)** Sponge and instrument counts are very important in vaginal procedures. Sponges should be secured on sticks in deep areas. This prevents loss in hard-to-see areas (Fortunato).

714. **(A)** The relief of either the scrub or the circulator by another person necessitates the verification of all counts before person being relieved leaves room. Persons taking final counts are held accountable and must sign record (Fortunato).

715. **(B)** During the closure count, the scrub person reports counts as correct or incorrect to the surgeon (Fortunato).

716. **(C)** If a sponge is intentionally retained for packing of an instrument remains with patient, this should be noted on operative record (Fortunato).

717. **(D)** If a pack contains an incorrect number of sponges, scrub hands pack to circulator. Attempts should not be made to correct errors or compensate for discrepancies. Pack is isolated and not used (Fortunato).

718. **(B)** Prep sponges are bagged in plastic and stored in the room. Never place in the kick bucket or trash receptacle until after completion of final count (Fortunato).

REFERENCES

Association of Surgical Technologists. *Surgical Technology for the Surgical Technologist: A Positive Approach.* Albany, NY: Delmar, 2001.

Ball KA. *Lasers, The Perioperative Challenge,* 2nd ed. St. Louis: Mosby-Year Book, 1995.

Fortunato, Nancymarie. *Berry and Kohn's Operating Room Technique,* 9th ed. St. Louis: Mosby, 2000.

Meeker M, Rothrock J. *Alexander's Care of the Patient in Surgery,* 11th ed. St. Louis: Mosby, 1999.

Mosby's Medical, Nursing, and Allied Health Dictionary, 5th ed. St. Louis: Mosby-Year Book, 1998.

Pilling Surgical: Instrument Catalogs (General and Specialty).

PART 3

Intraoperative and Postoperative Procedures
Questions

DIRECTIONS (Questions 719 through 1267): Each of the numbered items or incomplete statements in this section is followed by answers or by completions of the statement. Select the ONE lettered answer or completion that is BEST in each case. Check your answers with the correct answers at the end of the chapter.

I. GENERAL SURGERY

719. In a gastrointestinal closure, the mucosa of the intestinal tract is closed with

   (A) chromic 4–0 or 3–0
   (B) silk 4–0 or 3–0
   (C) Dacron 3–0 or 2–0
   (D) Novafil 3–0 or 2–0

720. Which type of suture would be used to invert the stump of an appendix?

   (A) buried
   (B) purse-string
   (C) mattress
   (D) tension

721. Why are bumpers or bolsters used on retention sutures?

   (A) to prevent the suture from cutting into the skin surface
   (B) to facilitate easy removal
   (C) to identify the order of suture removal
   (D) to prevent unequal tension on the wound edges

722. A Nissen Fundoplication procedure is done to correct

   (A) repeated attacks of volvulus
   (B) antireflux disease
   (C) bladder prolapse
   (D) gastroesophageal stenosis

723. A dissecting sponge that is a small roll of heavy cotton tape is a

   (A) Kitner
   (B) peanut
   (C) tonsil
   (D) tape

724. Which procedure would not require a pressure dressing?

   (A) plastic surgery
   (B) knee surgery
   (C) radical mastectomy
   (D) hysterectomy

725. Peanuts and dissecting sponges are generally

   (A) used dry
   (B) moistened with saline
   (C) moistened with water
   (D) moistened with antibiotic solution

726. Intraabdominally, lap pads are most often used

   (A) dry
   (B) moistened with saline
   (C) moistened with water
   (D) moistened with glycine solution

727. A catheter commonly used in a gastrostomy is a

(A) mushroom
(B) Rehfus
(C) Cantor
(D) Sengstaken–Blakemore

728. Before handing a Penrose drain to the surgeon

(A) place it on an Allis clamp
(B) attach a safety pin to it
(C) cut it to the desired length
(D) moisten it in saline

729. A closed-wound suction system works by

(A) positive pressure
(B) negative-pressure vacuum
(C) air displacement
(D) constant gravity drainage

730. Which condition regarding sterile technique is NOT recommended?

(A) sterile tables are set up just before the operation
(B) sterile tables may be set up and safely covered until time of surgery
(C) once sterile packs are open, someone must remain in the room to maintain vigilance
(D) sterile persons pass each other back to back

731. Which of the following conditions is not an acceptable aseptic technique?

(A) scrub nurse standing on a platform or standing stool
(B) scrub nurse keeps hands below shoulder level
(C) scrub nurse folds arms with hands at axillae
(D) scrub nurse's hands are at or above waist level

732. The disposable circular staple designed to hold two tubular structures together after resection is known as

(A) TA linear
(B) LDS
(C) EEA
(D) GIA

733. When a sterile item is hanging or extending over the sterile table edge, the scrub nurse

(A) must watch closely that no one comes near it
(B) does not touch the part hanging below table level
(C) should pull it back onto the table so it does not become contaminated
(D) may use the item

734. Which of the following is considered a break in technique?

(A) a sterile person turns his or her back to a nonsterile person or area when passing
(B) sterile persons face sterile areas
(C) a sterile person sits or leans against a nonsterile surface
(D) nonsterile persons avoid sterile areas

735. In which situation should sterility be questioned?

(A) if a sterilized pack is found in an unsterile workroom
(B) if the surgeon turns away from the sterile field for a brow wipe
(C) if the scrub drapes a nonsterile table, covering the edge nearest the body first
(D) if the lip of a pour bottle is held over the basin as close to the edge as possible

736. Transduodenal sphincterotomy refers to the incision made into the _____ to relieve stenosis.

(A) cardiac sphincter
(B) ileocecal sphincter
(C) sphincter of Oddi
(D) phyloric sphincter

737. When handing skin towels to the surgeon, where should the scrubperson stand in relation to the surgeon?

    (A) on the opposite side of the table
    (B) on the same side of the table
    (C) at the foot of the table
    (D) any position is acceptable

738. Irrigating fluid used to flush the organ between harvest and transplantation of a liver is known as

    (A) Ringer's Lactate
    (B) Physiosol
    (C) Collin's
    (D) normal saline

739. Each of the following actions by a scrubperson prevents wounds and punctures, according to CDC guidelines EXCEPT

    (A) use an instrument to remove blades
    (B) recap injection needles
    (C) account for each needle as surgeon finishes with it
    (D) protect sharp blades, edges, and tips

740. Which of the following is NOT an acceptable technique when draping a patient?

    (A) hold the drapes high until directly over the proper area
    (B) protect the gloved hands by cuffing the end of the drape over them
    (C) unfold the drapes before bringing them to the OR table
    (D) place the drapes on a dry area

741. The procedure to follow if a hair is found on the operative field is to

    (A) notify circulator
    (B) complete an incident report
    (C) remove it with a clamp, cover over area
    (D) no action is necessary

742. Cancer technique in surgery refers to

    (A) the administration of an anticancer drug directly into the cancer site
    (B) the discarding of instruments coming in contact with tumor after each use

    (C) the use of radiation therapy at the time of surgery
    (D) the identification of the lesion

743. Why are gowns, gloves, drapes, and instruments changed following a breast biopsy and before incision for a mastectomy?

    (A) to respect individual surgeon's choice
    (B) to follow aseptic principles
    (C) to accommodate two separate incisions
    (D) to protect margins of healthy tissue from tumor cells

744. A postoperative complication attributed to glove powder entering a wound is

    (A) granulomata
    (B) infection
    (C) inflammation
    (D) keloid formation

745. The correct procedure for sterile dressing application is

    (A) apply dressing after drape removal
    (B) apply dressing before drape removal
    (C) apply raytex sponges in thick layer
    (D) apply dressing in recovery room

746. When drop technique for an intestinal procedure is utilized

    (A) two Mayo stands are used
    (B) drapes and gloves do not need to be changed
    (C) contaminated instruments are discarded, gloves are changed
    (D) a separate setup is used for the closure

747. If the floor or wall becomes contaminated with organic debris during a case, the circulator

    (A) calls housekeeping stat
    (B) decontaminates promptly
    (C) decontaminates after case is complete
    (D) defers for terminal cleaning

748. The Sengstaken–Blakemore tube is used for

(A) esophageal hemorrhage
(B) tonsillar hemorrhage
(C) uterine hemorrhage
(D) nasal hemorrhage

749. A specially treated form of surgical gauze that has a hemostatic effect when buried in tissue is

(A) topical thrombin
(B) Gelfoam
(C) human fibrin foam
(D) Oxycel

750. An enzyme extract from bovine blood used as a topical hemostatic agent is

(A) oxytocin
(B) tannic acid
(C) thrombin
(D) collagen

751. A common complication of extubation is

(A) hypotension
(B) tachypnea
(C) hypoxia
(D) hypercapnia

752. The desirable position for better visualization in the lower abdomen or pelvis is

(A) Fowler's
(B) reverse Trendelenburg
(C) Trendelenburg
(D) Kraske

753. Another name for the Kraske position is

(A) prone on an adjustable arch
(B) lateral
(C) knee–chest
(D) jackknife

754. All of the following are helpful in keeping accurate account of sponges EXCEPT

(A) keep sponges separate from linen and instruments
(B) keep needles separate from sponges
(C) keep all sponges and tapes in a basin or close together on the field

(D) keep a mental count of the number of sponges on the field at any given time

755. Dark blood in the operative field may indicate that the patient is

(A) hyperkalemic
(B) hypovolemic
(C) hypotensive
(D) hypoxic

756. In an extreme patient emergency, a sponge count

(A) may be omitted
(B) may be done by the scrub alone
(C) must be done before the case is allowed to begin
(D) must be done before closure

757. Cultures obtained during surgery

(A) are handled as any other specimen
(B) are passed off the sterile field into a bag or container held by the circulator
(C) should be kept warm or sent to the lab immediately
(D) should be handled only by the scrub nurse

758. How is a frozen section sent to the lab?

(A) in formalin
(B) in saline
(C) in water
(D) dry

759. Which of the following specimens is NOT placed in preservative solution?

(A) stones
(B) curettings
(C) tonsils
(D) uterus

760. The term transduodenal sphincterotomy indicates surgery of the

(A) hepatic duct
(B) proximal end of the common bile duct
(C) distal end of the common bile duct
(D) pyloric sphincter

761. McBurney is an incision used for

    (A) appendectomy
    (B) cholecystectomy
    (C) herniorrhaphy
    (D) pilonidal cystectomy

762. The simplest abdominal incision offering good exposure to any part of the abdominal cavity is the

    (A) right subcostal
    (B) Kocher's
    (C) midabdominal transverse
    (D) vertical midline

763. During an appendectomy, a purse-string suture is placed around the appendix stump to

    (A) amputate the appendiceal base
    (B) retract the appendix
    (C) tie off the appendix
    (D) invert the stump of the appendix

764. Gastrointestinal technique is required in all of the following procedures EXCEPT

    (A) cholecystectomy
    (B) low anterior colon resection
    (C) appendectomy
    (D) hemicolectomy

765. A hernia occurring in Hesselback's triangle is called

    (A) indirect
    (B) spigelean
    (C) direct
    (D) femoral

766. Pathologic enlargement of the male breast is called

    (A) subcutaneous adenoma
    (B) gynecomastia
    (C) hypoplasia
    (D) cystic mastitis

767. Sutures placed in a wound to prevent wound evisceration are called

    (A) stent
    (B) fixation
    (C) retention
    (D) traction

768. Surgical enlargement of the passage between the prepylorus of the stomach and the duodenum is a

    (A) pyloromyotomy
    (B) pyloroplasty
    (C) Billroth I
    (D) Billroth II

769. A Whipple operation is surgically termed a

    (A) pancreatectomy
    (B) pancreatoduodenectomy
    (C) pancreatic cyst marsupialization
    (D) transduodenal sphincterotomy

770. A left subcostal incision indicates surgery of the

    (A) gallbladder
    (B) pancreas
    (C) spleen
    (D) common bile duct

771. A lower oblique incision is a(n)

    (A) Pfannenstiel
    (B) inguinal
    (C) paramedian
    (D) midabdominal

772. The curved transverse incision used for pelvic surgery is

    (A) midabdominal transverse
    (B) Poupart
    (C) Pfannenstiel
    (D) McVey

773. Which breast procedure removes the entire breast and axillary contents but preserves the pectoral muscles?

    (A) lumpectomy
    (B) wedge resection
    (C) modified radical mastectomy
    (D) radical mastectomy

774. The breast procedure performed to remove extensive benign disease is a(n)

    (A) axillary node dissection
    (B) simple mastectomy
    (C) radical mastectomy
    (D) modified radical mastectomy

775. What incision is indicated for an esophagogastrectomy?

    (A) left paramedian
    (B) upper vertical midline
    (C) thoracoabdominal
    (D) full midabdominal

776. In which incision could retention sutures be used?

    (A) vertical midline
    (B) McBurney
    (C) transverse
    (D) thoracoabdominal

777. In which hernia is the blood supply of the trapped sac contents compromised and in danger of necrosing?

    (A) direct
    (B) indirect
    (C) strangulated
    (D) reducible

778. In which hernia does the herniation protrude into the inguinal canal but NOT the cord?

    (A) incisional
    (B) femoral
    (C) direct
    (D) indirect

779. Which hernia leaves the abdominal cavity at the internal inguinal ring and passes with the cord structures down the inguinal canal?

    (A) direct
    (B) umbilical
    (C) spigelian
    (D) indirect

780. An abdominal wall defect may be reconstructed using

    (A) Gore-Tex patch
    (B) heavy interrupted silk
    (C) Shouldice repair
    (D) Bassini repair

781. Mersilene is a(n)

    (A) wire mesh
    (B) absorbable suture
    (C) nonabsorbable suture
    (D) synthetic mesh

782. In a cholecystectomy, which structures are ligated and divided?

    (A) cystic duct and cystic artery
    (B) common bile duct and hepatic duct
    (C) cystic duct and common bile duct
    (D) hepatic duct and cystic artery

783. All of the following statements refer to pilonidal cyst surgery EXCEPT

    (A) it is performed with an elliptical incision
    (B) the wound frequently heals by granulation
    (C) probes are required on setup
    (D) the cyst is removed, but the tract remains

784. An important consideration during cholangiogram is to

    (A) irrigate with distilled water
    (B) remove all air bubbles from the cholangiocath
    (C) flash sterilize the choledocoscope
    (D) dip the catheter in lubricating jelly

785. An instrument used to elevate the thyroid lobe during surgical excision is a

    (A) Babcock
    (B) Lahey
    (C) Green
    (D) Jackson

786. The intestinal layer in order, from inside to outside, is

    (A) serosa, mucosa, musculature
    (B) mucosa, submucosa, serosa
    (C) serosa, musculature, mucosa
    (D) mucosa, serosa, musculature

787. A common postoperative patient complaint following a laparoscopic procedure is

    (A) headache
    (B) diarrhea
    (C) gastric upset
    (D) shoulder pain

788. A subphrenic abscess occurs in the

    (A) pancreas
    (B) spleen
    (C) lung
    (D) liver

789. Portal pressure measurement is indicated in

    (A) liver transplant
    (B) splenectomy
    (C) hepatic resection
    (D) Whipple operation

790. Which organ is removed either because of trauma, a blood condition, or as a staging procedure for malignancy?

    (A) adrenals
    (B) spleen
    (C) liver
    (D) pancreas

791. Following a hemorrhoidectomy, a

    (A) dry dressing of 4 × 4s is packed in the rectum
    (B) petroleum gauze packing is placed in the anal canal
    (C) stent dressing is applied
    (D) steri-strip dressing is used

792. A benign anal wall "slit" type of lesion requiring excision is a(n)

    (A) hemorrhoid
    (B) anal fistula
    (C) anal fissure
    (D) pilonidal sinus

793. Which gallbladder procedure ALWAYS requires intraoperative x-rays?

    (A) choledochoscopy
    (B) cholelithotripsy
    (C) choledochoduodenostomy
    (D) cholangiogram

794. In a pilonidal cystectomy, the defect frequently is too large to close and requires use of a(n)

    (A) skin graft
    (B) traction suture
    (C) implant
    (D) packing and pressure dressing

795. The instrument most commonly used to grasp the mesoappendix during an appendectomy is a

    (A) Kelly
    (B) Kocher
    (C) Babcock
    (D) Allis

796. Vaporization and coagulation of hemorrhoidal tissue can be accomplished with

    (A) cautery, bipolar
    (B) cautery, monopolar
    (C) CO_2 laser
    (D) cryosurgery

797. An entire tumor/mass removal is termed

    (A) needle biopsy
    (B) staging biopsy
    (C) excisional biopsy
    (D) incisional biopsy

798. A surgical procedure performed to relieve esophageal obstruction caused by cardiospasm is an

    (A) esophagectomy
    (B) esophagogastrectomy
    (C) esophagomyotomy
    (D) esophagogastrostomy

799. Thrombosed vessels of the rectum are known surgically as

   (A) polyps
   (B) hemorrhoids
   (C) fistulas
   (D) anorectal tumors

800. A procedure done to give the colon a rest and is then reversed is

   (A) temporary colectomy
   (B) temporary colostomy
   (C) abdominoperineal resection
   (D) McVey procedure

801. A device that may obviate the need for an abdominoperineal resection because a low anterior anastomosis can be performed is a(n)

   (A) end-to-end anastomosis (EEA)
   (B) GIA
   (C) TA 55
   (D) LDS

802. An advanced inflammation of the bowel could be conservatively treated with which procedure?

   (A) temporary colostomy
   (B) anterior resection
   (C) hemicolectomy
   (D) abdominal perineal resection

803. Blunt dissection of the gallbladder from the sulcus of the liver requires the use of a

   (A) Metzenbaum
   (B) Kelly
   (C) tampon
   (D) peanut

804. Direct visualization of the common bile duct is accomplished with a

   (A) cholangiocath
   (B) cholangiogram
   (C) choledochoscope
   (D) trocar

805. "Scratch" marking is done in surgery of the

   (A) chin
   (B) eye
   (C) breast
   (D) thyroid

806. Fogarty biliary catheters are used to

   (A) drain the gallbladder
   (B) drain the common bile duct
   (C) instill contrast media
   (D) facilitate stone removal

807. In laparoscopy, tubal patency is checked by

   (A) irrigating with normal saline
   (B) injecting renografin into the tube
   (C) injecting methylene blue into the cervical canal
   (D) irrigating tube with Lugol's solution

808. In a thyroidectomy, a loop retractor retracts the

   (A) platysma muscle
   (B) cervical fascia
   (C) thyroid veins
   (D) sternocleidomastoid muscle

809. Which structure(s) are identified and preserved in thyroid surgery?

   (A) parathyroid glands
   (B) hyoid bone
   (C) thyroglossal duct
   (D) thyroid lobe

810. Bariatric surgery treats

   (A) ulcers
   (B) obesity
   (C) thyroid disease
   (D) carcinoma of the pancreas

811. Which incision would require cutting through Scarpa's fascia?

   (A) subcostal
   (B) inguinal
   (C) Pfannenstiel
   (D) McBurney

812. A gastroplasty

(A) reduces stomach size
(B) corrects gastric junction stenosis
(C) releases adhesions
(D) provides avenue for hyperalimentation

813. Which item retracts the spermatic cord structure in herniorrhaphy?

(A) army–navy retractor
(B) penrose drain
(C) Green retractor
(D) silk suture

814. After uterus removal in a hysterectomy

(A) cervical and vaginal instruments are isolated from the instrument set in a discard basin
(B) the cervix is cauterized
(C) new instruments are used on the cervical closure
(D) cervical instruments are returned to the basket

815. An irreducible hernia whose abdominal contents have become trapped in the extra-abdominal sac is called a(n)

(A) incarcerated hernia
(B) sliding hernia
(C) spigelean hernia
(D) strangulated hernia

816. Which type of endoscopy camera produces the truest color?

(A) one-chip
(B) two-chip
(C) three-chip
(D) four-chip

817. While balancing a video camera in endoscopy requires the scrub person to focus the camera on

(A) a white sponge
(B) a white wall
(C) a glove wrapper
(D) any of the above

818. Defogging the video camera is usually the responsibility of the

(A) circulator
(B) surgeon
(C) scrub person
(D) camera operator

819. A palliative invasive procedure done to prevent malnutrition or starvation is known as

(A) percutaneous endoscopic gastrostomy (PEG) procedure
(B) gastrotomy
(C) gastrostomy
(D) gastrojejunostomy

820. The use of noninvasive high-energy shock waves to pulverize gallstones into small fragments for easy passage through the common bile duct and out of the body is called

(A) choledochoscopy
(B) cholelithotripsy
(C) choledochostomy
(D) choledochotomy

821. Intraoperative cholangiograms can be performed either through open abdominal or laparoscopic procedures using a contrast medium directly into the common bile duct through a

(A) cystocath
(B) cholangiocath
(C) t-tube
(D) red rubber catheter

822. Intra-abdominal pressure during the instillation of CO_2 for creation of pneumoperitoneum is 8–10 mm Hg. A pressure reading higher than this may indicate that the needle may be

(A) buried in fatty tissue
(B) buried in the omentum
(C) in a lumen of intestines
(D) all of the above

823. The proper method of removing the gallbladder specimen after complete dissection and irrigation of the operative site in a laparoscopic cholecystectomy is to

(A) utilize an endobag
(B) pull gallbladder through the largest port
(C) decompress the gallbladder by suctioning bile before removal
(D) all of the above

824. All of the following are recommendations for actions necessary to support the aseptic principle of "confine and contain" EXCEPT

(A) restrict patient contacts to an area 3 feet around the patient
(B) discard sponges into plastic-lined pails
(C) clean spills immediately with broad-spectrum disinfectant
(D) all laundry should be discarded into impervious bags

825. All the following drains are considered active postoperative drains that are attached to an external force EXCEPT

(A) sump
(B) chest
(C) Penrose
(D) Hemovac

826. During a laparoscopic cholecystectomy the surgeon generally stands

(A) at the right side of the patient
(B) at the bottom of the patient's table
(C) at the left side of the patient
(D) in front of the first assistant

827. Gastrointestinal decompression during a general surgical procedure can be effected by the use of a

(A) Levine tube
(B) Miller–Abbot tube
(C) Vari-Dyne
(D) A and B

828. A selected alternative to a conventional ileostomy that denies spontaneous stool exiting from the stoma and requires catheterization of the stoma daily to evacuate the contents is a(n)

(A) cecostomy
(B) ileoanal pull-through
(C) ileal conduit
(D) Kock pouch

829. When both direct and indirect hernias occur in the same inguinal area, the defect is termed

(A) sliding
(B) pantaloon
(C) femoral
(D) spigelian

830. An inguinal hernia containing a Meckel's diverticulum is called a

(A) Richter's
(B) Littre's
(C) Maydl's
(D) spigelian

831. All of the following are designated options of laparoscopic hernia repair EXCEPT

(A) TAPP
(B) ERCP
(C) IPOM
(D) LEP

832. Which muscles are incised in the midline of the neck once the skin flaps are completed during a thyroidectomy?

(A) sternocleidomastoid
(B) strap
(C) sternothyroid
(D) sternoclavicular

833. Which bone is transected with bone-cutting forceps before removal of a thyroglossal cyst?

(A) ethmoid
(B) hyoid
(C) pterygoid
(D) zygomatic process

834. Drainage of an incision following a simple or modified radical mastectomy is accomplished by a

- (A) Penrose
- (B) sump
- (C) closed-wound drainage
- (D) cigarette drain

835. During laparoscopic cholecystectomy, the camera operator usually stands

- (A) across from the surgeon
- (B) to the right of the surgeon
- (C) to the right of the first assistant
- (D) behind the Mayo stand

836. The maximum pressure allowed to prevent the possible intraoperative complications of bradycardia, blood pressure changes, or potential gas emboli during a laparoscopic procedure is

- (A) 8 mm Hg
- (B) 10 mm Hg
- (C) 15 mm Hg
- (D) 20 mm Hg

II. OBSTETRICS AND GYNECOLOGY

837. During surgery, towel clips

- (A) may be removed only by the circulator
- (B) may not be removed once fastened
- (C) may be removed and discarded as long as the area is covered with sterile linen
- (D) may be removed and discarded from the field

838. As grossly soiled instruments are returned to the scrub, they should be

- (A) placed in a basin of sterile saline to soak off debris
- (B) wiped off with a sponge moistened with water or soaked in a basin of sterile distilled water
- (C) wiped off with a dry sponge
- (D) discarded so that the circulator can clean them thoroughly

839. Which of the following actions by the scrubperson is NOT an acceptable sterile technique principle?

- (A) discarding tubing that falls below sterile field edges without touching the contaminated part
- (B) reaching behind sterile team members to retrieve instruments so they do not collect on the patient
- (C) facing sterile areas when passing them
- (D) stepping away from the sterile field if contaminated

840. When the scrubperson is draping a nonsterile table, he or she must

- (A) cover the back edge of the table first
- (B) use a single-thickness drape
- (C) be sure the drape touches the floor
- (D) cuff the drape over his or her gloved hands

841. When covering a Mayo stand, the scrubperson should

- (A) use a wide cuff
- (B) use no cuff
- (C) open the cover fully before placement
- (D) ask the circulator to pull on the cover

842. If a sterile field becomes moistened during a case

- (A) nothing can be done
- (B) extra drapes are added to area
- (C) the wet sections are removed and replaced with dry sections
- (D) the wet sections are covered with a plastic adherent drape

843. The main purpose of the skin prep is to

- (A) remove resident and transient flora
- (B) remove dirt, oil, and microbes, and to reduce the microbial count
- (C) remove all bacteria from the skin
- (D) sterilize the patient's skin

844. Which is the antiseptic solution of choice for a skin prep?

(A) Cipex
(B) Staphene
(C) povidone–iodine
(D) Zephiran

845. When are counts done in the OR?

(A) at beginning and end of case
(B) before beginning of case, at beginning of wound closure, and at skin closure
(C) as case begins and when case is in progress
(D) before beginning of case and at end of case

846. Soiled sponges are

(A) never touched with bare hands
(B) left in the kick bucket until the count begins
(C) removed from the room once the peritoneum is closed
(D) counted and stacked on a towel or sheet on the OR floor

847. Specimens may be passed off the sterile OR table by the scrub person on all of the following items EXCEPT

(A) sponge
(B) towel
(C) basin
(D) paper

848. When handling uterine curettings

(A) never place them in preservative
(B) keep the endometrial and the endocervical curettings separate
(C) send the endometrial and the endocervical curettings to the lab in one container
(D) send them on a 4 × 4 to the lab because it is too difficult to remove them

849. Labor can be induced using

(A) ergotrate
(B) diazoxide
(C) Pitocin
(D) magnesium sulfate

850. The needle used to instill the gas during a laparoscopy is a

(A) Silverman
(B) Crile
(C) Hegar
(D) Verres

851. A Hulka forceps is used in

(A) gynecologic surgery
(B) urologic surgery
(C) thoracic surgery
(D) neurologic surgery

852. Which drug is given to aid in placental expulsion?

(A) oxytocic
(B) anticholinergic
(C) antihistamine
(D) hypoxic

853. A Humi cannula is used in

(A) eye surgery
(B) vascular surgery
(C) urologic surgery
(D) gynecologic surgery

854. The aim of stress incontinence operations includes all of the following EXCEPT

(A) to improve performance of a dislodged or dysfunctional vesical neck
(B) to restore normal urethral length
(C) to tighten and restore the anteriorurethral vesical angle
(D) to repair a congenital defect

855. A procedure done on young women who evidence benign uterine tumors but who wish to preserve fertility is a

(A) subtotal hysterectomy
(B) Wertheim procedure
(C) myomectomy
(D) Le Fort procedure

856. A procedure to prevent cervical dilatation that results in release of uterine contents is a

(A) Shirodkar
(B) LeFort
(C) Wertheim
(D) marsupialization

857. An endoscopic investigation of the uterus and tubes is a

(A) Rubin's test
(B) hysterogram
(C) hysterosalpingogram
(D) hysteroscopy

858. Sterility can be accomplished by all of the following procedures EXCEPT

(A) laparoscopy
(B) minilaparotomy
(C) posterior colpotomy
(D) culdoscopy

859. A scheduled procedure whose ultimate surgical goal involves abdominal, perineal, and groin dissection is a

(A) radical vulvectomy and lymphadenectomy
(B) Wertheim procedure
(C) pelvic exenteration
(D) Manchester procedure

860. An endoscopic approach to pelvic and intra-abdominal examination is

(A) culdocentesis
(B) hysteroscopy
(C) pelviscopy
(D) salpingogram

861. The procedure that provides visualization of the internal contour of the uterus is a

(A) laparoscopy
(B) pelviscopy
(C) hysteroscopy
(D) culposcopy

862. Extrauterine pregnancies can occur in the

(A) abdominal cavity and tube
(B) ovary and pelvic ligaments

(C) abdominal cavity and corpus luteum
(D) pelvic ligaments and tube

863. What gynecologic setup would include various sizes of sterile cannulas?

(A) cesarean
(B) hysterectomy
(C) oophorectomy
(D) suction curettage

864. A Foley catheter is placed into the presurgical hysterectomy patient to

(A) record accurate intake and output
(B) distend the bladder during surgery
(C) avoid injury to the bladder
(D) maintain a dry perineum postoperatively

865. What would an anterior and posterior repair accomplish?

(A) repair of cystocele and rectocele
(B) repair of vesicovaginal fistula
(C) repair of vesicourethral fistula
(D) repair of labial hernia

866. Reconstruction of the cervical canal is called

(A) cervicectomy
(B) trachelorrhaphy
(C) vulvectomy
(D) circlage

867. An incision made during normal labor to facilitate delivery with less trauma to the mother is a(n)

(A) colpotomy
(B) colporrhaphy
(C) episiotomy
(D) celiotomy

868. Cervical carcinoma in situ can be classified as

(A) limited to the epithelial layer, noninvasive
(B) microinvasive
(C) clinically obvious
(D) vaginal extension limitations

869. The fallopian tube is grasped with a

(A) Kocher
(B) Babcock
(C) Kelly
(D) Lahey

870. Reconstruction of the fallopian tube setup would include

(A) Bowman lacrimal probes
(B) Bakes dilators
(C) Hegar dilators
(D) VanBuren sounds

871. To confirm the diagnosis of ectopic pregnancy, it is sometimes necessary to perform a

(A) Rubin's test
(B) culdocentesis
(C) paracentesis
(D) laparotomy

872. Cervical conization is accomplished using all of the following EXCEPT

(A) scalpel
(B) cautery
(C) laser
(D) sclerosing solution

873. Laparoscopic tubal occlusion can be effected by all of the following methods EXCEPT

(A) silastic band
(B) bipolar coagulation
(C) spring clip
(D) chemical ablation

874. The most commonly identified ovarian cyst is the

(A) chocolate
(B) follicle
(C) serous cystadenoma
(D) dermoid

875. A herniation of the cul-de-sac of at the Pouch of Douglas is a(n)

(A) cystocele
(B) rectocele
(C) hydrocele
(D) enterocele

876. A vesicourethral abdominal suspension is known as a

(A) LeFort
(B) Wertheim
(C) Marshall–Marchetti
(D) Shirodkar

877. A condition causing leakage of urine into the vagina is a(n)

(A) ureterovaginal fistula
(B) cystocele
(C) vesicovaginal fistula
(D) rectovaginal fistula

878. What special technique is employed during a hysterectomy?

(A) discard instruments used on cervix and vagina
(B) use second set for closure
(C) redrape for closure
(D) remove Foley before uterus is removed

879. Papanicolaou indicates

(A) removal of small pieces of cervix for examination
(B) cytologic study of cervical smear
(C) staining of the cervix for study
(D) direct visualization of pelvic organs

880. A technique employed for cervical biopsy is

(A) random punches
(B) multiple punches at 3, 6, 9, and 12 o'clock
(C) one central punch at os
(D) one inferior and one superior punch

881. In a cesarean birth, the uterus is opened with a knife and extended with a(n)

(A) Metzenbaum
(B) Heaney
(C) iris scissor
(D) bandage scissor

882. At which point in a cesarean is a bulb syringe used?

(A) when the membranes are incised
(B) when the fetal head is delivered
(C) when the entire infant is delivered
(D) after placental delivery

883. Oxytocics are given in a cesarean after the baby's shoulders are delivered

(A) to contract the uterus
(B) to relax the uterus
(C) to prolong the contraction
(D) to facilitate membrane rupture

884. When closing a uterus in a cesarean, the edges of the uterine incision are clamped with which of the following?

(A) Allis
(B) Kocher
(C) Pennington
(D) Babcock

885. Intraoperative chromotubation can be effected by all of the following surgical cannulaes EXCEPT

(A) Humi
(B) Rubin
(C) Hui
(D) Hulka

886. What suture would be placed into the wall of a large ovarian cyst before aspiration of its contents and final removal?

(A) mattress
(B) suture ligature
(C) purse-string
(D) figure-of-eight

887. What is the preferred procedure for recurrent or persistent carcinoma of the cervix after radiation therapy has been completed?

(A) Wertheim's
(B) pelvic exenteration
(C) abdominal perineal resection
(D) low-anterior resection

888. Which of the following instruments would be used to grasp the anterior cervix of the uterus just before dissection from the vaginal vault during a total abdominal hysterectomy?

(A) Allis
(B) Heaney
(C) Phaneuff
(D) Kelly

889. Laparoscopic tubal occlusion may utilize all of the following methods of effecting sterilization EXCEPT

(A) bipolar coagulation
(B) Silastic bands
(C) Surgitie ligating loop
(D) spring clip

890. A holding instrument not found in a vaginal procedure is a

(A) Jacobs
(B) Lahey
(C) Staude
(D) Skene

891. Conization of the cervix may be accomplished by all of the following EXCEPT

(A) scalpel
(B) Thomas uterine curette
(C) laser
(D) electrosurgery

892. An enterocele differs diagnostically from a rectocele by its contents and its position in the perineum. Its location is in the

(A) Pouch of Douglas
(B) anterior vaginal wall
(C) posterior vaginal wall
(D) pelvic floor

893. Pelviscopy differs from laparoscopy in the

(A) utilization of a larger trocar and scope
(B) utilization of auxiliary ports for ancillary instrumentation
(C) utilization of a 30° angled scope
(D) A and C

894. A Stamey endoscopic procedure is performed to

(A) suspend the vesicle neck
(B) correct anterior wall prolapse
(C) correct posterior wall prolapse
(D) repair a bladder laceration

895. What is the name given to a radical vaginal hysterectomy?

(A) exenteration
(B) Schauta
(C) Wertheim's
(D) LeFort

896. What surgical procedure provides obliteration of the vagina by denuding and approximating the anterior and posterior walls of the vagina?

(A) vaginoplasty
(B) colpocleises
(C) colpoperinorrhaphy
(D) colporrhaphy

897. The hysteroscope may be used to identify or remove all of the following EXCEPT

(A) fallopian adhesions
(B) lost IUDs
(C) intrauterine adhesions
(D) submucosa fibroids

898. Needle aspiration of the cul-de-sac is surgically termed

(A) colpocleisis
(B) culdocentesis
(C) culdotomy
(D) colpotomy

899. An alternative to abdominal hysterectomy utilizing an endoscope is surgically termed a(n)

(A) laparoscopic-assisted vaginal hysterectomy (LAVH)
(B) LEEC
(C) pelviscopic-assisted vaginal hysterectomy (PAVH)
(D) A and C

900. What procedure cannot be performed through a pelviscope?

(A) ovarian cystectomy
(B) hysterectomy
(C) oophorectomy
(D) adhesiolysis

901. Endometrial ablation is performed to correct

(A) amenorrhea
(B) metrorrhagia
(C) menorrhagia
(D) endometriosis

902. Endoscopic visualization of the uterine cavity is called

(A) pelviscopy
(B) laparoscopy
(C) hysteroscopy
(D) colposcopy

903. Marsupialization of a Bartholin cyst involves the

(A) suturing the posterior wall of the cyst to the skin edges
(B) removal of anterior wall of cyst
(C) draining cyst contents
(D) A and B

904. What is the self-retaining retractor used in vaginal procedures?

(A) O'Sullivan–O'Conner
(B) Gelpi
(C) Graves
(D) Auvard

905. Extrauterine disease of the female reproductive system may utilize any of the following lasers via a colposcope or laparoscope EXCEPT

(A) CO_2
(B) Nd:YAG
(C) Candela
(D) argon

III. OPHTHALMOLOGY

906. A sponge used in brain surgery is a(n)

(A) cottonoid patty
(B) Kitner
(C) impregnated gauze
(D) porcine

907. A sponge that is cotton-filled gauze with a cotton thread attached is a

(A) patty
(B) tonsil
(C) Kitner
(D) peanut

908. In cataract surgery, a vesicoelastic drug sometimes used to occupy space in the posterior cavity of the eye is

(A) Alpha-chymotrypsin
(B) mannitol
(C) Healon
(D) Wydase

909. A miotic drug is

(A) pilocarpine
(B) homatropine
(C) atropine
(D) scopolamine

910. What topical anesthetic is used most frequently for preoperative ocular instillation?

(A) lidocaine
(B) tetracaine
(C) cocaine
(D) Dorsacaine

911. The drug added to a local ophthalmic anesthetic to increase diffusion is

(A) alpha-chymotrypsin
(B) hyaluronidase
(C) epinephrine
(D) Varidase

912. A solution used for eye irrigation is

(A) phenylephrine HCl
(B) normal saline
(C) alpha-chymotrypsin
(D) balanced salt solution

913. A synthetic local anesthetic that is effective on the mucous membrane and is used as a surface agent in ophthalmology is

(A) Miochol
(B) Zolyse
(C) Dibucaine
(D) tetracaine

914. Dilating eye drops are called

(A) mydriatics
(B) miotics
(C) myopics
(D) oxytocics

915. Which of the following uses ultrasonic energy to fragment the lens in extracapsular cataract extraction?

(A) keratome
(B) ocutome
(C) cystotome
(D) phacoemulsifier

916. A chalazion is a chronic inflammation of the

(A) lacrimal gland
(B) meibomian gland
(C) eyelid
(D) conjunctiva

917. What procedure is done for chronic dacrocystitis?

(A) extirpation
(B) lacrimal duct probing
(C) myectomy
(D) dacrocystorhinostomy

918. A procedure to treat retinal detachment is

(A) scleral buckling
(B) trabeculectomy
(C) goniotomy
(D) vitrectomy

919. Sagging and eversion of the lower lid is

   (A) entropion
   (B) blepharitis
   (C) ectropion
   (D) ptosis

920. Removal of the entire eyeball is

   (A) keratoplasty
   (B) exenteration
   (C) enucleation
   (D) evisceration

921. A noninvasive process to treat glaucoma by means of a slit lamp is a(n)

   (A) argon or Nd:YAG laser
   (B) Cavitron I&A
   (C) phacoemulsifier
   (D) cryoprobe

922. Removal of a portion of an ocular muscle with reattachment is called

   (A) recession
   (B) resection
   (C) strabismus
   (D) myomectomy

923. Opacity of the vitreous humor is treated by performing a

   (A) cataract removal
   (B) scleral buckling procedure
   (C) vitrectomy
   (D) goniotomy

924. Miocol solution is prepared for a cataract procedure no more than _____ minutes before the actual instillation.

   (A) 5
   (B) 15
   (C) 30
   (D) 60

925. Molteno implants are used surgically to reduce intraocular pressure during

   (A) goniotomy
   (B) trabeculectomy
   (C) argon laser iridotomy
   (D) laser trabeculoplasty

926. A drug used as a lubricant and as vesicoelastic support to maintain separation of tissues before removal of lens during cataract surgery is

   (A) 5-fluorouracil
   (B) Healon
   (C) Mitomycin
   (D) Miostat

927. A drug used to contract the sphincter of the iris during an intracapsular cataract extraction is

   (A) Zolyse
   (B) Healon
   (C) Miocol
   (D) Mitomycin

928. What procedure accomplishes correction of myopia?

   (A) keratoplasty
   (B) keratophakia
   (C) keratotomy
   (D) B and C

929. An enzymatic drug commonly used with anesthetic solutions to increase tissue diffusion is

   (A) Viscoat
   (B) epinephrine
   (C) Ophthaine
   (D) Wydase

930. Injection of anesthetic solution into the base of the eyelids or behind the eyeball to block the ciliary ganglion and nerves is known as

   (A) retrobulbar
   (B) Van Lint block
   (C) O'Brien akinesia
   (D) Bier block

931. A fleshy, triangular encroachment onto the cornea is surgically termed a(n)

   (A) pterygium
   (B) chalazion
   (C) ectropion
   (D) entropion

932. A procedure performed when the cornea is thickened or opacified is called a

(A) keratomileusis
(B) keratotomy
(C) corneal trephining
(D) keratoplasty

933. What is the procedure used to correct accidental vitreous loss during a cataract extraction?

(A) posterior vitrectomy
(B) anterior vitrectomy
(C) pars plana vitrectomy
(D) all of the above

934. A surgical treatment for chronic wide angle-closure glaucoma that re-establishes communication between the posterior and anterior chamber of the eye is

(A) iridectomy
(B) Elliot trephination
(C) cyclodialysis
(E) posterior lid sclerectomies

935. Which of the following hyperosmotic drugs is given preoperatively solely by oral administration to induce osmotic pressure and thereby reduce intraocular pressure in surgery?

(A) Diamox
(B) glycerol
(C) mannitol
(D) urea

936. What eye disease uses the argon slit lamp with a noninvasive procedure, which if successful, prevents the need for more invasive surgery?

(A) cataract
(B) retinal detachment
(C) glaucoma
(D) pterigium

IV. OTORHINOLARYNGOLOGY

937. Which dressing is used after nasal surgery?

(A) collodian
(B) moustache
(C) pressure
(D) telfa

938. What combination of lasers are particularly useful in surgery of the larynx and vocal cords?

(A) CO_2 and argon
(B) CO_2 and helium–neon
(C) CO_2 and Nd:YAG
(D) argon and helium–neon

939. The most common topical anesthetic agent used in ENT surgery is

(A) Xylocaine
(B) procaine
(C) cocaine
(D) Surfacaine

940. Irrigation is used with the ear drill

(A) to remove bone fragments
(B) to minimize transfer of heat from burr to surrounding structures
(C) to add moisture
(D) to control bleeding

941. A surgical schedule would describe the procedure to treat acute otitis media as a

(A) myringotomy
(B) stapes mobilization
(C) fenestration operation
(D) Wullstein procedure

942. In myringotomy, the tube to facilitate drainage is placed into the tympanic membrane with a(n)

(A) alligator forceps
(B) Castroviejo
(C) wire loop curette
(D) Tobey forceps

943. A perforated eardrum is corrected by

(A) myringotomy
(B) stapedectomy
(C) stapedotomy
(D) tympanoplasty

944. Severe vertigo may be relieved by

(A) stapedectomy
(B) myringotomy
(C) labyrinthectomy
(D) endolymphatic shunt

945. Middle ear ventilation is facilitated by

(A) antrostomy
(B) myringotomy
(C) stapedectomy
(D) turbinectomy

946. Cholesteatoma is treated by doing a

(A) tympanoplasty
(B) myringotomy
(C) stapedectomy
(D) mastoidectomy

947. A benign tumor arising from the eighth cranial nerve, which may grow to a size that produces neurologic symptoms is a(n)

(A) myoma
(B) acoustic neuroma
(C) teratoma
(D) fibroma

948. Facial nerve trauma can be decreased by use of

(A) computerized nerve monitor
(B) fluoroscopy
(C) Berman locator
(D) Doppler

949. Another name for submucous resection is

(A) septoplasty
(B) rhinoplasty
(C) antrostomy
(D) trephination

950. Surgical correction of a deviated septum is known as a(n)

(A) antrostomy
(B) submucous resection
(C) rhinoplasty
(D) turbinectomy

951. A forceps used in nasal surgery is a(n)

(A) bayonet
(B) Russian
(C) rat-tooth
(D) alligator

952. Which sinus is entered during an intranasal antrostomy (antral window)?

(A) ethmoid
(B) sphenoid
(C) maxillary
(D) frontal

953. Nasal polyps are removed with either a polyp forceps or a(n)

(A) antrum rasp
(B) Coakley curette
(C) Freer elevator
(D) nasal snare

954. Which of the following medications would be used as a topical anesthetic before nasal surgery?

(A) Numorphan
(B) codeine
(C) cocaine
(D) Marcaine

955. Which surgery requires an incision under the upper lip above the teeth?

(A) Caldwell–Luc
(B) submucous resection
(C) frontal sinus operation
(D) frontal sinus trephination

956. To establish a tracheostomy, a midline incision is created in the neck, below the

(A) suprasternal notch
(B) hyoid bone
(C) cricoid cartilage
(D) corniculate cartilage

957. Which medication is found on a tracheostomy setup to reduce the coughing reflex at tube insertion?

(A) cocaine 4%
(B) lidocaine 1%
(C) cocaine 10%
(D) lidocaine 10%

958. When a tracheostomy tube is inserted, the obturator is quickly removed and the trachea is suctioned with a

(A) catheter
(B) Frazier
(C) Poole
(D) Yankauer

959. The majority of benign salivary gland tumors occur in which gland?

(A) sublingual
(B) submaxillary
(C) parotid
(D) submandibular

960. Which position is used following a tonsillectomy?

(A) dorsal recumbent
(B) on side, horizontally
(C) reverse Trendelenburg
(D) supine

961. Total laryngectomy includes all of the following EXCEPT

(A) soft palate
(B) strap muscles
(C) hyoid bone
(D) larynx

962. What mode would be utilized to maintain drainage postoperatively in radical neck surgery?

(A) Penrose drain
(B) Hemovac
(C) sump drain
(D) t-tube

963. A trifurcate neck incision is done for a(n)

(A) parotidectomy
(B) submaxillary gland excision
(C) uvulopalatopharyngoplasty
(D) radical neck dissection

964. During ear surgery, pledgets generally used to control bleeding are soaked in

(A) saline
(B) heparin
(C) thrombin
(D) epinephrine

965. In cochlear implantation, the receiver is placed into which bone of the skull to gather impulses and send it along to the cerebral cortex?

(A) parietal
(B) mastoid
(C) occipital
(D) frontal

966. Facial nerve decompression is designed to identify an area of compression often seen in

(A) acoustic neuroma
(B) Bell's palsy
(C) vestibular schwannoma
(D) Ménière's disease

967. Which of the following endotracheal tubes can prevent a fire

(A) stainless steel
(B) silicone
(C) latex
(D) red rubber

968. Lesion of the larynx and vocal cords can be addressed surgically using which laser?

(A) Nd:Yag
(B) holmium
(C) CO_2
(D) argon

969. Which degree endoscope is used ONLY in maxillary sinus surgery?

(A) 30°
(B) 70°
(C) 90°
(D) 120°

970. What is the instrument used to effect removal of the septal cartilage in a rhinoplasty?

(A) Knight nasal scissor
(B) Joseph nasal scissor
(C) Jansen–Middleton forceps
(D) Freer septum knife

971. After the anterior pillar of a tonsil is incised with a #12 blade, the tonsil is freed from its attachments with a

(A) Sluder guillotine
(B) LaForce guillotine
(C) Hurd dissector
(D) Boettcher scissors

972. What is the most effective barrier to stop laser energy from penetrating healthy tissue?

(A) proper use of goggles
(B) covering reflective windows
(C) checking laser equipment after each use
(D) moist padding of surrounding tissue

973. A safer alternative laser retardant endotracheal tube used for CO_2 laser surgery of the larynx is made of

(A) copper
(B) stainless steel
(C) silicone
(D) A and B

V. PLASTIC AND RECONSTRUCTIVE SURGERY

---

974. A continuous suture placed beneath the epidermal layer of the skin in short lateral stitches is called a

(A) mattress suture
(B) transfixion suture
(C) retention suture
(D) subcuticular suture

975. An item used for padding that has smooth and clingy layers is called

(A) Webril
(B) stockingette
(C) telfa
(D) gypsum

976. A temporary biologic dressing is

(A) porcine
(B) telfa
(C) collagen
(D) mesh

977. Which of the following is NOT a reason for a pressure dressing?

(A) prevents edema
(B) conforms to body contour
(C) absorbs extensive drainage
(D) distributes pressure evenly

978. A dressing that is held in place by long suture ends criss-crossed and tied is called a

(A) passive
(B) strip closure
(C) Proxi-strip
(D) stent

979. When local anesthetic is passed to the surgeon

(A) hand syringe with cap on
(B) state kind and percentage of solution
(C) state amount being handed
(D) show surgeon the label

980. Which procedure is followed if the scrub is pricked with a needle?

(A) change glove only
(B) discard needle, change glove
(C) place new glove over old
(D) change gown and gloves

981. All of the following statements regarding the preparation for a skin graft are true EXCEPT

(A) the dermatome is placed on the recipient table
(B) the donor site is prepared with a colorless antiseptic agent

(C) separate setups are necessary for skin preparation of recipient and donor sites

(D) items used in preparation of the recipient site must not be permitted to contaminate the donor site

982. When using a sterile syringe, the scrub nurse should

(A) always let the surgeon attach the needle
(B) always use a Luer–Lok tip
(C) never use a Luer–Slip (plain) tip
(D) never touch the plunger except at the end

983. Which of the following is the LEAST desirable method for needle accountability?

(A) insert needle into original packet
(B) collect needles in a medicine cup
(C) place on an adhesive or magnetic board
(D) return to needle rack

984. Colorless prep solution may be indicated for

(A) orthopedic surgery
(B) vascular surgery
(C) plastic surgery
(D) urologic surgery

985. A graft containing epidermis and only a portion of the dermis is called a

(A) split-thickness graft
(B) full-thickness Wolfe graft
(C) composite graft
(D) full-thickness pinch graft

986. A progressive disease of the palmar fascia is termed

(A) Dupuytren's contracture
(B) tendinitis
(C) carpal tunnel syndrome
(D) synovitis

987. Microtia refers to

(A) protrusion of the external ear
(B) absence of the external ear
(C) abnormally small ear
(D) imperforate ear

988. Good contact between a skin graft and the recipient site is facilitated by use of a(n)

(A) stent dressing
(B) Elastoplast
(C) splint–Ace bandage dressing
(D) biologic dressing

989. Syndactyly refers to

(A) an extra digit
(B) an absent digit
(C) webbing of the digits
(D) an ear protrusion

990. A penile defect in which the urethra ends on the ventral surface of the penile shaft or in the perineum is termed

(A) epispadias
(B) chordee
(C) phimosis
(D) hypospadias

991. A face lift is termed a

(A) blepharoplasty
(B) mentoplasty
(C) rhytidectomy
(D) lipectomy

992. The intraoperative use of bone allografts requires all of the following responses from the scrub team EXCEPT

(A) culture before implant
(B) wash with an antibiotic solution
(C) completely thaw
(D) A and B

993. Bulky dressings added to the intermediate layer of a three-layer dressing are used to

(A) eliminate dead space
(B) concentrate pressure in one area
(C) immobilize a body part
(D) A and C

994. All of the following rules cover handling of prosthetic devices during plastic surgery procedures EXCEPT

(A) powder must be wiped from gloves before handling
(B) prosthesis must be dried completely before implant
(C) gloves must be used to prevent skin oils from causing inflammatory response
(D) prosthesis must be placed on lint-free surface to sterilize

995. Adherent, occlusive dressings that are used when slight or no drainage is expected are transparent polyurethane film such as

(A) telfa
(B) Bioclusive
(C) Opsite
(D) B and C

996. A method of applying dressings to an unstable area, such as the face or neck, utilizing long sutures tied over the dressing for stability is known as

(A) pressure
(B) stent
(C) one-layer
(D) three-layer

997. Free jejunal tissue transfers are frequently successful as adjunct surgical revisions following

(A) laryngoesophagectomy
(B) esophagectomy
(C) iliectomy
(D) A and B

998. What is the most commonly used donor tendon for a free flexor tendon graft?

(A) palmaris longus
(B) plantaris tendon
(C) abductor pollicis longus
(D) A and B

999. What bandage effects the process of exsanguination of a limb prior to the use of a tourniquet?

(A) Kling
(B) Elastoplast
(C) Esmarch
(D) Ace

1000. Which muscle is utilized to effect a TRAM flap in breast reconstruction?

(A) latissimus dorsi
(B) transrectus abdominis
(C) pectoralis major
(D) pectoralis minor

1001. The most widely used method of scar revision next to scar removal is

(A) chemical peel
(B) sanding
(C) Z-plasty
(D) planing

VI. GENITOURINARY SURGERY

1002. The Pereyra needle is used in which specialty area of surgery?

(A) neurology
(B) urology
(C) orthopedics
(D) ophthalmology

1003. Which ureteral catheter is used to dilate the ureter?

(A) Garceau tapered tip
(B) basket catheter
(C) Braasch bulb
(D) stent

1004. The use of distilled water during a highly invasive genitourinary procedure such as a transurethral resection of the prostate (TURP) is prohibited for irrigation because of the potential for

(A) hemolysis of RBC
(B) electrolytic dissipation of current
(C) increase of blood pressure
(D) body fluid shift

1005. Why is a 30-cc bag Foley used after a TURP?

(A) hemostasis
(B) decompression
(C) creation of negative pressure
(D) aspiration

1006. The three lumens of a Foley are used for inflation, drainage, and

(A) prevention of urine reflux
(B) access for sterile urine specimens
(C) continuous irrigation
(D) additional hemostasis

1007. The purpose of the kidney elevator is to

(A) increase the space between the lower ribs and iliac crest
(B) increase the space between the ribs
(C) stabilize the patient
(D) support the body in the flexed position

1008. Why is the table straightened before closing a kidney incision?

(A) to facilitate easier respirations
(B) to create better approximation of tissues
(C) to facilitate better circulation
(D) to prevent nerve damage

1009. Nonmalignant enlargement of the prostate is termed

(A) prostatitis
(B) benign prostatic hypertrophy (BPH)
(C) balanitis
(D) prostatism

1010. Urethral strictures can be dilated by use of each of the following EXCEPT

(A) Philips filiform and followers
(B) VanBuren sounds
(C) Braasch bulb
(D) McCarthy dilators

1011. A staghorn stone is one that lodges and continues to grow in the

(A) renal calyx
(B) space of Retzius
(C) ureter
(D) hilum

1012. In cystoscopy, the irrigating solution is

(A) distilled water
(B) glycine
(C) mannitol
(D) sorbitol

1013. Which of the following is NOT considered a permanent urinary diversion?

(A) ileal conduit
(B) ureterocystostomy
(C) cutaneous ureterostomy
(D) nephrostomy

1014. Rib removal for surgical exposure of the kidney requires all of the following EXCEPT a(n)

(A) Alexander periosteotome
(B) Doyen raspatory
(C) Heaney clamp
(D) Stille shears

1015. Penile condylomata are most successfully removed by

(A) dermabrasion
(B) laser
(C) cautery
(D) ultrasound

1016. Removal of a testis or the testes is called

(A) orchiopexy
(B) orchiectomy
(C) epididymectomy
(D) vasectomy

1017. Which solution is NOT used during a transurethral prostatectomy?

(A) normal saline
(B) sorbitol
(C) mannitol
(D) glycine

1018. Temporary diversion of urinary drainage by means of an external catheter that drains the renal pelvis is called

(A) vesicostomy
(B) nephrostomy
(C) pyelostomy
(D) cystostomy

1019. The procedure to treat organic sexual impotence is

(A) spermatocelectomy
(B) varicocelectomy
(C) testicular implant
(D) penile implant

1020. Which anomaly is corrected by the MAGPI procedure?

(A) epispadias
(B) hypospadias
(C) phimosis
(D) chordee

1021. Microscopic reversal of the male sterilization procedure is termed

(A) spermatogenesis
(B) orchiopexy
(C) vasovasostomy
(D) vasectomy

1022. A needle biopsy of the prostate may be accomplished with a(n)

(A) butterfly needle
(B) angiocatheter
(C) Tru-cut needle
(D) taper needle

1023. When the male penis is curved ventrally with the meatus and the glans in close proximity to each other it is called

(A) paraphimosis
(B) phimosis

(C) epispadias
(D) chordee

1024. An endoscopic procedure to treat stress incontinence is a

(A) Y–V-plasty
(B) stent procedure
(C) Stamey procedure
(D) colocystoplasty

1025. Continuous irrigation following TURP is accomplished by use of a

(A) suprapubic cystotomy tube
(B) 30-cc three-way Foley catheter
(C) 5-cc three-way Foley catheter
(D) 30-cc two-way Foley catheter

1026. Bladder drainage that diverts urine away from the urethral vaginal area is a(n)

(A) Foley catheterization
(B) ileal conduit
(C) cystostomy
(D) Stamey procedure

1027. When the prostate gland is removed through an abdominal incision into the anterior prostatic capsule, it is called a _____ prostatectomy.

(A) perineal
(B) suprapubic
(C) retropubic
(D) transurethral

1028. Kidney stones are sent to the lab in

(A) saline
(B) water
(C) dry state
(D) formalin

1029. A Pereyra procedure is done for

(A) stress incontinence
(B) chronic bladder infection
(C) drainage of the bladder
(D) impotence

1030. A percutaneous nephrolithotomy utilizes all of the following EXCEPT

(A) ultrasound wand
(B) flexible nephroscope
(C) lithotriptor
(D) lithotriptor tub

1031. Orchiopexy can be defined as

(A) fixation of an ovary
(B) uterine suspension
(C) testicle removal
(D) fixation of a testicle

1032. Abdominal resection of the prostate gland through an incision into the bladder is known surgically as a

(A) retropubic prostatectomy
(B) suprapubic prostatectomy
(C) transurethral prostatectomy
(D) suprapubic cystostomy

1033. A lumbar or simple flank incision for ureter or kidney surgery may include removal of which ribs?

(A) 5 and 6
(B) 7 and 8
(C) 9 and 10
(D) 11 and 12

1034. An abnormal accumulation of fluid in the scrotum is a(n)

(A) hydrocele
(B) enterocele
(C) varicocele
(D) hydronephrosis

1035. What is the alternative approach to surgical TURP that has resulted from advances in radiologic techniques and balloon catheter technology

(A) ureteroplasty
(B) tuboplasty
(C) urethroplasty
(D) prostatic dilation

1036. Bladder stones are crushed with a

(A) basket catheter
(B) lithotrite
(C) cautery
(D) resectoscope

1037. Urethral meatal stenosis is corrected by a(n)

(A) frenulotomy
(B) meatotomy
(C) urethral dilation
(D) extirpation of the penis

1038. In a penile implant, the inflation pump is located in the

(A) distal penis
(B) proximal penis
(C) scrotum
(D) groin

1039. Excision of the tunica vaginalis is a

(A) vagotomy
(B) vasectomy
(C) varicocelectomy
(D) hydrocelectomy

1040. Circumcision refers to

(A) removal of the foreskin
(B) removal of the glans
(C) widening of the urethral opening
(D) lengthening of the foreskin

1041. An alternative approach to surgical TURP utilizing a cystoscopic setup as its base is

(A) suprapubic prostatectomy
(B) transcystoscopic urethroplasty
(C) perineal prostatectomy
(D) retropubic prostatectomy

1042. The laser used to destroy small recurrent bladder tumors is the

(A) CO_2
(B) argon
(C) Nd:YAG
(D) A and B

1043. In creating a continent urinary diversion post-cystectomy, all of the following procedures are options for diversion EXCEPT

(A) Kock pouch
(B) Indiana pouch
(C) "Le bag"
(D) ileal conduit

1044. Stones removed during surgery should be sent to the laboratory

(A) dry
(B) in saline
(C) in formalin
(D) in distilled water

1045. Following anastomosis of a ureter during a ureteral reimplantation procedure, a _____ is left in place to ensure free drainage of the kidney postoperatively.

(A) Foley catheter
(B) ureteral catheter
(C) t-tube
(D) soft stent

1046. The combined correction of a redundant renal pelvis and resection of a stenotic portion of the ureteropelvic junctions is known as

(A) pyeloplasty
(B) Foley Y–V procedure
(C) ureteroplasty
(D) ureteropyeloscopy

1047. A reverse sterilization procedure in the male is called a(n)

(A) vasostomy
(B) vasovasostomy
(C) epididymovasostomy
(D) B and C

1048. Before insertion of a penile implant, the insertion site, as well as the implant itself, is irrigated with

(A) normal saline
(B) Betadine
(C) sterile water
(D) Kanamycin and Bacitracin

1049. To prevent thrombi from forming in the walls of the renal vein during transfer from the donor to the recipient, ———— is given just before clamping of the renal vessels.

(A) furosemide
(B) protamine sulfate
(C) heparin
(D) mannitol

1050. The drug of choice for adequate diuresis of a living donor before, during, and postremoval of the kidney is

(A) urea
(B) protamine sulfate
(C) Ringer's lactate solution
(D) mannitol

1051. All of the following are ideal requirements of cadaver donors EXCEPT

(A) any age
(B) free of infection or malignancy
(C) normotensive up until death
(D) under hospital observation before death

1052. Cooling and flushing of pancreas, liver, and kidneys of cadaver donors is accomplished by cannulation of the organ and infusion of large amounts of cold

(A) saline solution
(B) Ringer's lactate solution
(C) sterile water
(D) Sack's solution

1053. Nonconducting, isosmotic glycine irrigating solution must be used in the surgical presence of a

(A) cystoscope
(B) ureteroscope
(C) resectoscope
(D) nephroscope

1054. All of the following procedures may be completed through a cystoscope EXCEPT

(A) biopsy of bladder tumor
(B) removal of foreign body in bladder
(C) total removal of bladder tumor
(D) cystogram for diagnostic studies

1055. After incision is made into the scrotum during a vasectomy, the forceps used to grasp the vas and bring it to the surface for surgery is the

(A) Allis
(B) Babcock
(C) Kelly
(D) mosquito

1056. Extracorporeal shock wave lithotripsy (ESWL) disintegrates stones by introducing shock waves into the body through the medium of

(A) water
(B) air
(C) gas
(D) saline

1057. Laser lithotripsy utilizes the tunable pulse-dyed laser known as

(A) diode
(B) Nd:YAG
(C) Candela
(D) argon

VII. THORACIC SURGERY

1058. The tube that collects bronchial washings is

(A) Broyles
(B) Lukens
(C) Ellik
(D) Toomey

1059. What instrument is used to view lymph nodes or masses in the space that medially separates the pleural cavities?

(A) bronchoscope
(B) mediastinoscope
(C) endoscope
(D) colonoscope

1060. The procedure of choice for removal of a foreign body in a child's tracheobronchial tree is

(A) bronchoscopy
(B) mediastinoscopy
(C) fluoroscopy
(D) telemetry

1061. A cytologic specimen collector used in bronchoscopy is

(A) Ellik
(B) Toomey
(C) Jackson
(D) Lukens

1062. All of the following are true regarding disposable chest drainage units EXCEPT

(A) provides drainage collection from intrapleural space
(B) maintains a seal to prevent air from entering the pleural cavity
(C) provides suction control determined by water level
(D) aids in re-establishing positive pressure in the intrapleural space

1063. Compression of the subclavian vessels and the brachial plexus usually caused by the first rib is surgically known as

(A) cervical sympathectomy
(B) thoracic outlet syndrome
(C) thoracic sympathectomy
(D) decortication

1064. A reduction of negative pressure on one side of the thoracic cavity that causes the negative pressure on the normal side to pull in an effort to equalize pressure is called

(A) vital capacity
(B) mediastinal shift
(C) subatmospheric pressure
(D) pneumothorax

1065. Surgical removal of fibrinous deposits on the visceral and parietal pleura is called

(A) posteriolateral thoracoplasty
(B) talc poudrage
(C) decortication of the lung
(D) anterior thoracoplasty

1066. What substance is introduced through a thoracoscope to deal with recurrent pleural effusion attributable to advanced cancer?

(A) chemotherapeutics
(B) talc
(C) tetracycline
(D) hemostatic agents

1067. What instrument is used to reapproximate the ribs following an open thoracotomy?

(A) Doyen
(B) Bailey
(C) Alexander
(D) Bethune

1068. What cold solution is used to preserve a donor lung before transplant into a recipient?

(A) Ringer's lactate
(B) saline
(C) Collin's
(D) Physiosol

1069. How many anastomoses must be completed to effect a single-lung transplant?

(A) one
(B) two
(C) three
(D) four

VIII. CARDIOVASCULAR AND PERIPHERAL VASCULAR SURGERY

1070. Which of the following would be the suture of choice for a graft-to-tissue anastomosis in vascular surgery?

(A) collagen suture
(B) Maxon
(C) Ti-Cron
(D) Surgilon

1071. Which suture would be used on an aortic valve replacement?

(A) polypropylene
(B) Vicryl
(C) Dermalon
(D) Dexon

1072. In which procedure could a Fogarty catheter be utilized?

(A) embolectomy
(B) gastrectomy
(C) craniotomy
(D) thorocotomy

1073. Amputated extremities are

(A) sent to the pathology lab as are other specimens
(B) preserved in formaldehyde
(C) wrapped and refrigerated in the morgue
(D) placed in a dry container

1074. An anticoagulant given for its antagonistic effect on heparin is

(A) Dicumarol
(B) Coumadin sodium
(C) Protamine sulfate
(D) Dipaxin

1075. The action to be followed if a patient is experiencing a cardiac arrhythmia, specifically a ventricular fibrillation, would be to

(A) start an IV
(B) defibrillate
(C) order blood to replace blood volume
(D) administer intravenous lidocaine

1076. Dextran is used parenterally to

(A) expand blood plasma volume
(B) renourish vital tissue
(C) carry oxygen through the system
(D) decrease blood viscosity

1077. Which drug can be added to saline for irrigation during a vascular procedure?

(A) protamine
(B) epinephrine
(C) Sublimaze
(D) heparin

1078. The intraoperative diagnostic test that measures tissue perfusion is

(A) blood volume
(B) respiratory tidal volume
(C) arterial blood gases
(D) hematocrit

1079. Passage of a sterile catheter into the heart via the brachial or femoral artery for the purpose of image intensification is called

(A) angiography
(B) arteriography
(C) cardiac catheterization
(D) cardioscopy

1080. Hypothermia is employed in cardiac surgery

(A) to reduce oxygen consumption
(B) to reduce elevated temperature
(C) to slow metabolism
(D) to induce ventricular fibrillation

1081. Which vessels are harvested for a coronary artery bypass?

(A) pulmonary vein and external mammary vein
(B) portal vein and hepatic artery
(C) saphenous vein and internal mammary artery
(D) pulmonary artery and pulmonary vein

1082. If a knitted graph is preclotted, it

(A) minimizes bleeding
(B) makes a graft more pliable
(C) facilitates attachment
(D) prevents rejection

1083. The term used to denote the function accomplished by the cardiopulmonary bypass machine is

(A) diversion
(B) dialysis
(C) perfusion
(D) profusion

1084. A cardiopulmonary technique that employs the principle of counterpulsation that increases cardiac output is

(A) CPD
(B) IAPP
(C) VAD
(D) LVAD

1085. The antagonist to heparin sodium is

(A) epinephrine
(B) mannitol
(C) sodium bicarbonate
(D) Protamine sulfate

1086. Pedal pulses are assessed with a

(A) Berman locator
(B) Doppler
(C) Mobin–Uddin device
(D) PTFE

1087. Heparin is utilized during vascular surgery

(A) to coagulate blood
(B) to correct acidosis
(C) to constrict arteries
(D) to prevent thrombosis

1088. The prime consideration in a ruptured abdominal aortic aneurysmectomy is

(A) shunting blood flow
(B) hemorrhage control
(C) bypassing occlusion
(D) removal of thromboembolic material

1089. In which surgery would a tunneler be used?

(A) AAA
(B) angioplasty
(C) embolectomy
(D) femoral–popliteal bypass

1090. In balloon angioplasty, the dilating balloon is inflated with

(A) diluted heparin
(B) diluted solution of contrast media
(C) saline
(D) Ringer's lactate solution

1091. Which piece of equipment would be placed on an embolectomy setup for the purpose of removing clots through an arteriotomy?

(A) Wishard
(B) Swan–Ganz
(C) Fogarty
(D) Garceau

1092. The goal of a carotid endarterectomy is to

(A) remove a thrombus
(B) provide a shunt for blood flow
(C) bypass the affected area
(D) remove plaque

1093. Decompression of the portal circulation can be achieved by all of the following EXCEPT

(A) splenorenal shunt
(B) portocaval anastomosis
(C) arteriovenous shunt
(D) mesocaval shunt

1094. Plaque removal from a vessel is termed

(A) embolectomy
(B) thrombectomy
(C) shunt
(D) endarterectomy

1095. Placement of a vascular graft proximal to and inclusive of the common iliac vessels will necessitate the use of a(n)

(A) autogenous graft
(B) straight Teflon graft
(C) bifurcated graft
(D) polytetrafluorethylene graft

1096. The most common vessels used for access procedures to facilitate hemodialysis are

(A) radial artery and cephalic vein
(B) radial artery and cephalic artery
(C) brachial artery and cephalic vein
(D) cephalic artery and brachial vein

1097. Migrating clots that have formed in the lower extremities can be intercepted on the way to the heart or lungs by a

(A) Greenfield Filter
(B) Pudenz shunt
(C) Scribner shunt
(D) LeVeen shunt

1098. Retraction of fine structures and blood vessels during vascular surgery is accomplished by use of

(A) Senn retractor
(B) Penrose drain
(C) malleable ribbon retractor
(D) vessel loops

1099. Fluoroscopy is required for all of the following vascular procedures EXCEPT

(A) Greenfield filter
(B) endocardial pacing electrode
(C) myocardial pacing electrode
(D) A–V fistula creation

1100. A drug used intraoperatively for its antispasmodic effect on the smooth muscle of the vessel wall is

(A) Ringer's lactate
(B) papaverine hydrochloride
(C) Physiosol
(D) protamine sulfate

1101. Compression of subclavian vessels and brachial plexus at the superior aperture of the thorax is known as

(A) thymoma
(B) pectus excavatum
(C) thoracic outlet syndrome
(D) pectus carinatum

1102. In vascular surgery, the term in situ graft references the use of a(n)

(A) autogenous graft
(B) heterogeneous graft
(C) allograft
(D) synthetic graft

1103. The surgery scheduled as "Greenfield filter insertion" indicates a diagnosis of

(A) emboli formation
(B) venous stasis
(C) arteriovascular occlusion
(D) kidney failure

1104. The intraoperative endoscopic visualization of internal vessels is known as

(A) angiography
(B) angioplasty
(C) angioscopy
(D) arthrectomy

1105. During a vascular procedure, monitoring the activated clotting time intraoperatively provides useful data for judging the need for reversal or addition of

(A) Angiovist
(B) papaverine
(C) heparin
(D) Protamine sulfate

1106. A low-molecular-weight protein that, when combined with heparin, causes a loss of anticoagulant activity postoperatively is

(A) papaverine
(B) Protamine sulfate
(C) tromethamine
(D) Angiovist

1107. What is the purpose for the surgical creation of an arteriovenous fistula?

(A) hemodialysis
(B) insertion of Greenfield filter
(C) peritoneal dialysis
(D) placement of Javid shunt

1108. Conservative treatment of occlusive disease involving recanalization to restore the lumen of a vessel is called

(A) polytetrafluoroethylene prosthetic (PTFE)
(B) percutaneous transluminal angioplasty (PTA)
(C) Greenfield filter
(D) endarterectomy

1109. What catheter is used to remove thrombi or emboli from vascular structures?

(A) Gruntzig
(B) Fogarty
(C) Swan–Ganz
(D) Foley

1110. What procedure is used intraoperatively and postoperatively to determine blood flow in a vessel?

(A) arteriogram
(B) Swan–Ganz
(C) Doppler ultrasound
(D) angioscopy

1111. Removal of atherosclerotic plaque from a major artery is termed

(A) embolectomy
(B) aneurysmectomy
(C) endarterectomy
(D) thrombectomy

1112. An abnormal localized dilatation of an artery resulting from mechanical pressure of blood on a weakened wall is called

(A) atherosclerosis
(B) arteriosclerosis
(C) collateral circulation
(D) aneurysm

1113. What is the treatment of choice for capturing emboli that arise from the pelvis or lower extremities?

(A) Permacath
(B) Greenfield filter
(C) Vas-cath
(D) Porto-cath

1114. What intraoperative test determines the needed reversal or addition of heparin?

(A) arterial blood gases (ABGs)
(B) ACT
(C) APPT
(D) none of the above

1115. What drug is used intraoperatively in a topical manner for its direct effect on the muscle of the vessel wall?

(A) papaverine hydrochloride
(B) heparin
(C) topical thrombin
(D) Protamine sulfate

1116. The technique applied to the patient who is unable to be weaned from cardiopulmonary bypass is

(A) IAPB
(B) VADs
(C) pacemaker
(D) A and B

1117. What is the most common acquired valvular lesion?

    (A) mitral regurgitation
    (B) mitral stenosis
    (C) tricuspid valve regurgitation
    (D) aortic insufficiency

1118. What drug is used to effect coronary thrombolysis in the cardiac catheterization laboratory?

    (A) tissue plasminogen activator
    (B) heparin
    (C) streptokinase
    (D) A and C

1119. The term in situ graft represents the use of a(n)

    (A) autograft
    (B) biograft
    (C) dacron graft
    (D) filamentous velour

IX. ORTHOPEDIC SURGERY

1120. Which suture is commonly used to attach tendon to bone?

    (A) wire
    (B) cotton
    (C) chromic
    (D) Vicryl

1121. Seamless tubular cotton that stretches to fit a contour and is used for padding is called

    (A) Ace bandage
    (B) Webril
    (C) sheet wadding
    (D) stockinette

1122. What is the proper wrapping procedure utilizing an Esmarch bandage?

    (A) start at the distal end of the extremity
    (B) start at the proximal end of the extremity
    (C) start after the cuff is inflated
    (D) start at the incision site

1123. Fracture of the patella may be repaired with all of the following hardware EXCEPT

    (A) buttress plate
    (B) bone screws
    (C) tension band
    (D) circumferential loop

1124. A variation of bunionectomy, in which the surgeon includes resection of the proximal third of the phalanx and possible silicone implant is called a

    (A) McBride procedure
    (B) Keller arthroplasty
    (C) Bankart procedure
    (D) metatarsal osteotomy

1125. Baker's cysts are found in the

    (A) popliteal fossa
    (B) interdigital fossa
    (C) intercarpal joints
    (D) olecranon fossa

1126. Benign outpouchings of synovium from intercarpal joints are called

    (A) ganglia
    (B) exostosis
    (C) polyps
    (D) synovitis

1127. Compression of the median nerve at the volar surface of the wrist is known as

    (A) Dupuytren's contracture
    (B) carpal tunnel syndrome
    (C) ganglia
    (D) Volkmann's contracture

1128. A fixation device that provides maximum holding and rigid fixation of a fracture by tightening bone fragments together is called a(n)

    (A) compression plate and screws
    (B) intramedullary nailing
    (C) Ilizarov technique
    (D) interlocking nail fixation

1129. In a total hip replacement, which structure is reamed?

(A) acetabulum
(B) greater trochanter
(C) lesser trochanter
(D) femoral head

1130. A dorsal angulated fracture of the distal radius is commonly called a(n)

(A) Pott's fracture
(B) os calcis
(C) olecranon fracture
(D) Colles' fracture

1131. The ideal candidate for a noncemented total hip arthroplasty is

(A) young and healthy person
(B) young with arthritis
(C) old and healthy
(D) old with osteoporotic bone disease

1132. A total hip replacement would be indicated when the patient has

(A) degenerative hip joint disease
(B) hip fracture
(C) congenital hip dislocation
(D) hip cancer

1133. All of the following are frames used to attain the prone position during orthopedic surgery EXCEPT

(A) Alvarado
(B) Wilson
(C) Andres
(D) Hastings

1134. Which hardware could not be used to repair a tibial plateau fracture?

(A) Blade plate
(B) Buttress plate
(C) dynamic compression screws
(D) Ambi compression plate

1135. A flexion deformity at the proximal joint of the four lateral toes is called

(A) valgus
(B) exostosis

(C) hammer toe
(D) bunion

1136. Joint reconstruction is known as

(A) arthrodesis
(B) arthroplasty
(C) arthrotomy
(D) arthropexy

1137. What is the name of a shoulder positioning device used to position a shoulder for surgery?

(A) Alvarado
(B) McConnell
(C) Andres
(D) Hastings

1138. Osteogenesis or bone growth can be induced by

(A) bone grafting, autogenous
(B) bone grafting, homogeneous
(C) hormone installation
(D) electrical stimulation

1139. An infection in bone is termed

(A) osteomalacia
(B) osteomyelitis
(C) osteitis
(D) osteoporosis

1140. A surgical procedure designed to stiffen or fuse a joint is called

(A) arthropexy
(B) arthroplasty
(C) joint fixation
(D) arthrodesis

1141. A lateral curvature of the spine is

(A) kyphosis
(B) scoliosis
(C) lordosis
(D) orthosis

1142. Harrington rods are used to treat

(A) femoral fracture
(B) scoliosis
(C) talipes deformity
(D) congenital hip dislocation

1143. A rotator cuff repair is called a

(A) Bankart
(B) Keller
(C) McBride
(D) Silver

1144. The congenital deformity known as clubfoot is surgically referred to as

(A) talipes valgus
(B) talipes varus
(C) hallux valgus
(D) exostosis

1145. The most frequent site of cartilage tears in the knee joint are at the

(A) collateral ligament
(B) cruciate ligament
(C) lateral meniscus
(D) medial meniscus

1146. An abduction pillow would be used to

(A) immobilize hip joints after hip surgery
(B) stabilize a femoral fracture
(C) immobilize the tibia postsurgery
(D) rotate the hips outward after hip reconstruction

1147. A Free Lock compression screw system is indicated for correction of a(n) _____ fracture.

(A) hip
(B) wrist
(C) elbow
(D) cervical

1148. Decreased bone mass results in a condition called

(A) osteoporosis
(B) osteomyelitis
(C) ossification
(D) ecchymosis

1149. Place the stages of fracture healing in order: (1) hematoma formation, (2) remodeling, (3) fibrin network formation, (4) callus formation, (5) invasion of osteoblasts.

(A) 1, 3, 5, 4, 2
(B) 1, 2, 5, 4, 3
(C) 1, 3, 2, 4, 5
(D) 5, 3, 4, 1, 2

1150. An olecranon fracture occurs in the

(A) wrist
(B) knee
(C) elbow
(D) finger

1151. All of the following are considered good methods of maintaining strict asepsis within an orthopedic surgical suite EXCEPT

(A) isolation units
(B) laminar flow rooms
(C) charcoal masks
(D) isolation bubble systems

1152. Water temperature for plaster cast application is

(A) 50°–55°F
(B) 70°–75°F
(C) 85°–90°F
(D) 95°–100°F

1153. Orthopedic surgery prepping

(A) is done under sterile conditions
(B) is done the day before surgery
(C) is eliminated
(D) is increased in time only

1154. Limb exsanguination is accomplished by using

(A) limb elevation
(B) tourniquet application
(C) Kling bandage
(D) Esmarch bandage

1155. In orthopedic surgery, the viewing of the progression of a procedure on a television screen is known as

(A) image intensification
(B) radiography
(C) portable filming
(D) x-ray

1156. Surgery on the medial malleolus would be of the

(A) fibula
(B) jaw
(C) tibia
(D) radius

1157. Plaster is ready for application

(A) when air bubbles cease to rise
(B) when air bubbles begin to rise
(C) after 2 minutes of submersion
(D) after 10 minutes of submersion

1158. Which fracture most commonly occurs in childhood?

(A) spiral
(B) compound
(C) greenstick
(D) comminuted

1159. Which of the following is added to polymethylmethacrylate (PMMA), chemically similar to Plexiglas, to it to make it possible to assess distribution and changes at a later time?

(A) polymers
(B) barium sulfate
(C) polyethylene
(D) polypropylene

1160. Which orthopedic hip procedure is indicated for patients with degenerative joint disease or rheumatoid arthritis?

(A) AO external fixation
(B) total hip arthroplasty
(C) femoral endoprosthesis
(D) modular endoprosthesis

1161. Which total joint arthroplasty utilizes the Miller–Galante joint replacement prosthesis?

(A) elbow
(B) knee
(C) shoulder
(D) hip

1162. Which of the following is a disadvantage of arthroscopic surgery?

(A) less inflammatory response
(B) decreased recovery time
(C) reduced complications
(D) scarring of articular surface

1163. The proper positioning for a patient undergoing arthroscopic knee surgery is

(A) affected knee bent at 45° angle on table
(B) skeletal traction on fracture table
(C) degree flexion of foot of table
(D) Alvardo knee holder

1164. What skeletal traction requires the use of sterile supplies for application of a traction appliance?

(A) Thomas splint
(B) Russell
(C) Crutchfield
(D) Buck's extension

1165. Anterior spinal fusion is accomplished by use of which of the following instrumentations?

(A) TSRH cross-link
(B) Luque
(C) Cotrel-Dubousset
(D) Isola

1166. An infectious musculoskeletal condition affecting the bone and marrow is

(A) osteomalacia
(B) osteoporosis
(C) osteomyelitis
(D) Paget's disease

1167. An immobilization device used after total hip arthroplasty is

(A) adduction pillow
(B) abduction pillow
(C) sling
(D) splint

1168. Electrical stimulation is artificially applied postoperative electrical current that influences

(A) osteomalacia
(B) osteogenesis
(C) osteoporosis
(D) osteoarthritis

1169. All of the following are indications for external fixation EXCEPT

(A) infected joints
(B) clean long-bone fractures
(C) highly comminuted closed fractures
(D) major alignment and length deficits

1170. A procedure done to correct recurrent anterior dislocation of the shoulder that involves reattachment of the rim of the glenoid fossa is called a

(A) Bankart
(B) Putti–Platt
(C) Bristow
(D) Monteggia

1171. The most commonly fractured carpal bone is the

(A) scaphoid
(B) lunate
(C) trapezium
(D) capitate

1172. All of the following are intramedullary nails or rods EXCEPT

(A) Ender nail
(B) Sampson rods
(C) Harrington rods
(D) Russell–Taylor rods

1173. Compression force of the distal femur upon the tibia produces varying types of fractures of the

(A) patella
(B) tibia plateau
(C) femoral condyle
(D) head of the femur

1174. Fracture of the lateral malleolus can be treated with a

(A) Sampson rod
(B) Ender nail
(C) Lottes nail
(D) Rusch rod

1175. Surgery that requires incision of the long extensor tendon of the interphalangeal joint of the four lateral toes and subsequent fusion is called

(A) exostectomy
(B) Keller procedure
(C) hammer toe correction
(D) McBride procedure

1176. To maintain hydrostatic pressure against the joint wall during irrigation of an arthroscopic procedure the solution must be kept above the joint at least

(A) 1 foot
(B) 3 feet
(C) 5 feet
(D) 7 feet

1177. A prosthetic implant that allows gliding and shifting motions resembling normal range of motion is generally termed a

(A) nonconstrained implant
(B) constrained implant
(C) methylmethacrylate fixation
(D) biofixation

1178. Total wrist replacement indicates use of which of the following implants to replace the radiocarpal joint in the wrist?

(A) metal ball-to-plastic socket
(B) silicone rubber
(C) plastic-to-plastic
(D) high-density polyethylene

1179. The rare use of laser during orthopedic surgery may be seen in the use of the CO_2 laser during a revision arthroplasty to

(A) remove a cemented implant
(B) vaporize protein
(C) weld tissue for collagen bonding
(D) create hemostasis

1180. After surgery on a shoulder, the arm may be bound against the side of the arm for

(A) comfort
(B) abduction
(C) immobilization
(D) mobilization

1181. To provide decompression of the spinal roots and vertebral alignment following a thoracolumbar spinal fusion, which of the following may be used for fixation?

(A) Harrington rods
(B) Luque rods
(C) Dwyer devices
(D) A and B

1182. The most commonly used implants in hand surgery are made of flexible

(A) polypropylene
(B) Silastic
(C) tantellum
(D) polyethylene

1183. The procedure indicated by which of the following named prostheses tells one that a total hip arthroplasty is scheduled?

(A) Harris–Gallante
(B) Osteolok
(C) Miller–Galante
(D) Omnifit

1184. Before the insertion of cement into the femoral medullary canal during a total hip arthroplasty, which of the following is placed with an inserter to occlude the canal?

(A) polyethylene insert
(B) cement restrictor
(C) broach
(D) distal centralizer

1185. Femoral prostheses such as Austin Moore and Thompson are used to correct all of the following diagnoses EXCEPT

(A) avascular necrosis
(B) nonunion fractures
(C) displaced femoral neck fractures
(D) rheumatoid arthritis

1186. Before sterilizing unsterile Silastic or Teflon implants, they should be

(A) washed with mild soap
(B) rinsed with saline solution
(C) wrapped loosely with towels
(D) scrubbed with Betadine

1187. Orthopedic implants are covered by all of the following rules EXCEPT

(A) different metals should not be mixed because they may react chemically
(B) If the implant is driven by force, a driver with a metal head must be used
(C) a template must be used for sizing purposes
(D) handle as little as possible before insertion

1188. Galvanic corrosion is a process that occurs postoperatively because of

(A) poor handling of device during implant
(B) mixed use of metals for implant
(C) misplacement of implant
(D) damage of an implanted device

X. NEUROSURGERY

1189. Raney clips are

(A) skin clips
(B) hemostatic clips
(C) aneurysm clips
(D) hemostatic scalp clips

1190. Which of the following are tongs providing skeletal traction for cervical fracture/dislocation?

(A) Yasargil
(B) Cushing
(C) Gigli
(D) Crutchfield

1191. A surgical procedure used most frequently to control intractable pain of terminal cancer is called a

(A) sympathectomy
(B) neurectomy
(C) cordotomy
(D) thermocoagulation

1192. Which operative procedure facilitates the draining of a subdural hematoma?

(A) cranioplasty
(B) hypophysectomy
(C) craniosyntosis
(D) burr holes

1193. Hemostasis in neurosurgery is achieved by using Gelfoam saturated with saline solution or

(A) heparin
(B) topical thrombin
(C) mannitol
(D) epinephrine

1194. A tumor arising from the covering of the brain is a(n)

(A) hemangioblastoma
(B) angioma
(C) meningioma
(D) glioma

1195. Which of the following is used to control bleeding beneath the skull and around the spinal cord?

(A) Webril
(B) gauze sponges
(C) cottonoid
(D) Kitners

1196. A large, encapsulated collection of blood over one or both cerebral hemispheres that produces intracranial pressure is known as a(n)

(A) epidural hematoma
(B) intracerebral hematoma
(C) subdural hematoma
(D) subarachnoid hematoma

1197. A surgical procedure in which a nerve is freed from binding adhesion for relief of pain and restoration of function is termed a

(A) neurexeresis
(B) neurorrhaphy
(C) neurotomy
(D) neurolysis

1198. Surgical creation of a lesion in the treatment of a disease such as Parkinson's is called

(A) cryosurgery
(B) diathermy
(C) rhizotomy
(D) pallidotomy

1199. During neurosurgical procedures, venous stasis in the lower extremities and maintenance of blood pressure may be aided by all of the following EXCEPT

(A) Esmarch bandage wrapped groin to toe
(B) elastic bandages wrapped toe to groin
(C) sequential compression devices
(D) TED stockings

1200. Which of the following diseases CANNOT be treated by a sympathectomy?

(A) intractable nerve pain
(B) vascular extremity disorders
(C) hyperhydrosis
(D) neuroma

1201. All of the following are used for hemostasis in a neurosurgical procedure EXCEPT

(A) bone wax
(B) compressed cotton strips
(C) bipolar coagulation
(D) monopolar coagulation

1202. All of the following are permanent aneurysm clips EXCEPT

(A) Scoville
(B) McFadden
(C) Heifitz
(D) Olivecrona

1203. Upon craniotomy closure, the bone flap is sutured on with

(A) stainless steel suture
(B) silk
(C) absorbable suture
(D) nonabsorbable suture

1204. Removal of an anterior cervical disc with accompanying spinal fusion is termed a

(A) Schwartz procedure
(B) Cloward procedure
(C) Torkildsen operation
(D) stereotactic procedure

1205. In a laminectomy, herniated disc fragments are removed with a

(A) bayonet
(B) Cloward punch
(C) Scoville
(D) pituitary rongeur

1206. When using the perforator to create burr holes, heat is counteracted by

(A) irrigating drill site as hole is drilled
(B) surrounding the area with cool lap pads
(C) dipping perforator in water
(D) working quickly, stopping often

1207. A ventriculoperitoneal shunt treats

(A) Parkinson's disease
(B) hydrocephalus
(C) Ménière's disease
(D) trigeminal neuralgia

1208. The advantage of using a Javid Shunt during a carotid endarterectomy is

(A) continuous cerebral blood flow
(B) prevention of dislodging debris
(C) ease in securing patch to artery
(D) clearer view of surgical site

1209. Metal suction tips used during neurosurgery are used continuously to keep the field dry. They may be all of the following EXCEPT

(A) Cone
(B) Sacks
(C) Frazier
(D) Yankeur

1210. Neurosurgical sponges soaked in solution are placed within the reach of the surgeon and displayed on a(n)

(A) inverted emesis basin
(B) dry sterile towel
(C) plastic drape
(D) A and C

1211. All of the following statements are true about knee–chest positioning for laminectomy EXCEPT

(A) decreased bleeding
(B) better exposure of laminae
(C) increased operating time
(D) increased ease of ventilation

1212. What is the most common congenital lesion encountered, requiring neurosurgical intervention?

(A) meningomyelocele
(B) A-V malformation
(C) aneurysm
(D) neurofibromas

1213. To effect hemostasis during a neurosurgical procedure, small pieces of Gelfoam are cut into several different sizes and soaked in

(A) saline
(B) Avitene
(C) topical thrombin
(D) hydrogen peroxide

1214. What instrument is used to excise the laminae overlying the herniated disc during its removal in a laminectomy procedure?

(A) Cloward
(B) Leksell
(C) Schwartz–Kerrison
(D) Beckman–Adson

1215. Malabsorption of cerebrospinal fluid (CSF) and resultant hydrocephalus are corrected by a neurosurgical

(A) VP shunt
(B) AV shunt
(C) VA shunt
(D) A and C

1216. Neurosurgical procedures done for the purpose of locating and destroying target structures in the brain are called

(A) stereotactic
(B) cranioplasties
(C) craniosynostosis
(D) trigeminal rhizotomies

1217. What is the incisional approach used to effect a transsphenoidal hypophysectomy?

(A) middle of the upper gum
(B) bifrontal approach
(C) frontal approach
(D) frontotemporal approach

1218. Dorsal sympathectomy entails removal of which of the following chains of the sympathetic division of the autonomic nervous system?

(A) thoracolumbar
(B) cervicothoracic
(C) lumbar
(D) cervical

XI. PEDIATRIC AND GERIATRIC SURGERY

1219. A Hakim shunt is used to

(A) treat hydrocephalus
(B) aid in carotid nutrition

(C) access vessels for dialysis
(D) provide total parenteral nutrition (TPN) access

1220. The invagination of the proximal intestine into the lumen of the distal intestine is called

(A) volvulus
(B) intussusception
(C) pyloric stenosis
(D) ileal atresia

1221. An imperforation or closure of a normal opening is called a(n)

(A) hypertrophy
(B) atresia
(C) stenosis
(D) atrophy

1222. Failure of the intestines to encapsulate within the peritoneal cavity of a newborn is called

(A) umbilical hernia
(B) omphalocele
(C) hydrocele
(D) intestinal extrophy

1223. A congenital malformation of the chest wall with a pronounced funnel-shaped depression is called

(A) truncus arteriosus
(B) pectus excavatum
(C) pectus carinatum
(D) costochondral separation

1224. Newborn vomiting, free of bile and projectile in nature, is indicative of

(A) atresia of the esophagus
(B) pyloric stenosis
(C) volvulus
(D) intussusception

1225. The increased metabolic rate of a surgical pediatric patient establishes the need for all of the following EXCEPT

(A) oxygen
(B) caloric intake
(C) blood transfusions
(D) fluids

1226. Hirschsprung's disease is synonymous with

(A) congenital aganglionosis
(B) malrotation
(C) ileal stenosis
(D) Meckel's diverticulum

1227. The condition evidenced by incomplete closure of the vertebral arches in newborns is

(A) hydrocephalus
(B) encephalocele
(C) spina bifida
(D) myelomeningocele

1228. The condition involving premature closure of infant cranial suture lines is referred to as

(A) cranioplasty
(B) stereotactic surgery
(C) craniosynostosis
(D) transsphenoidal hypophysectomy

1229. An imperforate anus means

(A) anal opening is absent
(B) anus is closed
(C) anal sphincter is too tight
(D) anal sphincter is too loose

1230. Geriatric patients are more prone to each of the following EXCEPT

(A) infection
(B) poor wound healing
(C) cardiovascular problems
(D) gallbladder disease

1231. A Wilms' tumor, the most common intra-abdominal childhood tumor is known as a(n)

(A) nephroblastoma
(B) neuroblastoma
(C) aganglionic colon
(D) intussusception

1232. Incomplete closure of paired vertebral arches that can be treated surgically is known as

(A) spina bifida
(B) pectus excavatum
(C) spastic palsy
(D) encephalocele

1233. Nonclosure at birth of the duct that carries blood from the pulmonary artery directly to the aorta is termed

(A) tetralogy of Fallot
(B) coarctation of the aorta
(C) patent ductus arteriosus
(D) anomalous venous return

1234. The most common congenital cardiac anomaly in the cyanotic group is

(A) tricuspid atresia
(B) tetralogy of Fallot
(C) patent ductus arteriosus
(D) truncus arteriosus

1235. The mechanical strength of a weak eye muscle due to strabismus in a pediatric patient can be corrected by all of the following EXCEPT

(A) tucking
(B) advancement
(C) recession
(D) resection

1236. A cardiac procedure used primarily for anomalies associated with excessive pulmonary flow due to large intracardiac left-to-right shunt is called

(A) Glenn procedure
(B) Blalock–Taussig procedure
(C) pulmonary bonding
(D) Blalock–Hanlon procedure

1237. An abnormal communication between the aorta and the pulmonary artery of an infant is termed

(A) truncus arteriosus
(B) patent ductus arteriosus
(C) pulmonary stenosis
(D) hypoplastic left heart syndrome

1238. Failure of the abdominal viscera to become encapsulated within the peritoneal cavity during fetal development is known as a(n)

(A) umbilical hernia
(B) Meckel's diverticulum
(C) hiatal hernia
(D) omphalocele

1239. What surgery is performed to treat otitis media?

(A) myringotomy
(B) adenoidectomy
(C) tympanoplasty
(D) tonsillectomy

1240. What problem is most commonly seen in the pediatric postoperative patient?

(A) hypotension
(B) airway impairment
(C) hypothermia
(D) metabolic depression

1241. Which of the following is the primary indication for total joint arthroplasty of the hip and knee in elderly persons?

(A) osteoporosis
(B) osteoarthritis
(C) rheumatoid arthritis
(D) B and C

1242. What is the predominant reason for urological surgery in elderly men?

(A) prostatic malignancies
(B) benign prostatic hypertrophy (BPH)
(C) bladder malignancies
(D) nephritis

XII. EMERGENCY PROCEDURES AND MISCELLANEOUS

1243. An emergency drug useful in ventricular fibrillation or tachycardia is

(A) Aramine
(B) atropine
(C) Inderal
(D) calcium chloride

1244. An emergency drug that increases myocardial contractility is

(A) calcium chloride
(B) Levophed
(C) Lasix
(D) Isuprel

1245. The action of sodium bicarbonate in an advanced life support effort is to

(A) stimulate the heart muscle
(B) strengthen and slow heartbeat
(C) reduce ventricular excitement
(D) counteract metabolic acidosis

1246. Xylocaine is used intravenously for

(A) installation of local anesthesia
(B) treatment of cardiac arrhythmias
(C) diuretic action
(D) restoration of blood volume

1247. If cardiac arrest occurs in the OR, who is responsible for handling artificial ventilation?

(A) the anesthesiologist
(B) the circulating nurse
(C) the surgeon
(D) the scrub nurse

1248. Sudden shortness of breath in a postoperative patient may be indicative of

(A) pulmonary embolism
(B) pleural effusion
(C) emphysema
(D) asthma

1249. Which pulse is checked during a cardiac arrest effort?

(A) radial
(B) carotid
(C) pedal
(D) brachial

1250. Airways should be

(A) removed before the patient leaves the OR site
(B) left in until the patient is fully awake and ready to return to his or her room
(C) left in place until the patient breathes normally
(D) removed only by the anesthesiologist

1251. An anesthetic complication characterized by progressive elevation of body temperature is known as malignant

(A) hypothermia
(B) hypervolemia
(C) hypersalemia
(D) hyperthermia

1252. All of the following are results from aspiration of gastric contents during anesthesia EXCEPT

(A) impeded blood gas exchange
(B) impaired lung function
(C) gastric decompression
(D) chemical pneumonitis

1253. A telethermometer monitors the body temperature during surgery. It can be placed in all of the following areas EXCEPT the

(A) rectum
(B) esophagus
(C) axilla
(D) tympanic area

1254. Dark blood in the operative field may indicate that the patient is

(A) hyperkalemic
(B) hypovolemic
(C) hypotensive
(D) hypoxic

1255. The first and most important step for successful resuscitation in cardiac arrest is

(A) the precordial thump
(B) artificial ventilation
(C) immediate opening of the airway
(D) external cardiac compression

1256. The responsibility of the scrub nurse in cardiopulmonary resuscitation (CPR) is to

(A) bring in the emergency cart
(B) keep a record of all medication given
(C) help with the intravenous and monitoring lines
(D) give attention to the sterile field and the surgeon's needs

1257. A safety precaution used when a patient is being shocked with the defibrillator is

(A) no one is to touch the patient or anything metallic in contact with the patient
(B) available personnel gently but firmly support the extremities to protect the patient from injury
(C) the person holding the electrodes does not touch the patient but anyone else can
(D) the person holding the electrodes is the only one who may touch the patient

1258. When handing a syringe of medication to the surgeon for a local anesthetic, the scrub nurse should

(A) ask the circulating nurse what solution he or she has
(B) ask the circulator to show the vial to the surgeon
(C) show the surgeon the vial that it came from
(D) state the kind and percentage of the solution

1259. When cardiac arrest occurs, resuscitative measures must begin within

(A) 2 minutes
(B) 3–5 minutes
(C) 2–7 minutes
(D) 5–8 minutes

1260. Who is responsible for recording all medications given during CPR in the OR?

(A) the scrub nurse
(B) the circulating nurse
(C) the anesthesiologist
(D) the surgeon's assistant

1261. CPR is instituted if

   (A) the pulse is below 60, respirations are diminished, and blood pressure is dropping
   (B) there is no pulse or blood pressure, and the pupils contract
   (C) there is no pulse, respiration, or blood pressure, and the pupils are fixed and dilated
   (D) the pulse is weak and irregular, blood pressure is lowered, and pupils are dilated

1262. The first action to be taken in the event of a cardiac arrest in the OR is to

   (A) alert the OR supervisor and personnel
   (B) prepare medications
   (C) institute chest massage
   (D) apply fibrillator paddles

1263. Intraoperative and postoperative emergency procedures require the scrub person to

   (A) immediately intervene with patient care
   (B) attend the anesthesiologist during crisis
   (C) maintain sterile Mayo with instruments
   (D) A and B

1264. The following rules apply to needle use at the field EXCEPT

   (A) give needles to surgeon on an exchange basis
   (B) use needles and needleholders as a unit

   (C) keep needles away from sponges and laps
   (D) keep used needles in a medicine cup

1265. What is the disposition of all sharps that have been passed off the field intraoperatively?

   (A) keep off the field for final resolution of count
   (B) immediately place in sharp container on OR wall
   (C) roll in tape and discard
   (D) take from OR with original suture wrapper

1266. A washer–decontaminator, used after instruments are presoaked, uses which of the following processes to remove blood and protein?

   (A) impingement
   (B) cavitation
   (C) steam under pressure
   (D) chemicals

1267. What is the first step in handling the used and unused instruments after a case is completed?

   (A) washer–sterilizer
   (B) presoaking in a basin
   (C) ultrasonic cleaner
   (D) milking

Intraoperative
and Postoperative Procedures
Answers and Explanations

I. GENERAL SURGERY

719. (A) In a gastrointestinal closure, the mucosal layer is closed with chromic 4–0 or 3–0; the seromuscular layer is closed with chromic 3–0 or 2–0 and silk 4–0 or 3–0 (Meeker and Rothrock).

720. (B) A purse-string suture is a continuous suture placed around a lumen and tightened, drawstring fashion, to close the lumen. This is used, for example, when inverting the stump of an appendix or when closing the anus in the perineal stage of an abdominoperineal resection (Meeker and Rothrock).

721. (A) A bumper is passed over or through the exposed portion of suture in a retention suture to prevent the suture from cutting into the skin surface (Meeker and Rothrock).

722. (B) An antireflux procedure, which prevents reflux of gastric juices back into the esophagus. The three most frequently performed procedures are Nissen, Hill, and Belsy Mark IV (Meeker and Rothrock).

723. (A) Kitner dissecting sponges are small rolls of heavy cotton tape that are held in forceps (Fortunato).

724. (D) Pressure dressings are used frequently following extensive operations, especially in plastic surgery, knee operations, and radical mastectomies (Fortunato).

725. (B) Patties are moistened with saline and pressed out flat on a metal surface. They could pick up lint if placed on a towel (Fortunato).

726. (B) Normal saline is usually used to moisten sponges and tapes because it is an isotonic solution (Fortunato).

727. (A) Mushroom, Malecot, or Foley catheters are frequently used in the anterior gastric wall and are held in place by a purse-string suture (Meeker and Rothrock).

728. (D) Moisten the drain in saline before handing it to the surgeon (Fortunato).

729. (B) This portable system is used to apply suction to a large closed-wound site postoperatively. A constant, negative vacuum evacuates tissue fluid and blood to promote healing by reducing edema and media for microbial growth (Meeker and Rothrock).

730. (B) Covering sterile tables for later use is not recommended because it is difficult to uncover a table without contamination (Fortunato).

731. (C) Hands are kept at or above waist level, away from the face and arms, and never folded, because there may be perspiration in the axillary region (Fortunato).

732. (C) The end-to-end anastomoser (EEA) is designed to hold two tubular structures, to join the structures with staples and to cut the structures internally so proper lumen is provided (Meeker and Rothrock).

733. **(B)** Anything falling or extending over a table edge is unsterile. The scrub person does not touch the part hanging below table level (Fortunato).

734. **(C)** Sitting or leaning against a nonsterile surface is a break in technique because a sterile person should keep contact with nonsterile areas to a minimum (Fortunato).

735. **(A)** If sterility is doubtful, consider it not sterile. Do not use a pack, even if it appears to be sterile, if it is found in a nonsterile workroom (Fortunato).

736. **(C)** The sphincter of Oddi is located at the most distal end of the ampulla of vater. It may become scarred because of biliary obstruction, stones, or disease. Transecting the duodenum at the site of the sphincter allows the surgeon to reduce the stenosis and encourage the flow of bile and pancreatic juices into the gastrointestinal system (Meeker and Rothrock).

737. **(B)** The scrub who hands the drapes to the surgeon should stand on the same side of the table in order to avoid reaching over the unsterile OR table (Fortunato).

738. **(C)** Successful liver transplantation requires the cooperative efforts of the organ procurement team and the transplant team. The procurement team provides special Collin's solution for flushing the organ after harvest is complete and before delivery to transplant team (Meeker and Rothrock).

739. **(B)** Do not recap used injection needles (Fortunato).

740. **(C)** Drapes should be carried to the OR table folded to prevent them from coming in contact with unclean items in transport (Fortunato).

741. **(C)** A hair found on a drape must be removed with a hemostat; hand instrument off of field, and cover the area with a suitable drape (Fortunato).

742. **(B)** To minimize the risk of disseminating malignant tumor cells outside the operative area, some surgeons follow a special technique in which instruments in contact with tumor cells are discarded after use (Fortunato).

743. **(D)** Gown, gloves, drapes, and instruments are changed. The tumor is incised during biopsy for diagnosis. However, margins of healthy tissue surrounding a radical resection must not be inoculated with tumor cells (Fortunato).

744. **(A)** The postoperative complication of powder granulomata can result from powder that is not properly removed from gloves before surgery. This can be avoided by rinsing gloves before approaching the operative site (Fortunato).

745. **(B)** Sterile dressings should be applied before drapes are removed to reduce risk of the incision being touched by contaminated hands or objects (Fortunato).

746. **(C)** In drop technique, the contaminated instruments are discarded in a single basin. Gloves (and possibly gowns) are changed by the surgical team, and the incisional area is redraped with clean towels (Fortunato).

747. **(B)** Decontaminate floor and walls promptly during operation if contaminated by organic debris. Use a broad-spectrum detergent–disinfectant and wear gloves. This action helps prevent microorganisms from drying and becoming airborne (Fortunato).

748. **(A)** A Sengstaken–Blakemore tube is used to control esophageal hemorrhage. Pressure is exerted on the cardiac portion of the stomach and against bleeding esophageal varices by a double balloon tamponade. It is a three-element gastric tube (*Mosby's Medical, Nursing, and Allied Health Dictionary*).

749. **(D)** Oxycel's hemostatic action is caused by the formation of an artificial clot by cellulose action as it reacts with blood. It increases in size to form a gel and stops bleeding. It is used dry (Fortunato).

750. **(C)** Thrombin accelerates coagulation of blood and controls capillary bleeding. It is an enzyme derived from bovine blood (Fortunato).

751. **(C)** Extubation is precarious for the patient who may cough, jerk, or experience a spasm of the larynx from tracheal stimulation. Hypoxia is a common complication. It is a deficiency in oxygen (Fortunato).

752. **(C)** The Trendelenburg position is used for procedures in the lower abdomen or pelvis in which it is desirable to tilt the abdominal viscera away from the pelvic area for better exposure. The entire table is tilted downward (about 45 degrees at table head) while the foot is also lowered the desired amount (Fortunato).

753. **(D)** The Kraske position is also called the jackknife position. The patient is anesthetized in supine position. He or she is turned to the abdomen with the hips over the center break in the table (Fortunato).

754. **(C)** Sponges should be kept away from linen, instruments, and needles. Sponges and tapes should not be in a basin at the same time because a small sponge may be dragged unknowingly into the wound along with a tape. Keep a mental count of the number of sponges on the field (Fortunato).

755. **(D)** Hypoxia is lack of adequate amounts of oxygen; if prolonged, it can result in cardiac arrhythmia or irreversible brain, liver, kidney, and heart damage. The treatment is immediate adequate oxygen intake to stimulate the medullary centers and prevent respiratory system failure. Dark blood on the operative field is a symptom of hypoxia (Fortunato).

756. **(A)** Omitted counts because of extreme patient emergency must be documented on the operative record, and a patient incident report must be completed by the circulating nurse. This is only acceptable in a life-threatening emergency (Fortunato).

757. **(B)** Cultures are obtained under sterile conditions. The tips must not be contaminated by any other source. The circulating nurse can hold open a small bag for the scrub nurse to drop the tube into if it is handled on the sterile field. This protects personnel and prevents the spread of microorganisms (Fortunato).

758. **(D)** Frozen section specimens are not placed in solution because they can react with tissue and affect the pathologist's diagnosis. A frozen section is the cutting of a thin piece of tissue from a frozen specimen. This permits examination under a microscope (Fortunato).

759. **(A)** Stones are placed in a dry container to prevent dissolving. Stones are sent for additional study to determine their composition (Fortunato).

760. **(C)** The distal end of the common bile duct is called the sphincter of Oddi and is located where the duct enters the duodenum. A transduodenal sphincterotomy is done to treat recurrent attacks of pancreatitis because it is at this junction that the pancreatic duct enters and can be obstructed because of obstruction of the common bile duct (Meeker and Rothrock).

761. **(A)** The McBurney muscle-splitting incision is used for appendix removal. It is an 8-cm oblique incision that begins well below the umbilicus, goes through McBurney's point, and extends upward toward the right flank (Meeker and Rothrock).

762. **(D)** The vertical midline is the simplest abdominal incision to perform. It is an excellent primary incision offering good exposure to any part of the abdominal cavity (Meeker and Rothrock).

763. **(D)** A purse-string is a continuous suture placed around the lumen of the appendiceal stump to invert it. It is tightened, draw-string fashion, to close the lumen (Meeker and Rothrock).

764. **(A)** Whenever a portion of the gastrointestinal tract is entered, gastrointestinal technique must be carried out. Any instrument used after the lumen of the stomach or intestines has been entered cannot be used after it is closed. A cholecystectomy does not enter the gastrointestinal tract. An appendectomy, hemicolectomy, and an anterior resection of the sigmoid all require bowel technique (Meeker and Rothrock).

765. **(C)** Hesselback's triangle is formed by the boundaries of the deep epigastric vessels laterally, the inguinal ligament inferiorly, and the rectus abdominis muscle medially. Hernias occurring here are direct (Meeker and Rothrock).

766. **(B)** Gynecomastia is a relatively common pathologic lesion that consists of bilateral or unilateral enlargement of the male breast. Surgery consists of removal of all subareolar fibroglandular tissue and surgical reconstruction of the resultant defect (Meeker and Rothrock).

767. **(C)** Retention sutures may be used as a precautionary measure to prevent wound disruption and possible evisceration of the wound (Meeker and Rothrock).

768. **(B)** Pyloroplasty is the formation of a larger passage between the pylorus of the stomach and the duodenum. It may include the removal of a peptic ulcer if one is present (Meeker and Rothrock).

769. **(B)** A Whipple operation is a radical surgical excision of the head of the pancreas, the entire duodenum, a portion of the jejunum, the distal third of the stomach, and the lower half of the common bile duct. There is then re-establishment of continuity of the biliary, pancreatic, and gastrointestinal systems. This is done for carcinoma of the head of the pancreas and is a hazardous procedure (Meeker and Rothrock).

770. **(C)** A left subcostal incision is generally used for spleen surgery. The right subcostal is used for gallbladder, common bile duct, and pancreatic surgery (Meeker and Rothrock).

771. **(B)** A lower oblique incision, either right or left, is an inguinal incision. This incision gives access to the inguinal canal and cord structures (Meeker and Rothrock).

772. **(C)** The Pfannenstiel incision is frequently used for pelvic surgery. It is a curved transverse incision across the lower abdomen, 1½ inches above the symphysis pubis. It provides a strong closure (Meeker and Rothrock).

773. **(C)** A modified radical mastectomy involves removal of the involved breast and all three levels of axillary contents. The underlying pectoral muscles are not removed (Meeker and Rothrock).

774. **(B)** Simple mastectomy is removal of the entire breast without lymph node dissection, performed to remove extensive benign disease or a confined malignancy (Meeker and Rothrock).

775. **(C)** The diseased portion of the esophagus and stomach are removed through a left thoracoabdominal incision, including a resection of the seventh, eighth, or ninth ribs. Here, an anastomosis is accomplished between the disease-free ends of the stomach and the esophagus (Meeker and Rothrock).

776. **(A)** Retention or tension sutures may be used in a vertical midline incision to ensure strength of closure and support (Meeker and Rothrock).

777. **(C)** The great danger of an incarcerated hernia is that it may become strangulated—the blood supply of the trapped sac contents becomes compromised, and eventually the sac contents necrose (Meeker and Rothrock).

778. **(C)** Direct hernias protrude into the inguinal canal but not into the cord (Meeker and Rothrock).

779. **(D)** Indirect hernias leave the abdominal cavity at the internal ring and pass with the cord structures down the inguinal canal, thus the indirect hernia sac may be found in the scrotum (Meeker and Rothrock).

780. **(A)** A synthetic Gore-Tex patch is a popular method for reconstruction of abdominal wall defects. Mersilene, a synthetic, is also used for its strength and durability (Meeker and Rothrock).

781. **(D)** Synthetic meshes, such as Mersilene or Martex, are helpful in repair of recurrent hernias requiring a strong repair (Meeker and Rothrock).

782. **(A)** In cholecystectomy there is exposure of the neck of the gallbladder, the cystic duct, and the cystic artery. The cystic artery and duct are doubly ligated and divided, facilitating gallbladder removal (Meeker and Rothrock).

783. **(D)** In a pilonidal cystectomy, the cyst and sinus tract must be completely removed to prevent recurrence (Meeker and Rothrock).

784. **(B)** A cholangiocath is prepared using a 20-cc syringe of saline and a 20-cc syringe of contrast medium using a stopcock and Leuer-lock ports. All air bubbles are removed because they may be misinterpreted as gall duct stones on x-ray. The cholangiocath is irrigated with saline before and during the catheter insertion into the cystic duct and CBD (Meeker and Rothrock).

785. **(B)** A Lahey vulsellum forceps is used to grasp and elevate the thyroid lobe so that sharp dissection of the lobe away from the trachea can be accomplished (Meeker and Rothrock).

786. **(B)** The layers of the large intestine from inside to outside are: mucosa, submucosa, and serosa. Mucosa suture closure is most frequently absorbable suture, while the serosa layer is closed with nonabsorbable silk (Tortora and Grabowski).

787. **(D)** Postoperative shoulder pain may follow use of pneumoperitoneum. This is referred pain caused by pressure on the diaphragm, which is somewhat displaced by CO_2 during the procedure (Fortunato).

788. **(D)** A subphrenic abscess is a liver abscess that may require incision and drainage (Meeker and Rothrock).

789. **(C)** For hepatic resection, supplies and equipment should be available for hypothermia, electrosurgery, measurement of portal pressure, thorocotomy drainage, and replacement of blood loss (Meeker and Rothrock).

790. **(B)** Splenectomy is removal of the spleen, usually performed for trauma to the spleen, for specific conditions of the blood such as hemolytic jaundice or splenic anemia, or for tumors, cysts, or splenomegaly (Meeker and Rothrock).

791. **(B)** Petroleum gauze packing is placed in the anal canal. A dressing and a T-binder are applied (Meeker and Rothrock).

792. **(C)** Excision of an anal fissure involves the dilation of the anal sphincter and removal of the lesion. Anal fissures are benign lesions of the anal wall (Meeker and Rothrock).

793. **(D)** An intraoperative cholangiogram is usually performed in conjunction with cholecystectomy to visualize the common bile duct and the hepatic ductal branches and to assess patency of the common bile duct (Meeker and Rothrock).

794. **(D)** The defect resulting from recurrences may become too large for primary closure. In this case, the wound is left opened to heal by granulation. The wound is packed and a pressure dressing is applied (Meeker and Rothrock).

795. **(C)** After the abdomen is opened through a McBurney's incision, the mesoappendix is grasped with a Babcock and the appendix is gently dissected away from the cecum (Meeker and Rothrock).

796. **(C)**   The CO$_2$ laser may be used for vaporization and coagulation of hemorrhoidal tissue (Meeker and Rothrock).

797. **(C)**   In an excisional biopsy, the entire tumor mass is excised. In a needle biopsy, a plug of tissue is removed. In an incisional biopsy, a portion of the mass is excised (Meeker and Rothrock).

798. **(C)**   This myotomy of the esophagogastric junction relieves the stricture and allows food to pass unrestricted into the stomach (Meeker and Rothrock).

799. **(B)**   Varicosities of veins in the anus and rectum are called hemorrhoids. They may occur externally or internally. They must be ligated and ligatured after the sphincter of the anus is dilated (Fortunato).

800. **(B)**   A temporary colostomy is performed to decompress the bowel or give the bowel a rest and time to heal after inflammation (Meeker and Rothrock).

801. **(A)**   A low colon lesion may require an abdominoperineal resection and colostomy. The EEA (end-to-end anastomosis) is a stapling device that allows a very low anastomosis and thus avoids a colostomy (Meeker and Rothrock).

802. **(A)**   Advanced inflammation of the colon is frequently treated with a temporary colostomy, often done to decompress the bowel or give the bowel a rest (Meeker and Rothrock).

803. **(D)**   Blunt dissection, using a Kitner or peanut, is employed when removing the gallbladder from the infundibulum up to the fundal region (Meeker and Rothrock).

804. **(C)**   Choledochoscopy is direct visualization of the common bile duct by means of an instrument (choledochoscope) introduced into the common bile duct. This takes the place of cholangiography in difficult cases (Meeker and Rothrock).

805. **(D)**   The surgeon marks the incision site with a "scratch" of a scalpel in the normal neck creases and skin lines, which helps to ensure a wound line that blends with the patient's neck anatomy (Meeker and Rothrock).

806. **(D)**   A Fogarty-type balloon-tipped catheter is used to facilitate the removal of small stones and debris as well as to demonstrate patency of the common bile duct through the duodenum (Meeker and Rothrock).

807. **(C)**   To test for tubal patency during laparoscopy, diluted methylene blue or indigo carmine solution is injected through the intrauterine cannula in the cervical canal. If the fallopian tubes are patent, dye can be seen at fimbriated ends (Meeker and Rothrock).

808. **(D)**   The sternocleidomastoid muscle is retracted with loop retractors (Meeker and Rothrock).

809. **(A)**   Care is taken throughout thyroid surgery to identify and preserve parathyroid glands. Removal of all parathyroid tissue results in severe tetany or death (Meeker and Rothrock).

810. **(B)**   Morbid obesity and bariatric surgery have been developed for people who weigh more than 100 pounds over ideal weight (Fortunato).

811. **(B)**   The groin area contains the superficial group of muscles, the obliques, and Scarpa's fascia. An inguinal herniorrhaphy requires incision of Scarpa's fascia (Meeker and Rothrock).

812. **(A)**   A gastroplasty treats obesity by resecting the stomach to reduce its capacity (Fortunato).

813. **(B)**   A Penrose drain is used to retract the spermatic cord structures for better exposure (Meeker and Rothrock).

814. **(A)** After the cervix is dissected and amputated from the vagina, the uterus is then removed. Potentially contaminated instruments used on the cervix and vagina are placed in a discard basin and removed from the field (sponge sticks and suction as well) (Meeker and Rothrock).

815. **(A)** An irreducible hernia is one in which the contents of the hernia sac are trapped in the extraabdominal sac (incarcerated) (Meeker and Rothrock).

816. **(C)** With a three-chip camera, each chip picks up only one of the primary colors. Because each chip sees the entire image, there is no need to infer the color that should appear on the screen. Three-chip cameras provide truer color (Ball).

817. **(D)** To balance a video camera, the scrub person must focus the camera on a white sponge wrapper or wall to create a fixed point of reference for all other colors (Ball).

818. **(D)** Fogging occurs when the light going through the scope warms the air between the eyepiece and the coupler and causes trapped air to evaporate. To avoid fogging, the scrub person must make sure that the entire area is dry before assembling and uses an anti-fogging agent on the lens (Ball).

819. **(C)** Gastrostomy is a palliative procedure performed to prevent malnutrition or starvation. These may be caused by a lesion or stricture situated in the esophagus or cardia of the stomach (Meeker and Rothrock).

820. **(B)** Cholelithotripsy is a noninvasive procedure, done generally under IV sedation using spark-gap shockwaves generated by an electrode and passed on through the fluid medium into the body, focused at the stone with an ultrasound probe until they reach the stone (Fortunato).

821. **(B)** T-tubes are used to stent a common bile duct after common duct exploration. Red rubber catheters can be used to irrigate postoperatively. Cholangiocaths are plastic catheters used to insert dye into the common bile duct before x-ray or fluoroscopy (Fortunato).

822. **(D)** Gas flow is initiated at 1–2 L per minute. The intra-abdominal pressure is normally in the 8–10 mm Hg range and is used as an indicator for proper Verres needle placement. If the gauge indicates a higher pressure, the needle may be in a closed space such as fat, buried in omentum, or in a lumen of intestines (Meeker and Rothrock).

823. **(D)** Following irrigation of the liver bed, the scope and camera are moved to the upper midline sheath. Large grasping forceps are inserted into the umbilical sheath, and the gallbladder is pulled through. An endobag may be used to contain the specimen. If the gallbladder is too large to be extracted, the neck is brought to the surface, incised, and decompressed with a suction before removal (Meeker and Rothrock).

824. **(D)** The use of fluid-impervious bags eliminates potential contamination from wet linen soaking through. All linens from open packs, whether soiled or not, should be discarded in fluid-impervious bags (Meeker and Rothrock).

825. **(C)** Sump, chest, and Hemovac drains are all active drains attached to an external force of vacuum to create suction. The Penrose exits the wound and provides a path of least resistance for drainage into the dressing (Fortunato).

826. **(C)** The surgeon performing the laparoscopic procedure stands at the patient's left, while his or her assistant stands at the patient's right (*Stryker Endoscopy*).

827. **(D)** Both the Levine tube and the Miller–Abbot tube effect gastrointestinal decompression. The Levine tube is placed through the nasal passageway into the stomach, while the Miller–Abbot tube reaches into the small intestines (Fortunato).

828. **(D)** An alternative to a conventional ileostomy for selected patients is the Kock pouch, or continent ileostomy. The internal pouch is constructed of small intestine with an outlet to the skin. When it is functioning properly, no stool spontaneously exits from the stoma. A catheter is inserted several times a day to evacuate the contents (Meeker and Rothrock).

829. **(B)** When both direct and indirect hernias are present in the same patient, the defect is called a pantaloon hernia after the French word for pant, which the situation suggests (Meeker and Rothrock).

830. **(B)** An inguinal hernia containing Meckel's diverticulum is called Littre's hernia; one containing two loops of bowel is called Maydl's hernia. A special type of strangulated hernia is Richter's hernia. A spigelian hernia is usually located as a peritoneal sac that is between the different muscle layers of the abdominal wall (Meeker and Rothrock).

831. **(B)** All are references to a given method of laparoscopic hernia repair except ERCP is an endoscopic procedure referencing viewing of the biliary system (Meeker and Rothrock).

832. **(B)** After the upper and lower skin flaps are undermined at the level of the cricoid cartilage, the fascia in the midline is incised between the strap (sternohyoid) muscles with a knife. The sternocleidomastoid muscles are then retracted with loop retractors (Meeker and Rothrock).

833. **(B)** After the head is extended, the incision is made between the hyoid bone and the thyroid cartilage through the subcutaneous tissue. Sharp and blunt dissection is used to mobilize the cyst and duct, and the hyoid bone is transected twice with bone-cutting forceps, and the cyst is freed from adjacent structures (Meeker and Rothrock).

834. **(C)** Following meticulous hemostasis of the operative site, the wound is irrigated with normal saline, and closed wound drainage is instituted through a stab wound and secured to the skin with nonabsorbable suture and a cutting needle (Meeker and Rothrock).

835. **(C)** The camera operator stands to the right of the first assistant, across from the scrub person. He or she must closely follow the surgeon's actions (*Stryker Endoscopy*).

836. **(C)** During the procedure, the perioperative nurse should set the insufflation unit to a maximum pressure of 15 mm Hg. When intra-abdominal pressure reaches 15 mm Hg, the flow will stop. Pressure higher than 15 mm Hg may result in bradycardia, a change in blood pressure, or may force gas emboli into an exposed blood vessel during the procedure (Meeker and Rothrock).

II. OBSTETRICS AND GYNECOLOGY

837. **(C)** Once a clip has been fastened through a drape, do not remove it because the points are contaminated. If it is necessary to remove one during a case, discard it from the field and cover the area with a piece of sterile linen (Fortunato).

838. **(B)** Old blood and debris should be removed from instruments as soon as possible with water so that it does not dry on surfaces or crevices. Saline can damage surfaces, causing corrosion and pitting (Fortunato).

839. **(B)** Scrub persons should not reach behind a member of the sterile team. They may go around the person, passing back to back (Fortunato).

840. **(D)** In draping a nonsterile table, the scrub nurse should cuff the drape over his or her gloved hand in preparation for opening it. The side of the drape toward him or her is done first to minimize the possibility of contaminating the front of the gown (Fortunato).

841. **(A)** A wide cuff is used on the Mayo cover to protect the gloved hands (Fortunato).

842. **(B)** The table and sterile field should be kept as dry as possible. However, extra towels may be spread if a solution has soaked through a sterile drape (Fortunato).

843. **(B)** Methods of skin prep may vary, but the objectives are the same—to remove dirt, oil, and microbes from the skin so the incision can be made through the skin with a minimal danger of infection. It also reduces the resident microbial count and prevents the growth of microbes (Meeker and Rothrock).

844. **(C)** The current trend is toward a surgical scrub of antiseptic solution containing povidone–iodine. This reduces the number of bacteria on the skin and inhibits the growth. This process is eliminated in some ORs (Meeker and Rothrock).

845. **(B)** The first count is done by the instrument wrapper at assembly. The second count is done immediately before the operation begins by the scrub and the circulator. A third count is done when wound closure is started. A fourth is done for any discrepancy and at skin closure. An additional count may be done when a cavity within a cavity is closed, for example, uterus (Fortunato).

846. **(A)** Soiled sponges should never be touched with bare hands. Sponges should be counted in units and bagged in a waterproof plastic bag or transferred to a moisture-proof surface until the final count is completed. This is done to avoid hepatitis or pathogenic organism transmission (Fortunato).

847. **(A)** Hand specimen from the field in a basin, on a piece of paper wrapper, or on a towel. Never place specimen on a sponge that may leave the OR and disrupt the sponge count (Fortunato).

848. **(B)** The endometrial curettings should be kept separate from the endocervical curettings. Fractional curettage specimens differentiate between the endocervical and the endometrium of the corpus, which helps to locate a lesion more specifically (Fortunato).

849. **(C)** Pitocin is used to induce active labor or to increase the force or rate of existing contractions during delivery. It may be given postpartum to prevent or control hemorrhage. It acts on the uterus (Fortunato; *Mosby's Medical, Nursing, and Allied Health Dictionary*).

850. **(D)** A Verres needle is inserted into the peritoneal cavity to instill the CO_2 to effect a pneumoperitoneum (Meeker and Rothrock).

851. **(A)** In laparoscopy, a D & C may be done when indicated. After the cervix is exposed, and the position and depth of the uterus are confirmed, a Hulka forceps and uterine dilator may be introduced into the cervix to manipulate the uterus during the laparoscopy so the surgeon has better visibility (Meeker and Rothrock).

852. **(A)** As soon as the shoulders are delivered, about 20 units of oxytocic per liter of fluid are given intravenously so the uterus contracts, aiding in expulsion of the placenta and membranes (Meeker and Rothrock).

853. **(D)** A Humi cannula may be placed in the uterine cavity for intraoperative chromotubation with diluted methylene blue during microscopic reconstruction of the fallopian tube (Meeker and Rothrock).

854. **(D)** The aim of any operation for urinary stress incontinence is to improve the performance of a dislodged or dysfunctional vesical neck, to restore normal urethral length, and to tighten and restore the anterior urethral vesical angle (Meeker and Rothrock).

855. **(C)** Myomectomy is usually done on young women with symptoms that indicate the presence of benign tumors who wish to preserve fertility (Meeker and Rothrock).

856. **(A)** The postconceptional Shirodkar operation is placement of a collar-type ligature of Mersilene, Dacron tape, heavy nylon, or plastic-covered stainless steel at the internal os to close it when there is cervical incompetence characterized by habitual, spontaneous abortion (Meeker and Rothrock).

857. **(D)** A hysteroscopy is an endoscopic visualization of the uterine cavity and tubal orifices for evaluation of uterine bleeding, location and removal of IUDs, diagnosis, and so forth (Meeker and Rothrock).

858. **(D)** Laparoscopy, minilaparotomy, and posterior colpotomy are viable methods to create sterility. Culdoscopy cannot be used for this purpose (Meeker and Rothrock).

859. **(A)** A radical vulvectomy involves abdominal, perineal, and groin dissection; it requires a double setup (Meeker and Rothrock).

860. **(C)** Pelviscopy is an endoscopic approach to pelvic and intra-abdominal examination and/or surgery. Many procedures can be performed through the pelviscope (Meeker and Rothrock).

861. **(C)** Hysteroscopy is an endoscopic visualization of the uterine cavity and tubal orifices (internal) (Meeker and Rothrock).

862. **(A)** The abdominal cavity and the fallopian tube are sites of extrauterine pregnancies (ectopic). A salpingostomy done before rupture may preserve the tube (Fortunato).

863. **(D)** A, D, and C set plus added extras, including sterile cannulas for suction curettage, is used (for early pregnancy termination and for missed and incomplete abortions). The cannula is inserted into the uterus and suction is turned on to disrupt the sac and aspirate contents (Meeker and Rothrock).

864. **(C)** Because pelvic procedures involve manipulation of the ureters, bladder, and urethra, an indwelling Foley or suprapubic cystostomy catheter may be placed before or during operation (Meeker and Rothrock).

865. **(A)** Cystoceles (bulging bladder) and rectoceles (bulging rectum) occur because of weakened vaginal mucosa. Usually the cause is traumatic childbirth, and the cure is an anterior and posterior vaginal repair (Meeker and Rothrock).

866. **(B)** Trachelorrhaphy is done to treat deep lacerations of the cervix and reconstruct the cervical canal (Meeker and Rothrock).

867. **(C)** An episiotomy is an intentionally made perineal incision executed during a normal birth to facilitate delivery and prevent perineal laceration (Tortora and Grabowski).

868. **(A)** Carcinoma in situ is limited to the epithelial layer with no evidence of invasion (Fortunato).

869. **(B)** The fallopian tube is grasped with either an Allis or Babcock forceps (Meeker and Rothrock).

870. **(A)** Tuboplasty requires a basic gynecologic instrument set plus iris scissors, Adson forceps, mosquitos, Bowman lacrimal probes, Webster needle holder, and Frazier suction. A microsurgical set and laser may also be used (Meeker and Rothrock).

871. **(B)** Aspiration of fluid or blood from the cul-de-sac of Douglas (culdocentesis) confirms intraperitoneal bleeding caused by ectopic pregnancy (Meeker and Rothrock).

872. **(D)** Cervical conization may be performed by scalpel resection and suturing, by application of the cutting of cautery, or by use of a laser (Meeker and Rothrock).

873. **(D)** Tuboplasty is reconstruction of the fallopian tube to create patency and the possibility of fertilization. Intraoperative chromotubation with diluted methylene blue is used (Meeker and Rothrock).

874. **(B)** Functional cysts comprise the majority of ovarian enlargements. Follicle cysts are the most common (Meeker and Rothrock).

875. **(D)** An enterocele is a herniation of Douglas' cul-de-sac and almost always contains loops of the small intestine. It herniates into a weakened area between the anterior and posterior walls (Meeker and Rothrock).

876. (C) A Marshall–Marchetti procedure is an abdominal approach to repairing and elevating the fascial and the pubococcygeal muscle surrounding the urethra and the bladder neck for the correction of stress incontinence (Meeker and Rothrock).

877. (C) A vesicovaginal fistula may vary in size from a small opening that permits slight leakage of urine into the vagina to a large opening that permits all urine to pass to the vagina (Meeker and Rothrock).

878. (A) Once the cervix is dissected away from and is amputated from the vagina, all of the potentially contaminated instruments used on the cervix and vagina are placed in a discard basin and removed from the field (includes sponge sticks and suction) (Meeker and Rothrock).

879. (B) Papanicolaou is a cytologic study of smears of the cervical and endocervical tissue. Characteristic cellular changes can be identified (Tortora and Grabowski).

880. (B) Multiple punch biopsies of the cervical circumference (at the 3, 6, 9, and 12 o'clock positions) may be taken with a Gaylor biopsy forceps (Meeker and Rothrock).

881. (D) The uterus is opened with a knife and extended by cutting laterally with a large bandage scissor or by simply spreading with the fingers (Meeker and Rothrock).

882. (B) As soon as the head is delivered, a bulb syringe is used to aspirate the infant's exposed nares and mouth to minimize aspiration of amniotic fluid and its contents (Meeker and Rothrock).

883. (A) As soon as the shoulders are delivered, about 20 units of oxytocin per liter of fluid is administered intravenously so that the uterus contracts. This minimizes blood loss and aids in placenta and membrane expulsion (Meeker and Rothrock).

884. (C) The edges of the uterine incision are promptly clamped with Pean forceps, ring forceps, or Pennington clamps (Meeker and Rothrock).

885. (D) Once the vagina has been prepped and an indwelling catheter is placed into the bladder, chromotubation can be effected by placing a Kahn, Calvin, Hui, Humi, or Rubin cannulae into the cervical opening using diluted methylene blue dye to identify a nonpatent fallopian tube as visualized through a laparoscope (Meeker and Rothrock).

886. (C) For removal of a large ovarian cyst, a purse-string suture may be placed into the cyst wall, and a trocar is introduced into the center to aspirate its contents before the suture is tied (Meeker and Rothrock).

887. (B) Pelvic exenteration is preferred treatment for recurrent or persistent carcinoma of the cervix. It is considered the only surgical alternative after a thorough investigation of the patient and disease status to determine if there is a reasonable chance for a cure (Meeker and Rothrock).

888. (A) After the vaginal vault is incised close to the cervix during the removal of the uterus, an Allis, Kocher, or tenaculum may be used to grasp the anterior lip of the cervix (Meeker and Rothrock).

889. (C) Preknotted suture loops are used to ligate pedicle tissues. Bipolar coagulation, spring clips, and Silastic bands effect occlusion of fallopian tubes (Meeker and Rothrock).

890. (B) The Lahey vulsellum clamp is used to elevate the thyroid lobe during dissection. All of the others are holding instruments used to manipulate the cervix during vaginal surgery (Meeker and Rothrock).

891. **(B)** A Thomas uterine curette is used to remove endocervical as well as endometrial tissue scrapings from the internal lining of the uterus. All other options can be used to remove the endocervical cone to treat diseased tissue and preserve fertility (Meeker and Rothrock).

892. **(A)** An enterocele is a herniation of Douglas' cul-de-sac and almost always contains loops of the small intestine. An enterocele herniates into a weakened area between the anterior and posterior vaginal walls (Meeker and Rothrock).

893. **(D)** Pelviscopy differs from laparoscopy in two aspects: a 10-mm pelviscope with a 30° angle replaces the 7-mm laparoscope with a 0° angle. The larger lumen allows a wider field of range (Fortunato).

894. **(A)** Known as a Stamey procedure for female incontinence, the bladder neck is suspended by placing sutures on both sides of the vesicourethral junction from the anterior rectus fascia into the vagina. This is aided by insertion of a cystoscope to ascertain correct needle placement through an incision into the rectus fascia (Fortunato).

895. **(B)** An operative approach to early carcinoma of the cervix is a radical vaginal hysterectomy called a Schauta operation. It is useful in obese patients and removes the uterus, upper third of the vagina, parametria, fallopian tubes, and ovaries (Fortunato).

896. **(B)** Colpocleisis (LeFort) is obliteration of the vagina by denuding and approximating the anterior and posterior walls of the vagina and is generally reserved for elderly high-risk patients with uterine prolapse (Meeker and Rothrock).

897. **(A)** The hysteroscope is used most commonly for endometrial laser ablation. The hysteroscope also may be used to identify and remove polyps and submucous fibroids, retrieve lost uterine devices, or lyse intrauterine adhesions (Fortunato).

898. **(B)** Blood, fluid, or pus in the cul-de-sac is aspirated by needle via the posterior vaginal fornix for suspected intraperitoneal bleeding or ectopic pregnancy, or tubo-ovarian abscesses (Fortunato).

899. **(D)** Laparoscopic-assisted vaginal hysterectomy (LAVH) or pelviscopic-assisted vaginal hysterectomy (PAVH) offers an alternative to total abdominal hysterectomy and vaginal hysterectomy (Meeker and Rothrock).

900. **(B)** Procedures performed through a pelviscope include adhesiolysis, ovarian biopsy, ovarian cystectomy, oophorectomy, fimbrioplasty, and removal of ectopic pregnancies. Hysterectomies cannot be performed because of the solid size of the viscus (Meeker and Rothrock).

901. **(C)** Endometrial ablation is done to treat abnormal uterine bleeding. The overall goal is to create amenorrhea or to reduce menstrual bleeding to normal. It may be an alternative to hysterectomy in some patients with chronic menorrhagia (Meeker and Rothrock).

902. **(C)** Hysteroscopy is endoscopic visualization of the uterine cavity and tubal orifices. Laparoscopy may be done in association with hysteroscopy to assess the external contour of the uterus (Meeker and Rothrock).

903. **(D)** True marsupialization of the Bartholin's cyst involves the removal of the anterior wall of the cyst and suturing the cut edges of the remaining cyst to adjacent sides of the skin (Meeker and Rothrock).

904. **(C)** A Graves self-retaining speculum frequently is known as a duckbill speculum and is used for vaginal and cervical exposure (Meeker and Rothrock).

905. **(C)** The Candela laser is valuable to disintegrate stones in the urinary tract because it is tunable, and the wavelength can be adjusted. The CO_2, argon, and Nd:YAG are used to treat pelvic endometriosis, cervical dysplasia, condylomata, and premalignant

diseases of the vulva and the vagina (Meeker and Rothrock).

III. OPHTHALMOLOGY

906. **(A)** Cottonoid patties are compressed rayon or cotton sponges that are used moist on delicate such structures as nerves, brain, and spinal cord (Fortunato).

907. **(B)** Tonsil sponges are cotton-filled gauze with a cotton thread attached (Fortunato).

908. **(C)** Sodium hyaluronate (Healon) is a viscous jelly sometimes used to occupy space and prevent damage when opening the anterior capsule (Fortunato).

909. **(A)** Pilocarpine is a miotic. A miotic causes the pupil to contract (Fortunato).

910. **(B)** Tetracaine provides rapid, brief, and superficial anesthesia. It is widely used as a local ocular anesthetic. It is the generic name for Pontocaine (Fortunato).

911. **(B)** Hyaluronidase is commonly added to an anesthetic solution. This enzyme increases diffusion of the anesthetic through the tissue, thereby improving the effectiveness of the block (Fortunato).

912. **(D)** Balanced salt solution is an eye irritant. It is used to keep the eye moist during surgery. It is supplied in a sterile solution (Fortunato).

913. **(D)** Tetracaine produces surface anesthesia in eye surgery and is available in an 0.5% concentration for this use. Pontocaine is the trade name for this topical solution (Fortunato).

914. **(A)** Mydriatics dilate the pupil while allowing the patient to focus. A cycloplegic drug also can dilate the pupil, but it disturbs focusing ability (Meeker and Rothrock).

915. **(D)** In extracapsular extraction, the phacoemulsifier is used in a microsurgical technique to remove the lens. Ultrasonic energy fragments the hard lens, which can then be aspirated from the eye (Meeker and Rothrock).

916. **(B)** Removal of a chalazion is the incision and curettage of a chronic granulomatous inflammation of one or more of the meibomian glands of the eyelid (Meeker and Rothrock).

917. **(D)** Chronic dacrocystitis in adults requires dacrocystorhinostomy to establish a new tear passageway for drainage directly into the nasal cavity to correct deficient drainage with overflow of tears (Meeker and Rothrock).

918. **(A)** A scleral buckling is the operative treatment for retinal detachment. The procedure is aimed at preventing permanent vision loss by sealing off the area in which a hole or tear is located (Meeker and Rothrock).

919. **(C)** Ectropion is the sagging and eversion of the lower lid. It is common in older patients and is corrected by a plastic procedure that shortens the lower lid in a horizontal direction (Meeker and Rothrock).

920. **(C)** Enucleation is removal of the entire eyeball. Evisceration is removal of the contents of the eye, leaving the sclera intact (Meeker and Rothrock).

921. **(A)** Argon or Nd:Yag laser therapy is used to treat acute (angle-closure) glaucoma and open-angle glaucoma. It is uncomplicated and utilizes a slit lamp for laser beam delivery. It is noninvasive and a fairly uncomplicated outpatient procedure (Meeker and Rothrock).

922. **(B)** Resection of part of the ocular muscle rotates the eye toward the operated muscle, thereby strengthening it (Meeker and Rothrock).

923. **(C)** In its normal state, the vitreous gel of the eye is transparent. In certain disease states, it becomes opaque and must be removed (Meeker and Rothrock).

924. **(C)** Miocol solution is used to constrict the pupil to prevent vitreous loss during a cataract extraction. The Miocol solution must be used within 15 minutes after preparation. If complications arise, new solution should be prepared (Meeker and Rothrock).

925. **(B)** Of the devices used to increase drainage from the anterior chamber, the Molteno implant has become one of the most widely used drainage devices implanted after trabeculectomy (Meeker and Rothrock).

926. **(B)** Sodium hyaluronate functions as a lubricant and as a vesicoelastic support, maintaining a separation of tissues. It is used in intraocular procedures to protect the corneal epithelium and as a tamponade (Meeker and Rothrock).

927. **(C)** After the lens is removed slowly from the eye, the pupil is constricted with Miocol or Miostat if an IOL is to be inserted (Meeker and Rothrock).

928. **(D)** Radial keratotomy is a series of partial incisions in the cornea for reshaping and correction of the refractive power of the cornea. Keratophakia references a new procedure that utilizes a piece of donor corneal tissue to reshape the cornea (Meeker and Rothrock).

929. **(D)** Wydase, also referred to as hyaluronidase, is an enzyme that increases tissue diffusion and effectiveness of nerve blocks during ophthalmology procedures (Meeker and Rothrock).

930. **(A)** Retrobulbar anesthesia is an injection of anesthetic solution into the base of the orbital margins or behind the eyeball to block the ciliary ganglion and nerves (Meeker and Rothrock).

931. **(A)** Pterygiums tend to be bilateral. When a pterygium encroaches on the visual axis, it is removed surgically (Meeker and Rothrock).

932. **(D)** A corneal transplant is grafting of corneal tissue from one human eye to another.

This is known as keratoplasty and is performed when one's cornea is thickened or opaque because of disease or injury (Meeker and Rothrock).

933. **(B)** Vitreous humor may accidentally enter the anterior cavity of the eye if a miotic drug is not used during surgery. A vitreous catheter is placed through the cataract wound to remove vitreous humor and not allow it to fill the anterior chamber. It is then constricted with acetylcholine (Meeker and Rothrock).

934. **(A)** All of the procedures treat glaucoma. Iridectomy provides a communication between the anterior and posterior chambers to relieve intraocular pressure (Meeker and Rothrock).

935. **(B)** Glycerol and isosorbide are both given preoperatively to control intraocular pressure before ophthalmic surgery. Mannitol and urea are given parenterally, while Diamox may be given either parenterally or orally (Meeker and Rothrock).

936. **(C)** Argon or Nd:Yag laser therapy is being used to treat acute and open angle glaucoma. It is a noninvasive procedure and may, if successful, prevent more invasive procedures (Meeker and Rothrock).

IV. OTORHINOLARYNGOLOGY

937. **(B)** A moustache dressing may be applied under the nose (nares) to absorb any bleeding (Meeker and Rothrock).

938. **(B)** The CO_2 laser is efficient and has a high-power output. It uses a combination of CO_2, nitrogen, and helium. As energy levels subside, light beams are produced that form a single beam of light in the ultraviolet range that is invisible. For this reason, a red beam from a helium–neon laser is added so that it may be properly aimed at the affected tissue (Meeker and Rothrock).

939. **(C)** Cocaine is unrivaled in its power to penetrate the mucous membrane to produce surface anesthesia. Onset is immediate. It also causes vasoconstriction to reduce bleeding. Administration is only topical because of its high toxicity (Fortunato).

940. **(B)** The scrub cleans the burrs during the procedure. Continuous irrigation is necessary to minimize the transfer of heat from the burr to surrounding bone and structures. A suction irrigation may be used (Meeker and Rothrock).

941. **(A)** Incision of the tympanic membrane, known as myringotomy, is done to treat otitis media. By releasing the fluid behind the membrane, hearing is restored and infection controlled. Frequently, tubes are inserted through the tympanic membrane (Meeker and Rothrock).

942. **(A)** An alligator forceps is used to insert the tube into the incision (Meeker and Rothrock).

943. **(D)** Perforation of the eardrum (tympanic membrane) is the most common serious ear injury. Tympanoplasty using grafted tissue improves hearing and prevents recurrent infection (Meeker and Rothrock).

944. **(C)** Labyrinthectomy is a procedure that destroys the membranous labyrinth to relieve the patient of severe vertigo when other means have been tried. The operation leaves the ear deaf (Meeker and Rothrock).

945. **(B)** Myringotomy is incision into the tympanic membrane to ventilate the middle ear (Meeker and Rothrock).

946. **(D)** Mastoidectomy is the removal of the diseased bone of the mastoid, along with cholesteatoma that results from an accumulation of squamous epithelium and its products. This putty-like mass destroys the middle ear and mastoid, so diseased bone must be removed (Meeker and Rothrock).

947. **(B)** An acoustic neuroma arises in the eighth cranial nerve (acoustic). These tumors are benign but may grow to a size that produces neurologic symptoms. The main patient complaint is hearing loss (Meeker and Rothrock).

948. **(A)** Computerized facial nerve monitoring is used intraoperatively to decrease trauma during tumor dissection and to assess facial nerve status (Meeker and Rothrock).

949. **(A)** Submucous resection is also known as septoplasty—removal of either cartilage or bone portions of the septum that obstruct the sinus opening and prevent a clear airway (Meeker and Rothrock).

950. **(B)** A submucous resection is done for nasal septum deformity, fracture, or injury that has impaired normal respiratory function and has impaired drainage (Meeker and Rothrock).

951. **(A)** A bayonet forceps is used to introduce sponges into the nose (Meeker and Rothrock).

952. **(C)** This surgery is done to relieve edema or infection of the membrane lining the sinuses and resultant headaches. An opening is made into the maxillary sinus (Meeker and Rothrock).

953. **(D)** Polyps are removed with a snare, polyp forceps, and suction (Meeker and Rothrock).

954. **(C)** Frequently, a topical anesthetic is used before nasal surgery. The drug of choice is cocaine, 10% or 4%, and would be administered by means of soaked applicators introduced into the nasal cavity and absorbed by the mucous membrane (Meeker and Rothrock).

955. **(A)** A Caldwell–Luc (radical antrostomy) entails an incision under the upper lip above the teeth. It is done to ensure drainage and aeration and permit, under direct vision, removal of diseased sinus tissue (Meeker and Rothrock).

956. **(C)** Tracheostomy is the opening of the trachea and establishment of a new airway through a midline incision in the neck, below the cricoid cartilage. A cannula is put in place to maintain the airway. This is an emergency procedure (Meeker and Rothrock).

957. **(B)** Lidocaine 1% (1 or 2 mL) may be instilled into the trachea to reduce the coughing reflex when the tube is inserted (Meeker and Rothrock).

958. **(A)** A catheter is used to suction the trachea at tube insertion (Meeker and Rothrock).

959. **(C)** Most neoplasms of the salivary glands are benign mixed tumors; most of these affect the parotid gland (Meeker and Rothrock).

960. **(B)** The patient is placed in the semirecumbent (Fowler's) position or on one side, horizontally, to prevent aspiration of blood and venous engorgement postoperatively (Meeker and Rothrock).

961. **(A)** Total laryngectomy is complete removal of the larynx, hyoid bone, and the strap muscles (Meeker and Rothrock).

962. **(B)** To maintain hemostasis postoperatively in radical neck surgery, a Hemovac is generally employed. Continuous pressure from the gauze pressure dressings reduces the accumulation of serosanguineous fluid, which is removed by the Hemovac (Meeker and Rothrock).

963. **(D)** For radical neck, a Y-shaped or trifurcate incision is used in the affected side of the neck. A parotid incision is also a Y incision but on both sides of the ear and below the angle of the mandible (Meeker and Rothrock).

964. **(D)** During ear surgery, a local anesthetic with epinephrine is often the surgeon's choice because the epinephrine acts as a vasoconstrictor and prevents oozing in the wound. Epinephrine-soaked pledgets are also used to control bleeding (Meeker and Rothrock).

965. **(B)** The device is implanted in the cochlea, with the receiver resting in the mastoid bone. As the device receives sound through the receiver, it emits electrical impulses through the transmitter into the cochlea and along the acoustic nerve. These impulses are interpreted as a sound in the temporal cortex of the cerebrum (Meeker and Rothrock).

966. **(B)** Facial nerve decompression is a procedure designed to identify and relieve an area of compression of the facial nerve. The most common form of facial paralysis is Bell's palsy (Meeker and Rothrock).

967. **(A)** All choices except for A can cause fires if hit by a laser beam. To protect the patient, the endotracheal tube must be protected by wrapping it with adhesive sensitive tape. In addition, wet gauze is placed just above the cuff. Stainless steel, copper, and commercially prepared noncombustibles are better choices (Meeker and Rothrock).

968. **(C)** The advent of the CO_2 laser added a new dimension to the laryngologist's treatment of lesions of the larynx and vocal cords. The laser is efficient and has a high-power output. It uses a combination of CO_2, nitrogen, and helium gas (Meeker and Rothrock).

969. **(D)** The 120° endoscope is used only during maxillary sinus endoscopy. The 70° endoscope may occasionally be used in special maxillary procedure, but is a diagnostic scope generally (Meeker and Rothrock).

970. **(C)** During a rhinoplasty, the dorsal hump can be taken down with an osteotome. A cartilaginous hump can be removed by means of a cutting forcep, such as a Jansen–Middleton forcep (Meeker and Rothrock).

971. **(C)** During a tonsillectomy, the tonsil is grasped with a tonsil-grasping forcep, the mucous membrane of the anterior pillar is incised with a knife, and the tonsil lobe is freed from its attachments to the pillar with a tonsil dissector (Meeker and Rothrock).

972. **(D)** It is imperative that all gauze pads or patties be kept moistened during the surgery to prevent damage to healthy tissue from stray or reflected beams of light. Moisture is the most effective barrier to stop the laser energy from penetrating healthy tissue or igniting materials in the area (Meeker and Rothrock).

973. **(D)** Because regulation endotracheal tubes are combustible, they must be carefully wrapped with adhesive sensing tape. A safer alternative is the use of copper (Carden), stainless steel (Porch), or commercially prepared laser-retardant endotrachial tubes on a jet ventilation system (Meeker and Rothrock).

V. PLASTIC AND RECONSTRUCTIVE SURGERY

974. **(D)** A subcuticular suture is a continuous suture placed beneath the epithelial layer of the skin in short lateral stitches. It leaves a minimal scar (Meeker and Rothrock).

975. **(A)** Webril is a soft, lint-free cotton bandage. The surface is smooth but not glazed, so that each layer clings to the preceding one and the padding lies smoothly in place (Fortunato).

976. **(A)** Pigskin (porcine) is used as a temporary biologic dressing to cover large body surfaces denuded of skin (Fortunato).

977. **(B)** A pressure dressing prevents edema, distributes pressure evenly, absorbs excessive drainage, gives extra wound support, and provides comfort to the patient postoperatively (Fortunato).

978. **(D)** A stent dressing or fixation is a method of applying pressure and stabilizing tissues when it is impossible to dress an area. In the case of the nose, for example, long suture ends are criss-crossed over a small dressing and tied (Fortunato).

979. **(B)** After a syringe is filled and verification is established by the nurse and scrub, it is handed to the surgeon. The scrub states the kind and percentage of solution and keeps track of the amount used (Fortunato).

980. **(B)** Change a glove at once and discard needle or instrument if a glove is pricked by a needle or snagged by an instrument (Fortunato).

981. **(A)** Separate setups are used in skin preparation of the recipient and donor sites. Items used in preparation of the recipient site must not be permitted to contaminate the donor site. The donor site should be scrubbed with a colorless antiseptic agent so the surgeon can evaluate the vascularity of the graft postoperatively. Always place dermatome separately, never on recipient table (Fortunato).

982. **(D)** The scrub nurse should not touch the plunger except at the end, because glove powder can act as a contaminant. Contamination of the plunger can contaminate the inner wall of the barrel and the solution that is drawn into it (Fortunato).

983. **(B)** Needles are not safely stored in a medicine cup because of difficulty in counting them and the chance of puncturing the glove when removing them. Also by handling each needle individually, the potential for contamination increases (Fortunato).

984. **(C)** A colorless prep solution may be used in plastic surgery to facilitate observation of the true color of the skin (Fortunato).

985. **(A)** A split-thickness graft, or partial-thickness graft, contains epidermis and only a portion of the dermis (Meeker and Rothrock).

986. **(A)** Dupuytren's contracture is a progressive disease involving the palmar fascia and the digital extensions of the palmar fascia. The surgery required is a palmar fasciectomy (Meeker and Rothrock).

987. **(B)** Microtia refers to congenital total or subtotal absence of the external ear (Meeker and Rothrock).

988. **(A)**   A stent or tie-over dressing exerts even pressure, ensuring good contact between graft and recipient site (Meeker and Rothrock).

989. **(C)**   Syndactyly refers to webbing of the digits of the hand or foot (Meeker and Rothrock).

990. **(D)**   Hypospadias is a congenital anomaly in which the urethra ends on the ventral penile shaft or in the perineum. It is frequently accompanied by chordee (a downward curvature of the penis) (Meeker and Rothrock).

991. **(C)**   A rhytidectomy is a face lift designed to improve appearance by removing excess skin and sometimes excess fat of the neck (Meeker and Rothrock).

992. **(C)**   Frozen allografts are stored in plastic or cloth wraps to ensure sterility and prevent grafts from drying out. When requested for a procedure, the allograft is delivered to the field slightly thawed. It is then cultured and washed with an antibiotic solution (Meeker and Rothrock).

993. **(D)**   Pressure dressings are used mainly in general surgery or plastic procedures to eliminate dead space, absorb extensive drainage, distribute pressure evenly, and immobilize a body part when muscles are moved (Meeker and Rothrock).

994. **(B)**   Breast prostheses and tissue expanders should be placed in a container with sterile saline or antibiotic solution on the sterile field (Meeker and Rothrock).

995. **(D)**   Sterile, transparent occlusive dressings, such as Bioclusive and Opsite, are made of transparent polyethylene and may be used when slight or no drainage is expected. They are usually removed after 24–48 hours (Fortunato).

996. **(B)**   Stent fixation is a method of applying pressure and stabilizing tissues when it is impossible to dress an area such as the face or neck (Fortunato).

997. **(D)**   Reconstructive problems in patients undergoing laryngectomy and upper cervical esophagectomy can be adequately solved by a free jejunal transfer. Modern microscopic techniques greatly improve the success rate (Meeker and Rothrock).

998. **(D)**   The most commonly used donor tendon for a free graft is the palmaris longus tendon of the wrist and forearm. The plantaris tendon in the leg is also frequently used (Meeker and Rothrock).

999. **(C)**   An Esmarch bandage is used to exsanguinate the extremity before institution of a pneumatic tourniquet (Meeker and Rothrock).

1000. **(B)**   The TRAM flap is a single-stage reconstruction of a postmastectomy breast with the transverse rectus abdominis muscle of the lower abdomen (Meeker and Rothrock).

1001. **(C)**   The simplest form of scar revision is excision of an existing scar and simple resuturing of the wound. The Z-plasty is the most widely used method of scar revision. It breaks up linear scars, rearranging them so that all tissue lies in the same direction (Meeker and Rothrock).

VI. GENITOURINARY SURGERY

1002. **(B)**   A Pereyra needle suspension is used to treat stress incontinence, a urinary condition (Fortunato).

1003. **(A)**   The Garceau may be used to dilate the ureter (Meeker and Rothrock).

1004. **(A)**   When water is used for irrigation on an invasive surgical procedure, the pressure of the water against the exposed vessels creates a hemolytic reaction and therefore destroys red blood cells (Meeker and Rothrock).

1005. **(A)**   Pressure from a 30-cc catheter balloon inserted after closure of the urethra helps obtain hemostasis by controlling venous bleeding (Meeker and Rothrock).

1006. **(C)** The third lumen provides a means for continuous irrigation of the bladder for a time postoperatively to prevent formation of clots in the bladder (Meeker and Rothrock).

1007. **(A)** The OR table is flexed so that the kidney elevator can be raised the desired amount to increase the space between lower ribs and iliac crest. A body strap or tape is placed over the hips. The safety belt is over the legs (Fortunato).

1008. **(B)** When the kidney position is being used, the table is straightened before closure to afford better approximation of tissues. It is used for procedures on kidneys and ureters. This is done by the anesthesiologist (Fortunato).

1009. **(B)** As the male ages, the prostate gland may enlarge and gradually obstruct the urethra. This condition is known as benign prostatic hypertrophy (BPH) (Meeker and Rothrock).

1010. **(C)** A Braasch bulb is a ureteral catheter used to occlude the ureteral orifice during x-ray study. Urethral dilatation is accomplished using McCarthy dilators, Philips filiform and followers, and VanBuren sounds (Meeker and Rothrock).

1011. **(A)** A stone may lodge in a renal calyx and continue to enlarge, eventually filling the entire renal collecting system. It is known as a staghorn stone (Meeker and Rothrock).

1012. **(A)** For simple observation cystoscopy or retrograde pyelogram, sterile distilled water may be used (Meeker and Rothrock).

1013. **(D)** A nephrostomy temporarily drains the kidney with a Malecot or Pezzar catheter. In an ileal conduit, the ureter is implanted into the ileum, and an ileal stoma is created. The ureter diverted to the skin of the lower abdomen is a cutaneous ureterostomy. Repositioning the ureter is a ureterocystostomy (Meeker and Rothrock).

1014. **(C)** The Alexander periosteotome, Doyen raspatory, and Stille shears are all instruments required to remove a rib. A Heaney clamp is a hemostatic clamp used in gynecologic surgery (Meeker and Rothrock).

1015. **(B)** Laser ablation of condylomata is the eradication of diseased tissue by means of a laser beam. The recurrence rate with this technique is low (Meeker and Rothrock).

1016. **(B)** Removal of the testes (orchiectomy) renders the patient both sterile and hormone deficient. Bilateral orchiectomy usually denotes carcinoma. Unilateral orchiectomy may be indicated for cancer, infection, or trauma (Meeker and Rothrock).

1017. **(A)** Sorbitol, mannitol, and glycine do not produce hemolysis. They are nonelectrolytic and do not cause dispersion of high-frequency current with loss of cutting power as occurs with normal saline (Meeker and Rothrock).

1018. **(C)** The pelvis of the kidney is incised with a small blade. A catheter is placed through the incision into the renal pelvis to create a short-term urinary diversion (Meeker and Rothrock).

1019. **(D)** A penile prosthesis is implanted for treatment of organic sexual impotence (Meeker and Rothrock).

1020. **(D)** Radical lymphadenectomy is a bilateral resection of retroperitoneal lymph nodes to treat testicular tumors (Meeker and Rothrock).

1021. **(C)** Vasovasostomy is the surgical reanastomosis of the vas deferens, utilizing the operative microscope (Meeker and Rothrock).

1022. **(C)** The Tru-cut or Vim–Silverman biopsy needle is used to retrieve a prostate biopsy (Meeker and Rothrock).

1023. **(D)** Kidney transplant entails transplantation of a living related or cadaver donor kidney into the recipient's iliac fossa (Meeker and Rothrock).

1024.   **(C)**   Endoscopic suspension of the vesical neck for stress incontinence is a Stamey procedure (Meeker and Rothrock).

1025.   **(B)**   Following a TURP, the urologist may insert a 30-cc, three-way Foley catheter. The third lumen provides a means of continuous irrigation of the bladder for a period after surgery to prevent the formation of clots. The large balloon aids in hemostasis (Meeker and Rothrock).

1026.   **(C)**   Cystotomy (cystostomy) is an opening made into the urinary bladder through a low abdominal incision with insertion of a drainage tube (Meeker and Rothrock).

1027.   **(C)**   Retropubic prostatectomy is the enucleation of hypertrophied prostate tissue through an incision into the anterior prostatic capsule. Good exposure and excellent hemostasis are obtained (Meeker and Rothrock).

1028.   **(C)**   Stones removed during surgery are subjected to chemical analysis and thus are submitted in a dry state. Fixative agents invalidate the results of the analysis (Meeker and Rothrock).

1029.   **(A)**   A Pereyra procedure is a bladder neck suspension involving urethrovesical suspension with vaginourethroplasty (Meeker and Rothrock).

1030.   **(D)**   A percutaneous nephrolithotomy facilitates the removal of stones using a rigid or flexible nephroscope. Accessory instrumentation includes an ultrasonic wand (sonotrode), lithotriptor probe, stone basket, and stone grasper. A lithotriptor tub is used in extracorporeal shock wave lithotripsy (Meeker and Rothrock).

1031.   **(D)**   Orchiopexy is regarded as the transfer or fixation of an imperfectly descended testicle into the scrotum and suturing it in place (Meeker and Rothrock).

1032.   **(B)**   After a suprapubic incision is made abdominally, an opening is made into the

bladder, and the prostate is removed from above (Meeker and Rothrock).

1033.   **(D)**   The lumbar or simple flank incision may include removal of the 11th or 12th rib, thus a rib set should be available (Meeker and Rothrock).

1034.   **(A)**   A hydrocele is an abnormal accumulation of fluid within the scrotum, contained in the tunica vaginalis (Meeker and Rothrock).

1035.   **(C)**   Extracorporeal shock wave lithotripsy is a noninvasive approach to urolithiasis management. Shock waves disintegrate stones via a liquid medium visualized by an image intensifier (Meeker and Rothrock).

1036.   **(B)**   A lithotrite is used to crush large bladder calculi (Meeker and Rothrock).

1037.   **(B)**   Urethral meatotomy is an incisional enlargement of the external urethral meatus to relieve stenosis or stricture either congenital or acquired (Meeker and Rothrock).

1038.   **(C)**   The pump is placed in the most dependent portion of the scrotum (Meeker and Rothrock).

1039.   **(D)**   A hydrocelectomy is the excision of the tunica vaginalis of the testis to remove the enlarged fluid-filled sac (Meeker and Rothrock).

1040.   **(A)**   Surgical removal of the foreskin of the penis is frequently performed immediately after birth. At times, the condition known as phimosis (stricture of the foreskin) causes a circumcision to be done on an adult male who was not circumcised at birth (Meeker and Rothrock).

1041.   **(B)**   Balloon dilatation of the prosthetic urethra, also known as transcystoscopic urethroplasty, is an advanced alternative to transurethral prostatectomy. It is nonsurgical, and with a cystoscopic setup and balloon dilatation catheters, the urethra is stretched for a better urinary flow (Meeker and Rothrock).

1042. **(C)** The advantages of the Nd:YAG laser in the eradication of bladder tumors are that bleeding is minimized, only sedation is required, operating time is short, and there is minimal damage to healthy tissue (Meeker and Rothrock).

1043. **(D)** Ileal conduit is a cutaneous urinary diversion exteriorizing the urinary tract by creating a stoma. All of the other choices are continent urinary diversions forming a pouch to act as an intra-abdominal reservoir (Meeker and Rothrock).

1044. **(A)** During urologic surgery, stones removed from the system are sent to the lab in a dry state. Fixative agents may invalidate the analysis (Meeker and Rothrock).

1045. **(D)** The proximal stoma is transferred to the site of the anastomosis for reimplantation. Following anastomosis with fine atraumatic sutures, a stent is left in place until healing occurs (Meeker and Rothrock).

1046. **(B)** Foley Y–V is a surgical procedure done to create a better anatomic relationship between the renal pelvis and the proximal ureter, as well as resection of a stenotic portion of the ureteropelvic junction. A Silastic tubing may be used until adequate healing has occurred (Meeker and Rothrock).

1047. **(D)** Both vasovasostomy and epididymovasostomy are microscopic reanastomosis options for sterilization reversal in the male. Success rates vary from 40% to 70% (Meeker and Rothrock).

1048. **(D)** A serious complication to a penile implant is infection. Meticulous aseptic technique and careful draping are essential. Intraoperatively, and before insertion of the implant components, a prophylactic antibiotic irrigant of Bacitracin is used on the implants and in the insertion sites (Meeker and Rothrock).

1049. **(C)** Heparin is given IV to the donor just before clamping the renal vessels before removal of the kidney. Immediately after the kidney is removed (and only in a live donor), 50 mg of Protamine sulfate is given to reverse the action of the heparin in the donor (Meeker and Rothrock).

1050. **(D)** Forty-five minutes before surgery, 12.5 g of mannitol is given to the kidney donor to ensure diuresis during anesthesia induction. The dose is repeated 5 minutes before the renal vessel is clamped to maximize diuresis and once again at the end of the procedure (Meeker and Rothrock).

1051. **(A)** The ideal cadaver donor should be young, free of infection or cancer, and normotensive until just before death. There must also be family permission, and the medical examiner must unequivocally establish brain death (Meeker and Rothrock).

1052. **(B)** Just before completion of full dissection of the donor liver, the donor is heparinized and systemically cooled. Further cooling and flushing of the pancreas, liver, and kidneys is achieved by cannulation and infusion of cold Ringer's lactate solution via the inferior vena cava until properly cooled (Meeker and Rothrock).

1053. **(C)** The use of the resectoscope requires that irrigation be accomplished with a nonconducting, isosmotic solution to prevent conduction of current into the bladder, as well as to prevent hemolysis attributable to electroresection of tissue (Fortunato).

1054. **(C)** All of the following procedures can be accomplished through a cystoscope: bladder biopsy, removal of a foreign body, insertion of radionuclide seeds, coagulation of a hemangioma with argon laser, and cystographic studies. Excision of a bladder tumor requires the use of a resectoscope (Fortunato).

1055. **(A)** The vas is located by digital palpation of the upper part of the scrotum. A small incision is made over the vas. An Allis forceps is inserted into the scrotal incision to grasp the vas (Meeker and Rothrock).

1056. **(A)** A noninvasive approach to urolithiasis management is the use of ESWL. This device disintegrates stones by introducing shock waves into the body, utilizing a specially treated water as a medium (Meeker and Rothrock).

1057. **(C)** The Candela laser, a tunable dye laser, allows the operator to dial the desired wavelength within a limited range. It has the ability to disintegrate stones without damaging surrounding tissue. The technique may be used during a ureteropyeloscopy or nephroscopy (Meeker and Rothrock).

VII. THORACIC SURGERY

1058. **(B)** Suction tubing with a Lukens tube collects washing specimens during a bronchoscopy (Meeker and Rothrock).

1059. **(B)** The mediastinoscope is used to view the lymph nodes or masses in the superior mediastinum (Meeker and Rothrock).

1060. **(A)** A rigid bronchoscope is the instrument of choice for removal of foreign bodies in infants and children (Meeker and Rothrock).

1061. **(D)** A Lukens or a Clerf is used to hold secretions as they are sucked through the aspirating tube. They collect in this device permitting retrieval for cytologic study (Meeker and Rothrock).

1062. **(D)** Disposable chest drainage collects drainage, maintains a water seal, and provides suction control. It is aimed at providing a conduit for air, blood, and other fluids as well as the re-establishment of negative pressure in the intrapleural space (Meeker and Rothrock).

1063. **(B)** Decompression for thoracic outlet syndrome is done to correct either a congenital deformity or traumatic injury resulting in anatomical changes in the skeletal structure of the first rib (Meeker and Rothrock).

1064. **(B)** A reduction of negative pressure on one side causes the negative pressure on the normal side to pull on the mediastinum in an effort to equalize the pressure. This is referred to as mediastinal shift; it tends to compress the lung, causing dyspnea (Meeker and Rothrock).

1065. **(C)** Removal of the fibrinous deposit or restrictive membrane on the visceral and parietal pleura that interferes with pulmonary function is called decortication of the lung (Meeker and Rothrock).

1066. **(B)** Pleural effusions are a significant cause of morbidity, particularly in patients with advanced cancer. Pleurodesis with the instillation of talc can be accomplished through the thoracoscope for this purpose (Meeker and Rothrock).

1067. **(B)** All instruments are used to effect an open thoracotomy. A Doyen is a rib elevator, an Alexander is a rib raspatory, a Bethune is a rib shear, and a Bailey is a rib approximator (Meeker and Rothrock).

1068. **(C)** After harvesting of the lung is complete, the trachea is stapled shut, and the donor lung is placed in cold Collin's solution (Meeker and Rothrock).

1069. **(C)** Three anastomoses are completed for a single-lung transplant: bronchus to bronchus, pulmonary artery to pulmonary artery, and recipient pulmonary veins to donor atrial cuff (Meeker and Rothrock).

VIII. CARDIOVASCULAR AND PERIPHERAL VASCULAR SURGERY

1070. (C) Ti-Cron is a polyester fiber suture (coated with silicone) used in cardiovascular surgery for valve replacements, graft-to-tissue anastomosis, and revascularization procedures (Meeker and Rothrock).

1071. (A) A nonabsorbable synthetic suture of Teflon, Dacron, polyester, or polypropylene is usually selected for insertion of prosthesis and for vascular anastomosis. Most sutures are double armed. Alternate colors may help avoid confusion (Meeker and Rothrock).

1072. (A) In an embolectomy, a Fogarty catheter is inserted beyond the point of clot attachment. The balloon is inflated, and the catheter is withdrawn along with the detached clot (Meeker and Rothrock).

1073. (C) Amputated extremities are wrapped before sending them to a refrigerator. The morgue is the usual place that receives them, unless hospital policy dictates otherwise. They must be tagged and labeled properly (Fortunato).

1074. (C) Protamine sulfate is a protein-like substance that, by itself, is an anticoagulant. When given in the presence of heparin, each neutralizes the anticoagulant activity of the other. Thus, it is a heparin antagonist (Fortunato).

1075. (B) Ventricular fibrillation requires prompt defibrillation and CPR. It is rapidly fatal because respiratory and cardiac arrest follow quickly unless successful defibrillation is effected (Fortunato).

1076. (A) Dextran is used to expand plasma volume in emergency situations resulting from shock or hemorrhage. It acts by drawing fluid from the tissues. It remains in the circulatory system for several hours (Fortunato).

1077. (D) Heparin may be used locally or systemically to prevent thrombosis during vascular operative procedures. When a vessel is completely occluded during surgery, heparin is often injected directly. Heparinized saline irrigation may also be used. The dosage and concentration may vary according to the surgeon's preference. The saline used must be injectable saline (Fortunato).

1078. (C) Serial monitoring of blood gases is indispensable in evaluating pulmonary gas exchange and acid-base balance. Either or both arterial or venous blood gas determination can be monitored. It is a chemical analysis of the blood for concentrations of oxygen and carbon dioxide (Fortunato).

1079. (C) Cardiac catheterization is used to diagnose coronary artery disease. It involves a sterile setup and fluoroscopy to diagnose ischemic heart disease. The brachial or femoral artery is used to effect this procedure (Meeker and Rothrock).

1080. (A) Hypothermia deliberately reduces body temperature to permit reduction of oxygen consumption by about 50% (Meeker and Rothrock).

1081. (C) Coronary artery bypass grafting (CABG) involves harvesting of the saphenous vein and internal mammary artery (IMA) (Meeker and Rothrock).

1082. (A) A knitted graft is prepared before inserting to minimize blood loss from seepage through graft interstices. The patient's own blood may be used, immersing the graft in a small quantity (Meeker and Rothrock).

1083. (C) Perfusion is the technique of oxygenating and perfusing the blood by means of a mechanical pump-oxygenator (Fortunato).

1084. (B) The intraortic balloon pump increases cardiac output and permits the patient separation from the CPB.

1085. **(D)** Protamine sulfate reverses heparin (Meeker and Rothrock).

1086. **(B)** Pedal pulse can be assessed manually or with an ultrasonic instrument (Doppler). It assesses movement of blood through a vessel (Meeker and Rothrock).

1087. **(D)** Heparin may be used locally or systemically to prevent thrombosis during an operative procedure (vascular). It can be injected directly or used as a heparinized saline irrigation (e.g., 5000 units in 500 mL of saline) (Meeker and Rothrock).

1088. **(B)** The prime surgical consideration when a rupture or dissection occurs is the control of hemorrhage by occluding the aorta proximal to the point of rupture (Meeker and Rothrock).

1089. **(D)** A femoral–popliteal bypass is the restoration of blood flow to the leg with a graft bypassing the occluded section of the femoral artery with either a saphenous vein or a graft. The tunneler is passed from the popliteal fossa to the groin, and the graft is pulled through (Meeker and Rothrock).

1090. **(B)** The goal is to restore internal patency of a vessel by creating a channel through the diseased artery and then introducing a balloon catheter. The dilating balloon is inflated with fluid consisting of a dilute solution of the contrast media (Meeker and Rothrock).

1091. **(C)** During an arterial embolectomy, a Fogarty catheter is carefully inserted into an artery and placed beyond the point of the clot attachment. The balloon is inflated, and the catheter is withdrawn along with the attached clot (Meeker and Rothrock).

1092. **(D)** Carotid endarterectomy is the removal of an atheroma (plaque) at the carotid artery bifurcation. A temporary shunt or bypass can be used (Meeker and Rothrock).

1093. **(C)** Shunt operations for portal hypertension are splenorenal shunt, portocaval anastomosis, and mesocaval shunt. An arteriovenous shunt is used for dialysis (Meeker and Rothrock).

1094. **(D)** Endarterectomy is the removal of arteriosclerotic plaque from an obstructed artery. It occurs frequently at the bifurcation of the vessel (Meeker and Rothrock).

1095. **(C)** A graft placed proximal to and inclusive of the common iliac vessels will necessitate the use of a bifurcation into the common iliac branches (Meeker and Rothrock).

1096. **(A)** Either a shunting device or an arteriovenous fistula using the radial artery and cephalic vein are used to facilitate hemodialysis (Meeker and Rothrock).

1097. **(A)** A filter device may be inserted (in its collapsed form) through a cutdown in a large vein, usually the right internal jugular. The Greenfield filter is shaped like an umbrella. It is designed to allow blood to pass through the vena cava while filtering clots (Meeker and Rothrock).

1098. **(D)** To prevent undue trauma, umbilical tapes or vessel loops are used for retraction and vascular control (Meeker and Rothrock).

1099. **(C)** Vena cava filter insertion entails partial occlusion of the IVC with an intravascular filter, such as Greenfield, inserted under fluoroscopy. So too is an endocardial pacing electrode, which attaches to a pacemaker that is placed beneath the skin and powers the electrode. A seldom used myocardial pacing system requires a thoracotomy and direct visualization (Meeker and Rothrock).

1100. **(B)** Vasospasm may be of particular concern in working with small vessels during a procedure. Papaverine HCl may be added to saline solution for its direct antispasmodic effect on the smooth muscle of the vessel wall (Meeker and Rothrock).

1101. **(B)** The cause of this compression of the subclavian vessels, known as thoracic outlet syndrome, is usually congenital deformity or traumatic injury to the first rib (Meeker and Rothrock).

1102. (A) In situ femoral popliteal bypass is the restoration of blood flow to the leg bypassing an occluded portion of the femoral artery with a patient's own saphenous vein. The advantages of a vein bypass procedure include graft availability and improved patency (Meeker and Rothrock).

1103. (A) Greenfield vena cava filter insertion entails the partial occlusion of the inferior vena cava with an intravascular filter that maintains a patent vena cava but prevents pulmonary embolism by trapping emboli at the apex of the device (Meeker and Rothrock).

1104. (C) Angioscopy, the endoscopic visualization of vessels, began in the mid-1980s. Not a treatment in itself, it may be useful to predict the diagnoses of vascular access procedures or detect problems that lend themselves to correction intraoperatively (Meeker and Rothrock).

1105. (C) Heparin is the most common drug used in vascular surgery. It may be given as an intravenous bolus to systemically anticoagulate the patient. It is given just before the placement of the vascular clamp and is monitored regularly during surgery to determine its level in the body (Meeker and Rothrock).

1106. (B) A low-molecular-weight protein that, when combined with heparin, causes a loss of anticoagulant activity is called protamine sulfate. It is administered by the anesthesiologist IV after bypass is complete (Meeker and Rothrock).

1107. (A) A direct anatomic arteriovenous fistula provides a dilated vein valuable for direct cannulation with large-bore needles for hemodialysis (Meeker and Rothrock).

1108. (B) Percutaneous transluminal angioplasty (PTA) is a conservative treatment for localized or segmental stenosis or occlusive vascular disease. PTA recanalizes the vessel to allow for better flow. PTFE is a microporous graft for bypass. Greenfield filters are placed to catch venous thrombi, and endarterectomy requires the opening and scraping of a vessel to remove plaque (Fortunato).

1109. (B) Gruntzig catheters are used for angioplasty. Swan–Ganz arterial catheters provide monitoring of cardiac function. Foley catheters are indwelling urethral catheters. Fogarty catheters are balloon-tip catheters used to remove thrombi or emboli from a vessel (Fortunato).

1110. (C) After vascular closure is completed, a Doppler pulse detector (ultrasound) is used to check patency of a vessel and ultimate blood flow (Fortunato).

1111. (C) Endarterectomy is the excision of diseased endothelial lining of an artery and the occluding atheromatous deposits in the lumen (Fortunato).

1112. (D) Loss of structural integrity is implicit in this weakened structure. This localized abnormal dilatation results from mechanical pressure of blood on a vessel wall (Fortunato).

1113. (B) Vena cava filter insertion entails the partial occlusion of the inferior vena cava (IVC) with an intravascular filter, inserted under fluoroscopy. The Greenfield device offers the option of jugular or femoral vein insertion. It is the most widely successful device available (Meeker and Rothrock).

1114. (B) Monitoring the activated clotting time (ACT) intraoperatively provides useful data for judging the need for reversal or addition of heparin (Meeker and Rothrock).

1115. (A) Papaverine hydrochloride may be added to a heparinized saline for its direct antispasmodic effect on the smooth muscle of the vessel wall and its vasodilating properties (Meeker and Rothrock).

1116.   **(D)**   The intra-aortic balloon pump (IAPB) is a technique that employs the principle of counterpulsation. It increases the cardiac output and may permit separation of the patient from coronary bypass (CPB). Ventricular assist devices (VADs) are designed to augment cardiac output if patients cannot be weaned from CPB with IAPB (Meeker and Rothrock).

1117.   **(B)**   Mitral stenosis, the most common acquired valvular lesion, is usually caused by rheumatic fever. It causes a rise in pressure and dilatation of the left atrium (Meeker and Rothrock).

1118.   **(D)**   The cardiac catheterization laboratory has also become the site for more aggressive interventional therapies related to evolving and acute myocardial infarctions. Coronary thrombolysis with streptokinase and tissue plasminogen activator can dissolve fresh blood clots and reopen the artery (Meeker and Rothrock).

1119.   **(A)**   To vascularize a lower extremity, the saphenous vein is exposed but left in place. Using a valvutome or scissors, the valves are cut to allow reversal of blood flow. When a segment of vein is harvested, the vein is reversed so that valves will not obstruct blood flow (Fortunato).

IX. ORTHOPEDIC SURGERY

1120.   **(A)**   When attaching tendon to bone, wire suture is used. Most orthopedic tissues are very fibrous, contain few cells, and lack a rich blood supply and, thus, heal slowly. Nonabsorbable suture material is commonly preferred (Meeker and Rothrock).

1121.   **(D)**   Stockinette is a knitted, seamless tubing of cotton 1–12 inches wide. It stretches to fit any contour snugly (Fortunato).

1122.   **(A)**   Wrapping of an extremity begins at the distal end (Fortunato).

1123.   **(A)**   B, C, and D, are all options for repairing a fracture of the patella and can be anatomically reduced, if there are only two major pieces of the patella. A buttress plate is used to fixate a fracture of the tibia plateau (Meeker and Rothrock).

1124.   **(B)**   A Keller arthroplasty is a variation of a bunionectomy in which the proximal third of the phalanx is excised and replaced by a silicone implant (Fortunato).

1125.   **(A)**   Baker's cysts are found in the popliteal fossa. They are frequently painful and can become large. Excision requires prone position (Meeker and Rothrock).

1126.   **(A)**   Ganglia are benign outpouchings of synovium from the intercarpal joints that become filled with synovial fluid. They often resolve spontaneously but occasionally must be excised (Meeker and Rothrock).

1127.   **(B)**   In carpal tunnel syndrome, the median nerve becomes compressed at the volar surface of the wrist because of thickened synovium, fractures, or aberrant muscles (Meeker and Rothrock).

1128.   **(A)**   Rigid fixation by compression plate and screws uses heavy and strong compression plates to give maximum hold and rigid fixation. Tightening the nut on compression instruments brings bone fragments together (Fortunato).

1129.   **(A)**   The femoral head is removed and replaced with a prosthesis. The acetabulum is reamed to the configuration of the acetabulum component, which is then fixed in the socket (Fortunato).

1130.   **(D)**   A Colles' fracture is the most common and classic fracture. It is caused by breaking a fall with the outstretched hand (Meeker and Rothrock; Tortora and Grabowski).

1131.   **(A)**   Young active individuals with strong healthy bones are ideal candidates for noncemented total hip replacement. Elderly patients with osteoporotic and those patients with poor quality bone are usually candidates for cement because their bones may lack the compressive strength to support weight-bearing forces (Meeker and Rothrock).

1132. **(A)** Total hip replacement is indicated for patients with hip pain caused by degenerative joint diseases or rheumatoid arthritis (Fortunato; Meeker and Rothrock).

1133. **(A)** All of the frames are used to access a patient for surgery in the prone position except the Alvarado, which is a knee holder used for knee arthroplasties (Meeker and Rothrock).

1134. **(D)** A, B, and C are all options for tibial plateau fracture repair. The Ambi compression plate and lag screws are femoral hardware used for intertrochanteric fractures (Meeker and Rothrock).

1135. **(C)** Hammer toe deformity causes painful calluses on the dorsal joints of the four lateral toes, as the coiled-up digits rest against the shoes (Meeker and Rothrock).

1136. **(B)** Reconstruction of a joint (arthroplasty) may be necessary to restore or improve range of motion and stability or to relieve pain (Fortunato).

1137. **(B)** Many orthopedic procedures require a device for holding extremities. The McConnell is specifically designed to hold shoulders (Meeker and Rothrock).

1138. **(D)** Electrical stimulation is artificially applied electrical current that induces or influences osteogenesis. This accelerates fracture healing. Bone growth stimulations also are used in treating infected nonunions because the electrical stimulation retards bacterial growth (Meeker and Rothrock).

1139. **(B)** Osteomyelitis (infection in bone) occurs after bone is injured in an accident or is involved in surgical repair. It may cause nonunion of fractures. Microorganisms reach the bone via the bloodstream. *Staphylococcus aureus* is commonly the causative agent (Fortunato; Tortora and Grabowski).

1140. **(D)** Arthrodesis is most commonly employed to relieve pain by eliminating motion, to provide stability where normal ligament stability has been destroyed, or to correct deformity by realignment at the level of fusion (Fortunato).

1141. **(B)** Scoliosis is a lateral curve and rotation of the spine (Fortunato).

1142. **(B)** Harrington rods are used with spinal fusion to treat scoliosis (Fortunato).

1143. **(A)** A Bankart is done for a rotator cuff tear or recurrent anterior dislocation of the shoulder. Keller, McBride, and Silver are types of bunionectomies (Meeker and Rothrock).

1144. **(B)** Talipes varus, the condition known as clubfoot, refers to the inversion of the forefoot (Fortunato).

1145. **(D)** Tears in the menisci (semilunar cartilage) are the most common knee injuries occurring most frequently in the medial meniscus (Meeker and Rothrock).

1146. **(A)** An abduction pillow aids in immobilizing hip joints after surgery (Meeker and Rothrock).

1147. **(A)** Internal fixation of a hip can be accomplished with a free-lock compression hip screw fixation system allowing earlier ambulation and thus fewer complications (Meeker and Rothrock).

1148. **(A)** Osteoporosis is an age-related disorder characterized by increased susceptibility to fractures as a result of decreased levels of estrogen (Tortora and Grabowski).

1149. **(A)** The five stages of bone healing are hematoma formation, fibrin network formation, invasion of osteoblasts, callus formation, and remodeling (Meeker and Rothrock).

1150. **(C)** An olecranon fracture occurs in the elbow (Meeker and Rothrock).

1151. **(C)** Charcoal masks when used in the OR restrict inhaling vaporized particles of viruses such as venereal warts. All of the others are varying degrees of specialized units that address the principle of "strict surgical asepsis" for orthopedic surgery (Fortunato).

1152. **(B)** Water cast application is at room temperature: 70°–75°F (Fortunato).

1153. **(A)** A primary concern in orthopedic surgery is the prevention of infection, thus calling for meticulous technique with the operative scrub carried out under sterile conditions (Meeker and Rothrock).

1154. **(D)** An Esmarch rubber bandage is used to exsanguinate the limb; the tourniquet is then inflated (Meeker and Rothrock).

1155. **(A)** During orthopedic surgery, the mobile image intensification, also referred to as fluoroscopy or x-ray image, allows viewing of the case progression (Meeker and Rothrock).

1156. **(C)** Ankle fractures include fracture of the medial malleolus (tibia), lateral malleolus (fibula), and posterior malleolus (posterior distal fibia) (Meeker and Rothrock).

1157. **(A)** When preparing plaster rolls or splints, they are submerged in room temperature water (70–75°F). Water above this temperature will speed up the process and make the cast application ineffective. When bubbles cease to rise to the surface, the rolls are removed, lightly compressed, and used (Fortunato).

1158. **(C)** An incomplete fracture, only partly through the bone, is commonly found in children whose bones have not yet calcified. This is a greenstick fracture (Tortora and Grabowski).

1159. **(B)** Porosity can lead to fatigue and fracture, which ultimately can lead to implant loosening. PMMA, clinically similar to plexi-

glass, has barium sulfate added to make it possible to assess distribution and changes at a later time (Meeker and Rothrock).

1160. **(B)** The hip procedure indicated for degenerative joint disease or rheumatoid arthritis is total hip arthroplasty, cemented or noncemented. All of the others are femoral head components used to treat fractures that have not achieved union in a conventional manner (Meeker and Rothrock).

1161. **(B)** The Miller–Gallante joint replacement prosthesis is used in tricompartmental total knee replacement (Meeker and Rothrock).

1162. **(D)** Arthroscopic surgery has many advantages, including decreased recovery time, less inflammatory response, reduced complications, and more rapid surgery. A disadvantage is scoring of the articular surfaces based on reduced maneuverability (Meeker and Rothrock).

1163. **(C)** The patient is placed in the supine position on a standard OR bed. The foot of the table may be flexed at 90 degrees. The Alvarado knee holder is used for knee arthroplasty. Skeletal traction is used to reduce fractures prior to hardware application (Meeker and Rothrock).

1164. **(C)** Some cervical spine fractures or injuries may require Crutchfield or Gardner–Wells tongs inserted into the skull to stabilize the vertebrae and reduce spinal cord damage. Application of traction requires the use of sterile supplies, including a bow, pins, and drill (Meeker and Rothrock).

1165. **(D)** Isola instrumentation involves screw fixation into each vertebral body, complete disc excision with grafting, and segmental connection of the vertebrae. It is the preferred method for anterior spinal instrumentation (Meeker and Rothrock).

1166. **(C)** An infectious musculoskeletal condition affecting the bone and the marrow is osteomyelitis. This infection may develop from blood-borne pathogens deposited at the site. The infection develops as pathogenic organisms become trapped in small arteries in the metaphyseal area (Meeker and Rothrock).

1167. **(B)** Splints and slings are both immobilization devices used in orthopedics. The device used after total joint replacement is the abduction pillow. This prevents adduction, internal rotation, and hip flexion, which could dislocate the hip (Meeker and Rothrock).

1168. **(B)** Three types of stimulators that induce osteogenesis are implantable, percutaneous, and capacitance coupling (Meeker and Rothrock).

1169. **(B)** This method of fracture management provides rigid fixation and reduction with the ability to manage severe soft tissue wounds (Meeker and Rothrock).

1170. **(A)** A Bankart procedure involves reattachment of the anterior capsule to the rim of the glenoid fossa. A Putti–Platt is similar; in addition, it requires the lateral advancement of the subscapularis and produces a barrier against dislocation of the shoulder (Meeker and Rothrock).

1171. **(A)** The scaphoid is the most commonly fractured carpal bone. Internal fixation is generally accomplished with Kirschner wires, small compression screws, or minifragment compression plates and screws (Meeker and Rothrock).

1172. **(C)** Ender, Sampson, and Russell–Taylor are varieties of rods or nails available for femoral shaft fractures (Meeker and Rothrock).

1173. **(B)** Tibial plateau fractures have historically been attributed to bumper or fender injuries. Compression force of the distal femur upon the tibia produces varying types of plateau fractures (Meeker and Rothrock).

1174. **(D)** Fracture of the lateral malleolus can be treated with a Rusch rod, inserted through the fragment and into the fibular canal (Meeker and Rothrock).

1175. **(C)** A hammer toe flexion deformity develops at the proximal interphalangeal joint of the four lateral toes. It is treated by incising the long extensor tendon and fusing the middle joint (Meeker and Rothrock).

1176. **(B)** During an arthroscopic procedure, the circulating nurse hangs containers of solution at least 3 feet above the joint to ensure adequate hydrostatic pressure to keep the joint distended and to maintain flow of the irrigating solution (Fortunato).

1177. **(A)** A nonconstrained prosthesis, such as silicone rubber, allows shifting and gliding motions resembling normal range of motion, but is inherently unstable (Fortunato).

1178. **(B)** Silicone rubber implants are used to replace radiocarpal joints in the wrist, primarily to improve function. A resection arthroplasty is done usually from an anterior approach. Stems of the flexible, hinged implant are inserted into the intramedullary canals of the radius proximally and the capitate carpal bone distally. These are free sliding stems (Fortunato).

1179. **(A)** Although not used as commonly as in other surgical specialties, lasers are used in some orthopedic procedures. Methyl methacrylate can be vaporized with a carbon dioxide laser to remove a cemented implant. Nd:YAG laser can be used in arthroscopy to vaporize protein as well as to weld tissue by bonding collagen (Fortunato).

1180. **(C)** After a shoulder procedure, the arm may be bound against the side for immobilization. An absorbent pad or a large piece of cotton or sheet wadding is placed under the arm to keep skin surfaces from touching because they may macerate (Fortunato).

1181. **(D)** Dwyer and Duna rods are used only for an anterior approach to decompression. Many other devices, such as Harrington and Moe rods, Cotrel–Dubousset rods, Luque rods, and Wisonsin spinous process wires, may be used during a posterior approach to fixation (Fortunato).

1182. **(B)** The most commonly used implants in hand surgery are flexible implants made of Silastic. They are available for arthroplasty within the scope of hand surgery, such as finger joints, wrist joints, carpal trapezium, lunate, and navicular (Meeker and Rothrock).

1183. **(C)** The Miller–Gallante system is used to provide total knee replacement. Harris–Gallante, Osteolock, and Omnifit are all noncemented hip systems (Meeker and Rothrock).

1184. **(B)** After reaming of the femoral canal has been accomplished, a trial component is fitted. After removal of the trial, the canal is lavaged and brushed to accommodate the femoral component. A cement restrictor is inserted into the femoral canal. The cement is injected, and the femoral component with proximal and distal centralizers is inserted (Meeker and Rothrock).

1185. **(D)** These implants are a single unit including stem and head, which require limited rasping and canal preparation. Currently, this is the accepted treatment for nonunion fractures, avascular necrosis, and osteoarthritis. Total hip replacement is generally indicated for patients with degenerative joint disease or rheumatoid arthritis (Meeker and Rothrock).

1186. **(A)** If the materials to be implanted are Silastic or Teflon and are delivered unsterile, they should be washed with a mild soap (such as Ivory) and rinsed thoroughly before sterilization (Meeker and Rothrock).

1187. **(B)** Metal implants are extremely expensive. Once an implant has been scratched, it cannot be used. All personnel should follow these rules: store separately, handle as little as possible, use a driver with a Teflon head to drive the implant, do not bend, and use a template for sizing purposes (Fortunato).

1188. **(B)** Many different alloys are used in the manufacture of implants. However, the implantation of devices with different metallic composition must be avoided to prevent galvanic corrosion; internal fixation devices used during an orthopedic procedure should be of the same metal (Meeker and Rothrock).

X. NEUROSURGERY

1189. **(D)** Hemostatic scalp clips include Michel, Raney, Adson, and LeRoy clips (Meeker and Rothrock).

1190. **(D)** Head and neck stabilization in a patient with a cervical fracture and/or dislocation is effected by use of Vinke or Crutchfield tongs for skeletal traction (Fortunato).

1191. **(C)** Cordotomy is division of the spinothalamic tract for the treatment of intractable pain (Meeker and Rothrock).

1192. **(D)** Burr holes are placed to remove a localized fluid collection beneath the dura mater in a subdural hematoma (Meeker and Rothrock).

1193. **(B)** Gelfoam is supplied in powder and also a compressed sponge. The sponge form can be applied to an oozing surface dry or saturated with saline solution or topical thrombin (Meeker and Rothrock).

1194. **(C)** Meningioma arises from the arachnoid space tissue, the middle covering of the brain. It is slow growing and very vascular. Removal may be difficult (Meeker and Rothrock).

1195. **(C)** Cottonoid pledgets or strips or "patties" are used because they are gentler on the fragile tissue located here. They are counted items (Meeker and Rothrock).

1196. **(C)** A subdural hematoma, one that occurs between the dura and the arachnoid, is usually caused by a laceration of the veins that cross the subdural space (Fortunato).

1197. **(D)** Neurolysis is the freeing of an adhesed nerve to restore function and relieve pain. Carpal tunnel syndrome is an example in which the median nerve is entrapped in the carpal tunnel of the wrist (Fortunato).

1198. **(A)** Cryosurgery utilizes subfreezing temperatures to create a lesion in the treatment of disease, such as Parkinson's disease. This brain lesion destroys diseased cells of the brain and reduces the tremors associated with the disease (Meeker and Rothrock).

1199. **(A)** Preoperatively, elastic bandages (toe to groin), special tensor stockings (TED), or sequential compression stockings may be applied to help prevent venous stasis in lower extremities and also to help maintain blood pressure (Meeker and Rothrock).

1200. **(D)** Neuromas are frequently caused by retraction of nerve ends after trauma. The inability of regenerating axons to bridge the gap between both divided ends because of scar tissue requires that part of scar to be removed. This would not be accomplished by eliminating a neuropathway (Meeker and Rothrock).

1201. **(D)** Bipolar units are commonly used in neurosurgery. They provide a completely isolated output with negligible leakage of current between the tips of the forceps, permitting use of coagulation current in proximity to structures where ordinary unipolar coagulation would be hazardous (Meeker and Rothrock).

1202. **(B)** Temporary clips include Mayfield, McFadden, Drake, Yasargil, Sugita, and Schwartz. Permanent clips are Heifitz, Sundt–Kees, Olivecrona, Housepian, Scoville, Yasargil Phynox, and Sugita (Meeker and Rothrock).

1203. **(A)** In craniotomy the bone flap may be anchored with stainless steel suture (Fortunato).

1204. **(B)** A Cloward procedure is done to relieve pain in the neck, shoulder, or arm caused by cervical spondylosis or herniated disc. It involves removal of the disc with fusion of the vertebral bodies (Meeker and Rothrock).

1205. **(D)** Herniated disc fragments are removed in laminectomy with a pituitary rongeur (Meeker and Rothrock).

1206. **(A)** A great deal of heat is generated by the friction of the perforator against the bone. For this, irrigation of the drilling site counteracts the heat and removes bone dust (Meeker and Rothrock).

1207. **(B)** In hydrocephalus, there is an increase in CSF in the cranial cavity caused by excessive production, inadequate absorption, or obstruction of flow. The shunt procedures divert CSF from ventricles to other body cavities from which it is absorbed (Meeker and Rothrock).

1208. **(A)** The Javid or Argyle shunt, commonly used in carotid endarterectomy has as its main advantage continuous blood flow to the cerebrum during the surgery. It inhibits the surgeon's view during the surgery and during the repair (Meeker and Rothrock).

1209. **(D)** Metal suction tips such as the Cone, Sacks, Frazier, Bucy, and Adon are used because they not only keep the field dry but can be used to conduct coagulation current from a monopolar unit (Meeker and Rothrock).

1210. **(D)** Neurosurgical sponges, thoroughly soaked with saline or Ringer's lactate solution may be displayed near the surgeon's hand on an inverted basin, plastic drape, Vi-drape, or a small bowl. A dry towel absorbs the solution before its use (Meeker and Rothrock).

1211. **(C)** All are advantages of the knee–chest position except the increase in operating room time. Knee–chest actually reduces operating time (Meeker and Rothrock).

1212. **(A)** The most common congenital lesion encountered is a lumbar meningocele or meningomyelocele. The fluid-filled, thin-walled sac often contains neural elements. Surgical correction is necessary when the sac wall is so thin that there is a potential or actual CSF leak (Meeker and Rothrock).

1213. **(C)** Gelfoam will be cut into assorted sizes and soaked in topical thrombin for placement on the brain (Meeker and Rothrock).

1214. **(C)** The edges of the laminae overlapping the interspace with a herniated disc are defined with a curette. A partial hemilaminectomy of these laminal edges extending out into the lateral gutter of the spinal canal is performed with a Schwartz–Kerrison rongeur (Meeker and Rothrock).

1215. **(D)** Hydrocephalus is a pathologic condition in which there is an increase in the amount of CSF in the cranial cavity because of inadequate absorption or obstruction through the ventricular system. Ventriculoatrial (VA) shunts and ventriculoperitoneal (VP) shunts are used for absorption of excess cerebrospinal fluid (Meeker and Rothrock).

1216. **(A)** The use of complex mechanisms to locate and destroy target structures in the brain is known as stereotactics. Common target areas include obliterating tumors, aneurysms, abolishing movement disorders, and alleviating pain (Meeker and Rothrock).

1217. **(A)** Bifrontal, frontal, and frontotemporal approaches are frequently used for removal or craniopharyngiomas, optic gliomas, and other suprasellar and parasellar tumors. A transsphenoidal hypophysectomy approaches the pituitary gland through the upper gum margin into the floor of the sella tunica (Meeker and Rothrock).

1218. **(B)** Sympathetic denervation of the upper extremities and heart may be accomplished by cervicothoracic sympathectomy (dorsal). The vasospastic phenomenon of Raynaud's disease is relieved by this procedure (Meeker and Rothrock).

XI. PEDIATRIC AND GERIATRIC SURGERY

1219. **(A)** A valve system such as Holter, Hakim, or Denver directs the flow of CSF in children with hydrocephalus (Meeker and Rothrock).

1220. **(B)** Intussusception is the telescopic invagination of a portion of intestine into an adjacent part with mechanical and vascular impairment frequently at ileocecal junction (Meeker and Rothrock).

1221. **(B)** Atresia is an imperforation or closure of an opening. Atresia and stenosis (a narrowing of an opening) are the most common causes of obstruction in a newborn (Meeker and Rothrock; Tortora and Grabowski).

1222. **(B)** Failure of the intestines to become encapsulated within the peritoneal cavity during fetal development results in herniation through a midline defect in the abdominal wall at the umbilicus. This is termed omphalocele (Meeker and Rothrock).

1223. **(B)** A congenital malformation of the chest wall, pectus excavatum, is characterized by a pronounced funnel-shaped depression over the lower end of the sternum (Meeker and Rothrock).

1224. **(B)** The first sign of pyloric stenosis is projectile vomiting free of bile. The surgical procedure for repair is a pyloromyotomy. The muscles of the pylorus are incised to relieve the stenosis (Meeker and Rothrock).

1225. **(C)** Oxygen, calories, and fluids must be increased because of the increased demands of surgical stress. Blood is not given unless there is a need (Meeker and Rothrock).

1226. **(A)** Hirschsprung's disease is characterized by the presence of a segment of colon that lacks ganglia (congenital aganglionosis). Surgery for this anomaly requires several biopsies to locate the section of bowel with normal ganglia, followed by resection of the portion that is aganglionic (Meeker and Rothrock).

1227. **(C)** A newborn anomaly that is evidenced by incomplete closure of the vertebral arches, with or without herniation of the meninges, is called spina bifida (Tortora and Grabowski).

1228. **(C)** In craniosynostosis, the suture line of an infant has closed prematurely. A synthetic material (such as silicone) is used to keep the edges of the cranial sutures from reuniting and preventing brain growth (Meeker and Rothrock).

1229. **(B)** In imperforate anus, the anus remains closed during fetal development and must be opened soon after birth (Fortunato).

1230. **(D)** Geriatric patients are prone to infection, poor wound healing, and cardiovascular problems. Obesity is a greater contributing factor to liver and biliary disease (Fortunato).

1231. **(A)** A Wilms' tumor, also known as nephroblastoma, is the most common intra-abdominal childhood tumor. It presents as a painless mass whose enlargement may laterally distend the abdomen (Meeker and Rothrock).

1232. **(A)** Incomplete closure of the paired vertebral arches in the midline of the vertebral column may occur without herniation of the meninges. A spina bifida may be covered with intact skin. Laminectomy may be indicated to repair the underlying defect (Fortunato).

1233. **(C)** During fetal life, the ductus arteriosus carries blood from the pulmonary artery to the aorta, bypassing the lungs. After birth, this duct closes in the first hours. Nonclosure is termed patent ductus arteriosis and requires surgical closure (Fortunato).

1234. **(B)** Tetralogy of Fallot is the most common congenital cardiac anomaly in the cyanotic group. It is the result of shunting unoxygenated blood into the systemic circulation (Meeker and Rothrock).

1235. **(C)** Recession is a procedure done for strabismus where the muscle is overactive. All other procedures listed deal with the underactive (weak) eye muscle (Meeker and Rothrock).

1236. **(C)** Pulmonary artery bonding is used for anomalies associated with excessive pulmonary blood flow caused by large intra-cardiac left-to-right shunts. These include ventricular septal defect, truncus arteriosus, and others (Meeker and Rothrock).

1237. **(B)** Closure of the patent ductus arteriosus, an abnormal communication between the aorta and the pulmonary artery, is achieved by suture ligation or by division of the ductus. Although the ductus is important during fetal life, it normally closes immediately following birth (Meeker and Rothrock).

1238. **(D)** Failure of the abdominal viscera to become encapsulated within the peritoneal cavity during fetal development results in herniation through a midline defect in the abdominal wall of the umbilicus (Fortunato).

1239. **(A)** Secretory otitis media is the most common chronic condition of childhood. Fluid accumulates in the middle ear from eustachian tube obstruction. This condition is corrected by myringotomy, an incision in the tympanic membrane (Fortunato).

1240. **(B)** Airway problems are the most common concern on emergence from surgery and immediately postoperative. At the conclusion of the operation, the oropharynx and stomach are suctioned. All monitors are left in place until the patient is fully awake and extubated (Fortunato).

1241. **(D)** Degenerative joint disease (osteoarthritis) and inflammatory polyarticular disease (rheumatoid arthritis) are the primary indications for total joint replacement of hips and knees in the elderly (Meeker and Rothrock).

1242. **(B)** The predominant reason for urologic surgery in elderly men is benign prostatic hypertrophy (BPH) (Meeker and Rothrock).

XII. EMERGENCY PROCEDURES AND MISCELLANEOUS

1243. **(C)** Propranolol hydrochloride (Inderal) is useful in ventricular fibrillations or tachycardia. It is hazardous when cardiac function is depressed. It is also used in treating hypertension (Fortunato).

1244. **(A)** Calcium chloride is useful in profound cardiovascular collapse. It increases myocardial contractility, enhances ventricular excitability, and prolongs systole. Calcium cannot be given together with sodium bicarbonate because a precipitate forms from the mixture (Fortunato).

1245. **(D)** Sodium bicarbonate counteracts metabolic acidosis generated during time without oxygen. It elevates the pH of the blood. It restores the bicarbonate ion (Fortunato).

1246. **(B)** Lidocaine (xylocaine) is used intravenously for treatment of cardiac arrhythmias, particularly ventricular in nature. It is used before, during, and after cardiac procedures, in cardiac arrest, and in treatment and prevention of irritability in myocardial infarct (Fortunato).

1247. **(A)** When a cardiac arrest occurs in the OR, the anesthesiologist handles the artificial respiration. He or she may already have an endotracheal tube in place or in an airway (Fortunato).

1248. **(A)** Pulmonary embolus is an obstruction of one or more of the pulmonary arteries by a thrombus that becomes dislodged and is carried to the lung. This may be accompanied by sudden substernal pain, rapid and weak pulse, shock, syncope, and sudden death. It is often associated with advanced age and postoperative states (Fortunato).

1249. **(B)** The carotid pulse is palpated in CPR. The carotid arises from the aorta. It is the principal blood supply to the head and neck and is palpable in the neck (Fortunato).

1250. **(C)** Often the anesthesiologist leaves a hard rubber or plastic airway in the mouth. This should remain in place until the patient recovers sufficiently to breathe normally. It should not be removed until the patient expresses a desire to have it removed (Fortunato).

1251. **(D)** Malignant hyperthermia is an often fatal complication, characterized by progressive elevation of the body temperature monitored as high as 109°F. It occurs most often during general anesthesia, and its exact cause is unknown. If untreated, it can result in cardiovascular collapse (Fortunato).

1252. **(C)** Aspiration of gastric contents into the lungs may occur during throat reflexes when the patient is unconscious, or in conscious patients when the throat is anesthetized, as in bronchoscopy. Residual effects are impaired lung function and blood gas exchange, pneumonitis, atelectasis, and lung abscesses (Fortunato).

1253. **(C)** The telethermometer monitors the body temperature during an operation. It is electronic, connects to a probe, and provides direct temperature readouts on a dial. Rectal, esophageal, or tympanic probes are used. This is frequently used in pediatric surgery (Fortunato).

1254. **(D)** Hypoxia is lack of adequate amounts of oxygen; if prolonged, it can result in cardiac arrhythmia or irreversible brain, liver, kidney, and heart damage. The treatment is immediate adequate oxygen intake to stimulate the medullary centers and prevent respiratory system failure. Dark blood on the operative field is a symptom of hypoxia (Fortunato).

1255. **(C)** Immediate opening of the airway is the most important factor for successful resuscitation. The back of the tongue is the most common obstruction. Because the tongue is attached to the lower jaw, moving the jaw forward lifts the tongue from the back of the throat and opens the airway (Fortunato).

1256. **(D)** The scrub nurse should pay attention to the field and the surgeon's needs. The scrub nurse should also keep syringes of medications filled and ready for use, keep track of sponges, and be prepared to close the wound rapidly. If arrest occurs during the operation, the wound is packed and the patient repositioned for CPR (Fortunato).

1257. **(A)** When using the defibrillator, neither the person holding the electrodes nor anyone else may touch the patient or anything metallic that is in contact with the patient. This is done to prevent self-electrocution. No part of the operator's body should touch the paste or insulated electrodes (Fortunato).

1258. **(D)** When handing a syringe with a local anesthetic to the surgeon, the scrub nurse should state the kind and percentage of the solution. This action prevents errors (Fortunato).

1259. **(B)** Resuscitative measures must be instituted immediately (within 3–5 minutes) to prevent irreversible brain damage. Time of arrest should be noted. A clock should be started to check time lapse (Fortunato).

1260. **(B)** It is the circulating nurse's responsibility to keep a record of all medications given, including the time and the amount. One person, usually the anesthesiologist, commands the effort with support from others (Fortunato).

1261. **(C)** The patient is in cardiopulmonary arrest if there is no pulse, respiration, or blood pressure and the pupils are dilated. If unconscious, check airway; if not breathing, check resuscitation; if there is no pulse and pupils are dilated, massage heart (Fortunato).

1262. **(A)** Most hospitals are equipped with a special code switch or foot pedal that sets off an alarm indicating an arrest in the room in which it occurs. Within seconds, additional personnel will be available to aid in resuscitation efforts (Fortunato).

1263. **(C)** Hospital policy usually requires that a Mayo stand remain sterile until the patient has left the room. This may provide a field and instruments for surgical intervention if a crisis occurs (Fortunato).

1264. **(D)** Needles should be given on an exchange basis, never leaving any free needle on the field. Keep all needles away from sponges and laps. All used needles should be kept in a magnetic or adhesive count pad for ease of counting. Needles kept in a medicine cup is not a desirable method because each needle must be handled for the count, and this may puncture the glove of the scrub person (Fortunato).

1265. **(A)** Counted sharps should not be taken from the OR during the procedure. If one falls from the field or is passed off the field, it must remain in the room to be added to the final count (Fortunato).

1266. **(A)** The process of impingement is the strong spray force found in a washer–decontaminator. Cavitation is the process utilized by the ultrasonic cleaner (Fortunato).

1267. **(B)** The purpose of presoaking instruments is to prevent blood and debris from drying, or to soften and remove dry blood and debris. The circulating nurse can prepare a basin of solution for the scrub person. Demineralized water or proteolytic enzymatic detergent is a good choice. Do not use saline because it is corrosive (Fortunato).

REFERENCES

Ball KA. *Lasers, The Perioperative Challenge,* 2nd ed. St. Louis: Mosby-Year Book, 1995.

Fortunato L. *Berry and Kohn's Operating Room Technique,* 9th ed. St. Louis: Mosby, 2000.

Meeker M, Rothrock J. *Alexander's Care of the Patient in Surgery,* 11th ed. St. Louis: Mosby-Year Book, 1999.

Mosby's Medical, Nursing, and Allied Health Dictionary, 5th ed. St. Louis: Mosby-Year Book, 1998.

Stryker Endoscopy: Video Endoscopy for Perioperative Nurses—A Study Guide. Denver, CO.

Tortora G, Grabowski S. *Principles of Anatomy and Physiology,* 9th ed. New York: Wiley & Sons, 2000.

PART 4

Technological Sciences for the Operating Room
Questions

DIRECTIONS (Questions 1268 through 1343): Each of the numbered items or incomplete statements in this section is followed by answers or by completions of the statement. Select the ONE lettered answer or completion that is BEST in each case. Check your answers with the correct answers at the end of the chapter.

I. COMPUTER USE

1268. Located on the back of the CPU are special openings called _____ for plugging in cables for adding additional computer components.

(A) drives
(B) cords
(C) ports
(D) networks

1269. The largest storage capacity for portable saved information is the

(A) Zip Drive 100
(B) Zip Drive 250
(C) CD-Rom
(D) DVD

1270. The device that enables a computer to send and receive information by phone line is called a

(A) modem
(B) scanner
(C) USB port
(D) lateral port

1271. The largest memory size of information in the following list is the

(A) megabyte
(B) kilobyte
(C) gigabyte
(D) terabyte

1272. Visual display on the desktop of shortcuts to available programs are called

(A) topics
(B) windows
(C) displays
(D) icons

1273. When open to the internet, what function can be used to return to a recently opened site that you have not saved on your computer?

(A) search
(B) history
(C) favorites
(D) address book

1274. Web research is generally conducted with the help of

(A) cursors
(B) search engines
(C) browser
(D) instant access

1275. A product used to buffer the computer hardware against high electrical voltages is called a

(A) zip drive
(B) surge protector
(C) modem
(D) lateral port

1276. A hardware component that converts printed text or picture to digital information for use in documents is called the

(A) scanner
(B) printer
(C) modem
(D) Ethernet card

1277. The arrow or small hand, which appears on the screen to identify the location of currently addressed information is known as a

(A) scanner
(B) cursor
(C) icon
(D) taskbar

1278. The component part of the computer that controls the cursor is called the

(A) scroller
(B) mouse
(C) index
(D) scanner

II. SURGICAL APPLICATIONS OF ELECTRICITY

1279. All of the following applications can be performed through an endoscope EXCEPT

(A) cavity washings for diagnosis
(B) video monitoring
(C) biopsy
(D) resection of malignant tumors

1280. Anything that has mass and occupies space is termed

(A) element
(B) matter
(C) conductor
(D) insulator

1281. The center of an atom is called the

(A) matter
(B) mass
(C) nucleus
(D) charge

1282. The movement of electrical charge through a conductor is called

(A) migration
(B) electrical current
(C) conduct
(D) insulation

1283. An ESU unit used in the operating room completes an electric circuit by carrying the current from the machine to the patient by way of the

(A) inactive electrode
(B) active electrode
(C) ground pad
(D) patient plate

1284. Current is measured in

(A) volts
(B) amps
(C) circuits
(D) loads

1285. The path which electricity travels from its energy source and back again is called

(A) resistor
(B) circuit
(C) conductor
(D) ampere

1286. A mathematical equation that shows the relationship between voltage and resistance is known as

(A) Bohr's Theory
(B) Ohm's Law
(C) magnetic fields
(D) periodic table

1287. Restriction of the flow of current to a source is called

(A) magnetism
(B) resistance
(C) force field
(D) power

1288. The device that transforms electrical energy into a useful function is the

(A) source
(B) power
(C) load
(D) switch

1289. In a simple electrical circuit, the wire that connects to the switch is

(A) neutral
(B) ground
(C) hot
(D) none of the above

1290. A separate wire that is essential protection against an electric shock is

(A) hot
(B) neutral
(C) ground
(D) active

1291. How many types of electrical systems exist?

(A) 1
(B) 2
(C) 3
(D) 4

1292. Most outlets in the operating room run on

(A) 220 V
(B) 110 V
(C) 120 V
(D) 60 V

1293. When current moves in one direction, and then reverses to return to the source it is known as

(A) alternating current
(B) electrical current
(C) direct current
(D) optional current

1294. One example of DC (direct current) is

(A) an electrosurgical unit
(B) a flashlight
(C) a surgical room light
(D) an x-ray machine

1295. Alternating current has the ability to

(A) step down voltage
(B) step up voltage
(C) alternate voltage
(D) all of the above

1296. A device that transmits an impulse to a wave-transmitting system is

(A) an optical fiber
(B) a radio transmitter
(C) an isolated circuit
(D) a resistor

1297. An ESU used for delicate surgery is a

(A) monopolar unit
(B) disposable unit
(C) bipolar unit
(D) dispersive electrode unit

1298. A plume of vaporized tissue may contain residual _____ and is, therefore, important to protect the staff.

(A) carcinogens
(B) blood-borne pathogens
(C) mutagens
(D) all of the above

1299. An alternating current cycle is termed a

(A) wave
(B) volt
(C) amp
(D) hertz

1300. Radio waves are considered _____ waves.

(A) isolated
(B) direct
(C) simple
(D) magnetic

1301. When current passes from the ESU through the active electrode, the energy is converted from electrical to _____.

(A) mechanical
(B) chemical
(C) thermal
(D) magnetic

1302. What material forms the best conductor of electricity?

(A) rubber
(B) saltwater
(C) copper
(D) lead

1303. What device is used to control the flow of electricity at the will of the operator?

(A) load
(B) resistor
(C) switch
(D) conductor

1304. When operating a piece of electrical OR equipment the most vital prong for safety purposes is the

(A) ground
(B) negative
(C) positive
(D) safety

1305. Which theory explains the flow of electricity?

(A) Ohm's
(B) electron
(C) Kirchhoff's
(D) atomic

1306. The standard metric unit of power is

(A) amp
(B) volt
(C) watt
(D) hertz

1307. A medical imaging technique that reveals the bodies dynamic activities is

(A) CT
(B) PET
(C) tomogram
(D) ultrasound

III. THE RELATIONSHIP BETWEEN PHYSICS AND MEDICINE

1308. Motion is known as _____ energy.

(A) mechanical
(B) total

(C) potential
(D) kinetic

1309. The rate at which work is done is known as

(A) velocity
(B) energy
(C) power
(D) watt

1310. _____ borders the outer perimeter of an atom and is _____ charged.

(A) neutron, positively
(B) electron, negatively
(C) electron, positively
(D) proton, negatively

1311. The gain or loss of electrons in an atom is termed

(A) hydraulic pressure
(B) Boyle's Law
(C) ionization
(D) consolidation

1312. The transfer of thermal energy by contact is called

(A) greenhouse effect
(B) radiation
(C) convention
(D) conduction

1313. A repeated periodic disturbance or variation of energy, carried through a medium from point to point is called

(A) transfer energy
(B) wave
(C) oscillations
(D) molecular change

1314. The frequency of sound is stated in a measurement of

(A) amps
(B) hertz
(C) waves
(D) compressions

1315. The study of objects in motion is

(A) mechanics
(B) velocity
(C) speed
(D) acceleration

1316. The study that focuses on the forces which cause motion is

(A) kinematics
(B) dynamics
(C) statics
(D) inertia

1317. The three laws of motion that are the basics of classical mechanics are the work of

(A) Hooke
(B) Newton
(C) Bohr
(D) Ohm

1318. Any time that an object's velocity is changing we say it is

(A) accelerating
(B) projecting
(C) orbiting
(D) static

1319. The property of matter that causes matter to resist change in motion is called

(A) speed
(B) inertia
(C) momentum
(D) range

1320. What is the measure of the amount of inertia an object possesses?

(A) momentum
(B) range
(C) equilibrium
(D) mass

1321. For every action there is an equal and opposite reaction references _____ law.

(A) Newton's first law
(B) Newton's second law
(C) Newton's third law
(D) Hooke's law

1322. If an object returns to its original position after force has been applied and then removed is said to be

(A) dynamic
(B) static
(C) elastic
(D) periodic

1323. The maximum distance that an object moves from its central position (equilibrium) is called

(A) frequency
(B) amplitude
(C) cycle
(D) momentum

1324. The bending of a light ray as it passes from one substance to another is called

(A) reflection
(B) refraction
(C) vibration
(D) incidence

1325. What scientist, expanding Hooke's wave theory, theorized that light can bend because it is a wave?

(A) Ohm
(B) Einstein
(C) Newton
(D) Young

1326. The longer wavelengths of the color spectrum are seen in what color?

(A) violet
(B) green
(C) blue
(D) red

1327. Who first identified a collection of particles of light as "photons"?

(A) Einstein
(B) Newton
(C) Bohr
(D) Young

1328. The device that transforms energy from other forms into electromagnetic radiation is called

(A) prism
(B) laser
(C) medium
(D) resonator

1329. On the surface of the Earth, what causes objects to accelerate downward?

(A) energy
(B) excitation
(C) gravity
(D) electrical charges

1330. What laser has the most power output?

(A) liquid
(B) semiconductor
(C) gas
(D) solid state

1331. The fourth force found only in nature, and not in the nucleus, is known as

(A) electromagnetic force
(B) gravitational force
(C) binding energy
(D) kinetic energy

1332. Nucleons are composed of subatomic particles known as

(A) isotopes
(B) quarks
(C) protons
(D) neutrons

IV. SURGICAL ROBOTS

1333. What term identifies the arms of a robot in surgery?

(A) articulations
(B) ratchets
(C) graspers
(D) manipulators

1334. Voice-controlled robots are provided with binaural hearing by

(A) sound transducers
(B) waveforms
(C) manipulators
(D) pitch

1335. An "up and down" movement of a robot's arm is known as

(A) roll
(B) yaw
(C) pitch
(D) rotation

1336. What is the "right to left" movement of a robotic arm called?

(A) yaw
(B) roll
(C) pitch
(D) x-y-z-axis rotation

1337. The technical terms for the robot's three dimensional movement is called

(A) micromanipulation
(B) remote manipulation
(C) binocular machine vision
(D) Cartesian geometry

1338. What term is used when likening "robotic vision" to "human vision"?

(A) sensitivity
(B) binocular vision
(C) depth perception
(D) resolution

1339. What allows the robotic computer to create and record 3-D data of the surgical site?

(A) magnetic resonance sites
(B) image planning
(C) laser scanning
(D) CT scan

1340. Which of the following parts for robotic surgery SHOULD NOT be sterilized?

(A) manipulators
(B) the collar that connects the endoscope
(C) the endoscope
(D) surgical instrumentation

1341. Realistic simulation of bones and tissues using computational models of the behavior of human joints and tissue is called

(A) external simulation
(B) deformable modeling
(C) surgical planning
(D) surfaced based registration

1342. Sterilization of component parts for endoscopic robotic surgery is best accomplished by

(A) STERIS system
(B) steam sterilization
(C) hydrogen peroxide sterilizer
(D) ETO gas sterilization

1343. The most popular robotic system used today is

(A) AESOP HR
(B) Da Vinci system
(C) surgical navigation system
(D) both A and B

Technological Sciences for the Operating Room
Answers and Explanations

I. COMPUTER USE

1268. **(C)** Located at the back of the computer are ports that allow us to access a connection to the hard drive to attach scanners, printer and other components to the system (Frey and Price).

1269. **(D)** All of the choices have increasing megabytes for storage of information. The DVD has the capacity to hold 7 gigabytes, as opposed to 100 megabytes on the Zip Drive 100 (Frey and Price).

1270. **(A)** A modem is the communications device that sends and receives information over a telephone line, thereby, connecting us to the internet (Frey and Price).

1271. **(D)** A terabyte is equivalent to 1 trillion characters. As the megabyte contains 1024 bytes (characters) (Frey and Price).

1272. **(D)** Icons that appear on the desktop screen are shortcuts to programs that also can be accessed through the start menu (Frey and Price).

1273. **(B)** The computer holds the most recently visited sites in a history menu. Clicking on history will return the site to the screen for viewing (Frey and Price).

1274. **(B)** There are several search engines available to reach the web; for example, Google, Alta Vista, and Yahoo (Frey and Price).

1275. **(B)** A surge protector is a buffer against damaging high voltage surges of energy (Frey and Price).

1276. **(A)** A scanner resembles a printer, but reproduces the image electronically rather than duplicating the print (Frey and Price).

1277. **(A)** The cursor is a small arrow that appears on the screen to identify the information to be addressed (Frey and Price).

1278. **(B)** The mouse moves the cursor to different areas on the screen and selects commands (Frey and Price).

II. SURGICAL APPLICATIONS OF ELECTRICITY

1279. **(D)** Resections of malignant tumors are usually approached through large open incisions because the cavity must also be explored after removal of the tumor (Frey and Price).

1280. **(B)** Matter is anything that has mass and occupies space. All matter consists of atoms, and all atoms contain protons, neutrons, and electrons (Frey and Price).

1281. **(C)** The center of an atom contains the nucleus, which contains in its center, protons and neutrons (Frey and Price).

1282. **(B)** The electrical current moves through conductors by movement of free electrons (Frey and Price).

1283. **(B)** The active electrode carries the energy to the patient, goes through the ground pad on the patient into the inactive cord and back to the machine (Frey and Price).

1284. **(B)** Current is measured in amperes (amps) (Frey and Price).

1285. **(B)** The path of electricity from energy source to the piece of equipment and back again is called a circuit (Frey and Price).

1286. **(B)** Ohm's law is a mathematical equation that shows relationship between voltage, current, and resistance (Frey and Price).

1287. **(B)** Restriction of the flow of current to a source is called resistance (Frey and Price).

1288. **(C)** In a simple electric circuit, the device that transforms the electrical energy into a useful function is called the load (Frey and Price).

1289. **(C)** In a simple electric circuit, the wire that connects to the switch is hot (Frey and Price).

1290. **(C)** A separate wire that is essential protection against electric shock is the ground wire (Frey and Price).

1291. **(B)** There are two types of electrical systems. The first is alternating current, which sends the electric current and reverses to the source when it has completed its task. The other is direct current, which leaves the source and flows in only one direction (Frey and Price).

1292. **(B)** Most outlets in the operating room run on 110 V current. X-ray units require the use of 220 V lines (Frey and Price).

1293. **(A)** Alternating current (AC) describes the flow of current that reverses direction periodically. Direct current (DC) indicates current that flows in only one directions. (e.g., a flashlight) (Frey and Price).

1294. **(B)** A flashlight is an example of one way current or direct current (Frey and Price).

1295. **(D)** Alternating current has the ability to step-down, step-up, or alternate voltage continuously. Hospitals use a reduced current (Frey and Price).

1296. **(B)** A device called a radio transmitter carries an impulse or signal to a wave transmitting antennae system (Frey and Price).

1297. **(C)** The unit used to perform electrosurgery in delicate areas, such as ophthalmology, plastic, and neurosurgery is the bipolar unit. It has reduced power. The circuit is completed within the handpiece (Frey and Price).

1298. **(D)** Certain surgical procedures than employ the use of electrocautery, laser, and drills can produce a plume of vaporized tissue that may include carcinogens, bloodborne pathogens, and mutagens. Smoke evacuators are frequently used to remove the potentially hazardous smoke (Frey and Price).

1299. **(D)** An alternating current cycle is a hertz. The number of cycles per second is a frequency (Frey and Price).

1300. **(D)** Radio waves are magnetic waves. The number of wave cycles is also called a frequency (Frey and Price).

1301. **(C)** When electrical current passes through the active electrode, it converts electrical energy to thermal (Frey and Price).

1302. **(C)** The best conductor of electricity is copper. Examples that use copper wire as a conductor in the OR are surgical lamps, electrosurgical units, and power drills (Frey and Price).

1303. **(C)** A simple electrical circuit is composed of a source of power, conductor, load, and switch. The switch allows the operator to turn the piece of equipment on and off (Frey and Price).

1304. **(A)** When operating a piece of equipment in the OR, the most important prong is the ground. It safely transfers any leaking electrons to the ground and prevents injury (Frey and Price).

1305. **(A)** The scientific theory that explains electricity is Ohm's Law. It is a mathematical equation that shows the relationship between voltage, current, and resistance (Frey and Price).

1306. **(C)** Power is defined as the rate at which work is done. Power is measured in watts (Frey and Price).

1307. **(B)** Positron emission tomography (PET) is the medical imaging of dynamic activities in the body such as blood flow and glucose uptake in tissues (Frey and Price).

III. THE RELATIONSHIP BETWEEN PHYSICS AND MEDICINE

1308. **(D)** Motion is known as kinetic energy. The mechanical energy of an object can be a result of its motion (Frey and Price).

1309. **(C)** The rate at which work is done is called power. It is expressed as the amount of work per unit of time (Frey and Price).

1310. **(B)** Electrons border the outer perimeter of an atom and are negatively charged. These outer electrons are known as free electrons, and it is the movement of free electrons that produces electric current (Frey and Price).

1311. **(C)** The gain or loss of electrons in an atom is termed ionization. A loss converts an atom into a positively charged ion; whereas, a gain converts an atom into a negatively charged ion (Frey and Price).

1312. **(D)** The transfer of thermal energy by contact is called conduction. Some energy is transferred to molecules of a second object when they collide. Certain substances are better used for this transfer, such as metals, rather than wood or paper (Frey and Price).

1313. **(B)** A wave may be composed of light, sound, heat, or water (Frey and Price).

1314. **(B)** The frequency of sound can be measured in hertz. Multiples of sound are measured megahertz (Frey and Price).

1315. **(A)** Mechanics is the study of objects in motion, and is normally restricted to a small number of very large objects (Frey and Price).

1316. **(B)** Dynamics is the study of motion; whereas, kinematics is the study of objects in motion with little concern for the forces that cause it (Frey and Price).

1317. **(B)** Isaac Newton's three laws of motion are the basis of classical mechanics, or Newtonian mechanics (Frey and Price).

1318. **(A)** Acceleration is defined as a change in velocity over time (Frey and Price).

1319. **(B)** Newton's first of three laws states that "inertia is a property of matter that causes matter to resist change in motion" (Frey and Price).

1320. **(D)** Newton's first law on the nature of inertia, then states that the mass is the measure of the amount of inertia an object possesses (Frey and Price).

1321. **(C)** Also known as the "law of conservation of momentum" states that whenever a force is exerted an equal or opposite force arises in reaction (Frey and Price).

1322. **(C)** If an object returns to its original position after a force is applied or removed, then it is said to be elastic. An example is a coiled spring (Frey and Price).

1323. **(B)** Amplitude is the maximum distance that an object moves from its central position (called equilibrium) (Frey and Price).

1324. **(B)**   Refraction is the bending of a light ray as it passes from one substance to another. Light travels at differing speeds as it travels through one medium or another (such as water or glass) (Frey and Price).

1325. **(C)**   Hooke proposed that light was a wave, but it was Sir Isaac Newton who posited that if light were a wave, it would bend around corners (Frey and Price).

1326. **(D)**   The red wavelengths of light are the longest; whereas, the violet are the shortest. The view along the color spectrum changes with each color. White is not a color, but is perceived when all colors hit the eye at the same time (Frey and Price).

1327. **(A)**   In 1905, Einstein explained details of the photoelectric effect, which requires that light be a collection of particles called "photons." Young continued his work and Neils Bohr of the University of Copenhagen further refined the research to establish the "Complimentary Principle of Light" (Frey and Price).

1328. **(B)**   The three main components of a laser are the resonator cavity, the pump force, and the gain medium (Frey and Price).

1329. **(C)**   In situation near the surface of the Earth gravity causes objects to accelerate downward (Frey and Price).

1330. **(D)**   A solid-state laser creates the most powerful output (Frey and Price).

1331. **(B)**   The gravitational force, found only in nature and one of the four forces affecting matter does not affect the nucleus of an atom (Frey and Price).

1332. **(B)**   Protons and neutrons act as if they are identical articles and differ only in their electrical charge. The nucleons themselves are made of subatomic particles called "quarks" (Frey and Price).

IV. SURGICAL ROBOTS

1333. **(D)**   The term used to identify the robotic arms that control the surgical efforts is manipulators (Frey and Price).

1334. **(A)**   The voice-controlled robots utilize binaural hearing, which is much like human hearing. It differentiates direction and person (Frey and Price).

1335. **(C)**   Pitch identifies the up and down movement of the arms jaw, and yaw identifies right and left movement of the jaw. The rotating movement of the shaft is called a roll (Frey and Price).

1336. **(A)**   A "right to left" movement of a jaw is called a yaw (Frey and Price).

1337. **(D)**   Cartesian coordinate geometry is applied as a mathematical equation to move the manipulators in a fashion that resembles the movements of the human arm (Frey and Price).

1338. **(B)**   Binocular machine vision is analogous to human vision which is also known as stereovision. This vision is similar to the robot's binaural hearing (Frey and Price).

1339. **(C)**   Once an MRI or CAT scan is performed to retrieve a layout of the person's anatomy, a laser scan is then done to achieve a set of three-dimensional coordinates on the patients skin (Frey and Price).

1340. **(A)**   The manipulators that hold the endoscope and the instrumentation are not sterilized, they are covered with a sterile sleeve (Frey and Price).

1341. **(B)**   The goal of deformable modeling is to achieve realistic three-dimensional simulation of soft tissue behavior under the effect of external simulation (Frey and Price).

1342. **(A)**   The "STERIS System" (paracetic acid) sterilizer is ideal for sterilization of camera, light cord, and other delicate components used for the procedure (Frey and Price).

1343. **(D)**   The primary robotic systems used in the operating room today are the AESOP HR and the da Vinci System (Frey and Price).

REFERENCES

Frey, K, Price, P. *Technological Sciences for the Operating Room,* 1st ed. Centennial, CO: Association of Surgical Technologists, 2002.

Practice Test

---

1. This exam consists of 250 questions. You will be required to take the entire exam in 3 hours. As on the Certifying Examination, this gives you an average of 40 to 45 seconds per question.
2. Be certain to have an adequate number of pencils and erasers with you.
3. Schedule the test to be taken in a quiet, *uninterrupted* atmosphere. Be certain a clock is in sight to help you pace yourself.
4. Remove the answer grid at the end of the book and fill out properly.
5. Be certain that the number on the answer sheet corresponds to the question number on the test.
6. When the test is completed, compare the responses with those supplied at the end of the test section.
7. An additional sheet has been provided at the end of the test section that identifies which questions are reflective of a particular subject.
8. Additional study emphasis may be required in a particular area if you have not correctly completed at least 75% of the identified questions on a particular subject.

Questions

1. In an inguinal herniorrhaphy the spermatic cord is

   (A) ligated with a hemoclip
   (B) retracted with a Penrose drain
   (C) incised for ease of access
   (D) clamped with a Kelly

2. Polyglycolic acid sutures are

   (A) absorbed by an enzyme action
   (B) absorbed by the process of hydrolysis
   (C) nonabsorbable
   (D) encapsulated by body tissue

3. The pounds of pressure necessary in a flash steam sterilizer set at 270°F is

   (A) 15
   (B) 17
   (C) 20
   (D) 27

4. A patient is having elective surgery. The nurse notes that her white cell count is 14,000 cu mm. This would indicate that

   (A) there may be an inflammation or infection present
   (B) the count is within normal range, and surgery can proceed
   (C) the count is below normal
   (D) there may be an anemic condition present, and surgery should be canceled

5. Distal refers to

   (A) closer to the body
   (B) away from the body
   (C) in the center of the body
   (D) toward the feet

6. Meckel's diverticulum is found in the

   (A) esophagus
   (B) sigmoid colon
   (C) ileum
   (D) duodenum

7. In which case would a Frazier suction be used?

   (A) eye
   (B) ear
   (C) gynecology
   (D) general

8. Airborne contamination is reduced by recirculation of filtered outside air at a rate of

   (A) 12 air exchanges per minute
   (B) 12 air exchanges per hour
   (C) 20 air exchanges per minute
   (D) 25 air exchanges per hour

9. The purpose of OSHA is to

   (A) ensure safe and healthful working conditions
   (B) provide a mechanism for peer review
   (C) establish quality assurance
   (D) provide standards of patient care

10. Body heat in pediatric patients is controlled with all of the following EXCEPT

    (A) wrapping child in plastic materials
    (B) warming blanket
    (C) increasing room temperature
    (D) hot water bottles

11. If a family is contacted but cannot come in to sign a permission for emergency surgery, the surgeon should

    (A) wait until they arrive
    (B) accept permission by phone, telegram, or in written communication
    (C) ask another physician to sign
    (D) refuse to do the case

12. Unwrapped instruments are sterilized at 270°F (132°C) for a minimum of

    (A) 3 minutes
    (B) 5 minutes
    (C) 7 minutes
    (D) 10 minutes

13. A retention suture passes through all of the following EXCEPT

    (A) mesentery tissue
    (B) rectus muscle
    (C) fascial tissue
    (D) subcutaneous tissue

14. A hernia that passes through the inguinal ring into the inguinal canal is termed

    (A) direct
    (B) indirect
    (C) pantaloon
    (D) sliding

15. Dead space is the space

    (A) that has no blood supply
    (B) caused by separation of wound edges that have not been closely approximated
    (C) where the tissue has been approximated with sutures
    (D) where the suture line has broken down

16. Wrapped tubing can be sterilized at 250°F for a minimum of

    (A) 5 minutes
    (B) 10 minutes
    (C) 20 minutes
    (D) 30 minutes

17. Funnel chest is also known as

    (A) pectus carinatum
    (B) pectus excavatum
    (C) atresia
    (D) Ramstedt–Fredet

18. Which term denotes low or decreased blood volume?

    (A) anoxia
    (B) hypovolemia
    (C) hypoxia
    (D) hypocapnia

19. Injection of contrast media into the brachial, carotid, or vertebral artery to study the intracranial vessels is called

    (A) myelography
    (B) pneumoencephalography
    (C) computed axial tomography (CAT) scan
    (D) angiography

20. Instruments and other items sterilized together in the flash autoclave require

    (A) 3 minutes at 270°F
    (B) 53 minutes at 250°F
    (C) 10 minutes at 270°F
    (D) 30 minutes at 250°F

21. Suture material that becomes encapsulated with fibrous tissue during the healing process is

    (A) nonabsorbable suture
    (B) absorbable suture
    (C) synthetic absorbable suture
    (D) gut suture

22. A right hemicolectomy is performed to remove pathology of the

    (A) descending colon
    (B) ascending colon
    (C) sigmoid colon
    (D) mesocolon

23. Dacryo refers to

    (A) eyelid
    (B) eyeball
    (C) cornea
    (D) lacrimal gland

24. When transporting a patient, drainage systems should be placed

    (A) at stretcher level
    (B) below stretcher level
    (C) above stretcher level
    (D) optionally

25. The maximum size of a linen pack must not exceed

    (A) $8 \times 10 \times 16$ inches
    (B) $10 \times 14 \times 18$ inches
    (C) $12 \times 12 \times 20$ inches
    (D) $14 \times 16 \times 36$ inches

26. Another name for a stay suture is a(n)

    (A) tension suture
    (B) retention suture
    (C) interrupted suture
    (D) buried suture

27. Which two anatomic structures are ligated and divided to effect a cholecystectomy?

    (A) common hepatic duct, common bile duct
    (B) cystic duct, cystic artery
    (C) common bile duct, cystic artery
    (D) cystic duct, hepatic artery

28. Adeno means

    (A) lymph
    (B) gland
    (C) joint
    (D) bone

29. When the patient is being transferred from the OR table after surgery, the action should be

    (A) swift but cautious in order to get the patient to the recovery room as quickly as possible
    (B) performed with comfort of the patient as the prime concern
    (C) gentle and rapid so that the patient does not wake up
    (D) gentle and slow in order to prevent circulatory depression

30. In steam sterilization, the function of pressure is to

    (A) destroy microorganisms
    (B) increase the temperature of the steam
    (C) lower the exposure time
    (D) create condensation

31. Which of the following suture materials is not generally used in the presence of infection?

    (A) silk
    (B) surgical gut
    (C) polypropylene
    (D) stainless steel

32. Radical surgery done for lower sigmoid or rectal malignancy is a(n)

    (A) Wertheim's procedure
    (B) abdominal perineal resection
    (C) Whipple procedure
    (D) pelvic exenteration

33. The term for fluid or water in the ventricles of the brain is

    (A) hydrophobia
    (B) hydrocephalus
    (C) hydrocele
    (D) hydronephrosis

34. The patient may be left on the transport stretcher unattended

    (A) under no circumstances
    (B) if he or she is alert and responsible
    (C) if he or she is sound asleep
    (D) if he or she can be observed by passing personnel

35. 212°F is equivalent to

(A) 32°C
(B) 98.6°C
(C) 100°C
(D) 175°C

36. An anti-inflammatory drug whose effect is useful in reversing early rejection of organ transplants is

(A) Cyclosporine
(B) Polyclonal
(C) Prednisone
(D) Orthoclone

37. A congenital abnormality of the musculature between the stomach and the duodenum is called

(A) esophageal atresia
(B) pyloric stenosis
(C) intestinal atresia
(D) duodenal atresia

38. A fossa is a

(A) ridge
(B) basin-like depression
(C) projection
(D) seam

39. A procedure performed to treat myasthenia gravis is a(n)

(A) adrenalectomy
(B) splenectomy
(C) thymectomy
(D) parathyroidectomy

40. The purpose of lidocaine installation during a tracheotomy is to

(A) extend anesthesia
(B) decrease coughing
(C) decrease gag reflex
(D) reduce edema

41. A procedure that is done to give the bowel a rest when there is advanced inflammation is

(A) abdominoperineal resection (APR)
(B) right hemicolectomy
(C) anterior sigmoid resection
(D) temporary colostomy

42. A forceps used to grasp lung tissue is a(n)

(A) Crile
(B) Adson
(C) Duval
(D) Walton

43. Heat-sensitive items that can be completely immersed can be processed via the _____ in 30 minutes.

(A) ethylene oxide (ETO) sterilizer
(B) Endoflush
(C) gravity displacement sterilizer
(D) STERIS

44. The maximum recommended dosage of local anesthetic drug per hour is

(A) 10 mL of 1% solution
(B) 50 mL of 1% solution
(C) 150 mL of 1% solution
(D) 250 mL of 1% solution

45. Ischemia can be defined as

(A) excessive blood supply to a part
(B) deficient blood supply to a part
(C) abnormal condition of the hipbone
(D) abnormal condition of the ischium and the anus

46. The person transporting the patient on a stretcher should

(A) push the stretcher from the head
(B) pull the stretcher by the foot
(C) guide the stretcher from either side
(D) guide the stretcher from any position that is comfortable

47. Activated glutaraldehyde

(A) is corrosive to instruments
(B) causes damage to lenses or the cement on lensed instruments
(C) is absorbed by rubber and plastic
(D) can be reused

48. A Weitlaner is a

(A) dissector
(B) grasper
(C) forceps
(D) retractor

49. Which part of the pancreas is the most common site of malignant tumors?

    (A) head
    (B) body
    (C) tail
    (D) splenic portion

50. The purpose of the two-way stopcock on a Verres needle is

    (A) to deflate pneumoperitoneum
    (B) to control gas flow
    (C) to release excess gas
    (D) to permit passage of accessory items

51. An abnormal communication between two parts occurring in the anorectal area is called

    (A) fissure in ano
    (B) fistula in ano
    (C) ischiorectal abscess
    (D) hemorrhoid

52. Burn removal of tissue down to fascia where all superficial layers are denuded is called

    (A) escharectomy
    (B) debridement
    (C) tangential excision
    (D) fasciotomy

53. The method of sterilization used for liquids is

    (A) slow exhaust
    (B) fast exhaust
    (C) gas
    (D) dry heat

54. Medullary canal reamers are used to insert

    (A) Smith–Petersen nails
    (B) Richards nails
    (C) Jewett nails
    (D) Kuntschner nails

55. A protrusion of fat through an abdominal wall defect between the xiphoid process and umbilicus is a(n)

    (A) umbilical hernia
    (B) diaphragmatic hernia
    (C) epigastric hernia
    (D) Spigelian hernia

56. The position frequently utilized in thyroid and gallbladder surgery is

    (A) supine
    (B) Trendelenburg
    (C) reverse Trendelenburg
    (D) dorsal recumbent

57. What part of the cell is destroyed in steam sterilization?

    (A) cell protein
    (B) ovum
    (C) monocyte
    (D) basophil

58. Which scope has a trocar?

    (A) cystoscope
    (B) laparoscope
    (C) laryngoscope
    (D) bronchoscope

59. Laminar air flow provides

    (A) ultraclean air
    (B) controlled filter, dilution, and distribution of air
    (C) unidirectional positive-pressure stream of air
    (D) all of the above

60. A rotator cuff tear would occur in the

    (A) hip
    (B) shoulder
    (C) ankle
    (D) knee

61. Which position would be chosen for a pneumonectomy?

    (A) supine
    (B) dorsal
    (C) lateral
    (D) Kraske

62. When preparing tubing or any item with a lumen for gas sterilization

    (A) a residual of distilled water should be left in the lumen
    (B) the lumen should be blown out with air to force-dry before packaging
    (C) a residual of saline should be left in the lumen
    (D) it does not matter if it is moist or dry

63. A rib raspatory is a

    (A) Sauerbruck
    (B) Alexander
    (C) Josephs
    (D) Stille–Luer

64. A right-angled gallbladder forceps is a

    (A) Crile
    (B) mixter
    (C) Jackson
    (D) Rochester–Pean

65. A self-retaining mouth gag is a

    (A) Jennings
    (B) Hurd
    (C) Castro
    (D) Cushing

66. The maximum storage life for a muslin-wrapped item on open shelving is

    (A) 7 days
    (B) 14 days
    (C) 30 days
    (D) indefinite

67. How are the legs placed in the lateral position?

    (A) both legs are straight
    (B) both legs are flexed
    (C) the lower leg is flexed with the upper leg straight
    (D) the lower leg is straight with the upper leg flexed

68. Which statement regarding the changing of a glove during an operation is TRUE?

    (A) closed-glove technique is used
    (B) open-glove technique is used

    (C) another team member assists in regloving
    (D) either B or C

69. Each statement regarding OR room ventilation is true EXCEPT

    (A) ventilation provides a minimum of 20–30 air exchanges in an hour
    (B) scavenger systems prevent buildup of anesthetic gases
    (C) humidity is kept at 20–30%
    (D) room temperature is 68–76%

70. How many thoracic vertebrae are there?

    (A) 4
    (B) 5
    (C) 7
    (D) 12

71. When moving a patient from lithotomy position

    (A) lower legs together quickly
    (B) lower legs together slowly
    (C) lower each leg separately and slowly
    (D) lower each leg separately and quickly

72. If a sterile muslin package drops to the floor

    (A) it may never be used
    (B) it may be used if it is carefully checked
    (C) it may be used if the floor is dry
    (D) it may be used if it is dusted off

73. A tonsil suction is a

    (A) Young
    (B) Poole
    (C) Frazier
    (D) Yankauer

74. The most susceptible organ to laser injury is the

    (A) nasopharynx
    (B) ovaries
    (C) testes
    (D) eyes

75. The principal hazard encountered in splenectomy is

(A) trauma to adjacent structures
(B) hypertension
(C) hemorrhage
(D) poor visualization of organs

76. When assisting with a cast application one must

(A) handle cast with flat open hands
(B) hold plaster bandage under water horizontally to allow air bubble to escape
(C) provide water in bucket at body temperature
(D) place all rolls to be used in water and remove as surgeon requests each

77. The most common postoperative complication of orthopedic surgery is

(A) nonunion
(B) osteomyelitis
(C) thromboembolism
(D) urinary tract infection

78. Which is an acceptable means of pouring a sterile solution onto a sterile field?

(A) the scrub nurse holds a receptacle away from the table as the circulator pours
(B) the scrub nurse sets the receptacle near the edge of a waterproof-draped table
(C) all solutions are poured over the ring stand by the circulator
(D) A and B

79. Which nerve is affected by pressure on the lower leg or knee?

(A) phrenic
(B) pudendal
(C) perineal
(D) peroneal

80. What advantage is phacoemulsification for cataract removal?

(A) shortened convalescence
(B) superior cosmetic effect
(C) employs small incision
(D) A and C

81. The structure that covers the entrance of the larynx when one swallows, thus preventing food from entering the airway (trachea) is called

(A) glottis
(B) vocal fold
(C) epiglottis
(D) oropharynx

82. Physiologic salt solution used intravenously when the body needs additional sodium, calcium, and potassium is

(A) Dextran
(B) normal saline
(C) dextrose in saline
(D) Ringer's lactate

83. In the lateral chest position, a sandbag or padding is placed under the chest at axillary level to

(A) facilitate respiration
(B) aid in position stability
(C) prevent pressure on the lower arm
(D) create good body alignment

84. A viscous jelly used to occupy space, thus preventing damage, in anterior segment surgery of the eye is

(A) Healon
(B) Chymar
(C) Miocol
(D) Wydase

85. Which of the following is frequently used over an incision following pediatric surgery?

(A) collodian
(B) benzoin
(C) pressure dressing
(D) cotton-elastic bandage

86. An agent used for epidural, spinal, or local providing good relaxation is

(A) Marcaine
(B) Norcuron
(C) Ketalar
(D) Sublimaze

87. The instrument used to measure the depth of the uterus during a dilation and curettage is a

   (A) Sim's curette
   (B) Jacob's forceps
   (C) Boseman forceps
   (D) uterine sound

88. Vagotomy is performed for peptic ulcer disease to

   (A) decrease transmission of pain stimuli
   (B) increase secretion of gastrin
   (C) increase circulation to the greater curvature
   (D) decrease secretion of gastric acid

89. Before surgery, elastic bandages or special stockings are sometimes applied to the lower extremities to

   (A) prevent pressure areas
   (B) prevent skin irritation
   (C) prevent venous stasis
   (D) prevent chilling

90. Surgical masks should be changed

   (A) after each case
   (B) daily
   (C) twice a day
   (D) every 2 hours

91. Why would benzoin be applied to the skin before dressing application?

   (A) to facilitate easier removal
   (B) to increase adhesiveness
   (C) to add a microbial film to the skin
   (D) to prevent allergic reaction to tape

92. Closing the internal os of an incompetent cervix with a ligature of tape is called

   (A) Manchester
   (B) Wertheim
   (C) Shirodkar
   (D) Le Fort

93. Pneumoperitoneum is effected by instilling gas into the peritoneal cavity by way of a

   (A) Silverman needle
   (B) Verres needle

   (C) trocar
   (D) Craig needle

94. In addition to providing bladder drainage following a suprapubic prostatectomy, a Foley catheter

   (A) exerts pressure to obtain hemostasis
   (B) provides for bladder expansion
   (C) prevents nosocomial infection
   (D) prevents bladder atrophy

95. Electrical connection of the patient to the conductive floor is assured by

   (A) a conductive strap over the sheet covering the patient
   (B) a conductive table mattress
   (C) a conductive strap in direct contact with the patient's skin, with one end of the strap fastened to the OR table metal frame
   (D) a ground plate under the patient

96. Safety during use of the defibrillator includes all of the following EXCEPT

   (A) maintaining contact with OR table and the patient
   (B) keeping hands dry
   (C) standing on dry floor
   (D) pressing paddle switches simultaneously

97. A drug that may be used as an IV flush or as a flush for a blood vessel lumen is

   (A) vitamin K
   (B) heparin
   (C) Coumarin
   (D) desmopressin acetate

98. Nipple reconstruction can be enhanced by the use of a(n)

   (A) tattoo
   (B) flap technique
   (C) laser
   (D) TRAM

99. Where are the adrenal glands located?

(A) in the brain
(B) above the kidney
(C) in the pancreas
(D) alongside the thyroid

100. The following are all contraindications to vaginal hysterectomy EXCEPT

(A) large uterus
(B) malignancy
(C) adnexal mass
(D) presence of a cystocele

101. Instruments used to close the vaginal vault in an abdominal hysterectomy must be

(A) kept separate from the setup before use
(B) considered contaminated after use
(C) noncrushing clamps
(D) kept on the Mayo stand after use

102. The addition of adrenalin to a local anesthetic provides

(A) vasodilatation, heightened anesthesia, decreased bleeding
(B) vasodilatation, increased oxygenation of tissue, decreased bleeding
(C) vasoconstriction, increased absorption, decreased bleeding
(D) vasoconstriction, prolonged anesthesia, decreased bleeding

103. During laser surgery, each of the following policies must be adhered to EXCEPT

(A) signs are placed on doors
(B) prescription glasses are approved protection mechanisms
(C) patient's eyes are protected with moistened pads or goggles
(D) all persons within the treatment area wear protective eyewear

104. There are _____ parathyroids

(A) 2
(B) 3
(C) 4
(D) 5

105. A constant closed suction that utilizes a plastic container serving as both a suction and a receptacle for blood is a

(A) Hemovac
(B) Robinson
(C) Sengstaken–Blakemore
(D) Potts–Smith

106. The sphincter at the junction of the small and large intestine is the

(A) sphincter of Oddi
(B) ileocecal sphincter
(C) pyloric sphincter
(D) duodenal sphincter

107. Which hepatitis poses a threat to health care workers?

(A) A
(B) B
(C) C
(D) D

108. A dye used in gynecology to test tubal patency is

(A) methylene blue
(B) fluorescein
(C) gentian violet
(D) anilene

109. Which stage of wound healing takes place when there is tissue loss with an inability to approximate wound edge?

(A) first (primary)
(B) second (granulation)
(C) third
(D) delayed primary

110. An abnormal accumulation of fluid in the tunica vaginalis is referred to as a

(A) cystocele
(B) hydrocele
(C) spermatocele
(D) varicocele

111. Periosteum is lifted from the surface of the bone with a(n)

(A) rongeur
(B) curette
(C) osteotome
(D) elevator

112. Repair of a cranial defect is surgically represented by the term

(A) trephination
(B) cranioplasty
(C) craniosynostosis
(D) craniectomy

113. For surgery on a known AIDS patient, all of the following precautions should be followed EXCEPT

(A) wear double gloves
(B) masks and protective eyewear worn
(C) needles resheathed
(D) universal precautions undertaken

114. Health care workers who are potentially exposed to blood, can be vaccinated to prevent

(A) hepatitis A virus (HAV)
(B) hepatitis B virus (HBV)
(C) non-A and non-B hepatitis
(D) delta hepatitis

115. An alternative indwelling urinary drainage system diverting urine away from the urethra is a

(A) suprapubic cystostomy catheterization
(B) French catheterization
(C) ureteral catheterization
(D) urethral catheterization

116. A common radiopaque contrast medium used in the OR is

(A) barium sulfate
(B) Ritalin
(C) Baralyme
(D) Renografin

117. What is the purpose of a chest tube and water-seal drainage?

(A) evacuate fluid and air
(B) evacuate lung secretions
(C) oxygenate the lung
(D) plug the hole in the chest wall

118. Extreme flexion of the thighs in the lithotomy position impairs

(A) circulatory function
(B) respiratory function
(C) nerve continuity
(D) operative ability

119. A femoral–popliteal bypass is scheduled. Which self-retaining retractor would be used to facilitate exploration of the femoral artery?

(A) Mason–Judd
(B) DeBakey
(C) Weitlaner
(D) Craford

120. A double-bowl-shaped glass evacuator used to irrigate the bladder during transurethral surgery is called a(n)

(A) Robb
(B) Valentine
(C) Ellik
(D) Toomey

121. An approach to infection control designed to prevent transmission of blood-borne diseases in health care settings is called

(A) aseptic technique
(B) sanitization
(C) universal precautions
(D) disinfection

122. An elevated PSA test could be indicative of cancer of the

(A) lung
(B) prostate
(C) lymph nodes
(D) cervix

123. In which intention of healing is there a wide, fibrous scar?

    (A) primary
    (B) secondary
    (C) third
    (D) fourth

124. Which Gram-positive bacteria can cause abscesses?

    (A) *Escherichia coli*
    (B) *Salmonella*
    (C) *Proteus*
    (D) *Staphylococcus aureus*

125. Mannitol is a(n)

    (A) anticholinergic
    (B) osmotic diuretic
    (C) stimulant
    (D) beta-blocker

126. The organism causing hepatitis B is a

    (A) virus
    (B) bacteria
    (C) fungus
    (D) protozoa

127. An example of an anti-inflammatory is

    (A) cortisone
    (B) cyclosporine
    (C) Isuprel
    (D) Levophed

128. Hemorrhage is suspected if

    (A) the blood pressure drops in direct relationship to the drop in the pulse
    (B) the blood pressure drops and pulse rate rises
    (C) there is no change in the blood pressure, only in the pulse rate
    (D) the blood pressure elevates and the pulse drops

129. How many feet above the ground is considered safe for electrical outlets and fixtures that are not explosion-proof?

    (A) 1
    (B) 3
    (C) 5
    (D) 7

130. Carpal tunnel syndrome affects the

    (A) elbow
    (B) wrist
    (C) knee
    (D) ankle

131. Documenting, tracking, and registering are mandated for

    (A) anesthesia
    (B) implants
    (C) medications
    (D) inventory

132. When the foreskin of the penis cannot be retracted over the glans it is called

    (A) hypospadias
    (B) ptosis
    (C) phimosis
    (D) balanitis

133. The burn characterized by blister formation, pain, and a moist and mottled red appearance is

    (A) first
    (B) second
    (C) third
    (D) fourth

134. Microorganisms that grow in the absence of oxygen are

    (A) spores
    (B) aerobes
    (C) facultative bacteria
    (D) anaerobes

135. The islets of Langerhans are located in the

    (A) adrenals
    (B) parathyroids
    (C) pituitary
    (D) pancreas

136. The master gland is the

    (A) thyroid
    (B) pituitary
    (C) adrenal
    (D) parathyroid

137. A condition that can occur as a result of gross bone contamination or improper surgical technique is

    (A) osteoporosis
    (B) osteomalacia
    (C) osteomyelitis
    (D) osteoarthritis

138. Oxytocics are used to

    (A) relax the uterus
    (B) contract the uterus
    (C) treat bronchospasm
    (D) increase renal flow

139. Which of the following instruments would be used to retract the bladder walls during a suprapubic prostatectomy?

    (A) Weitlaner
    (B) O'Sullivan–O'Connor
    (C) Mason–Judd
    (D) Dennis–Brown

140. Maintenance of bony exposure during a lumbar laminectomy is effected by the use of a

    (A) Gelpi
    (B) Finochietto
    (C) Cloward
    (D) Beckman–Adson

141. A common abdominal complication caused by previous abdominal or pelvic surgery is

    (A) adenomyosis
    (B) endometriosis
    (C) adhesions
    (D) vaginal discharge

142. Which of the following shunts would be used surgically to correct hydrocephalus?

    (A) Scribner
    (B) Brisman–Nova
    (C) Le Veen
    (D) Hakim

143. A spinal fusion is usually effected by autogenous grafts taken from the patient's

    (A) ischium
    (B) ileum
    (C) ilium
    (D) lamina

144. A complication of orthopedic surgery is

    (A) thromboembolism
    (B) fat embolism
    (C) infection
    (D) all of the above

145. Nonunion of bone can be treated with

    (A) artificially applied electric current
    (B) medication
    (C) traction
    (D) casting

146. The word which best describes "staging" is

    (A) reproduction criteria
    (B) categorization
    (C) series
    (D) B and C

147. Nosocomial infection refers to

    (A) hospital-acquired infection
    (B) infection in the nose
    (C) infection in the wound
    (D) surgery-related infection

148. During a CPR effort in the OR, the scrub nurse

    (A) starts time clock and records arrest time
    (B) remains sterile and keeps tables sterile
    (C) assists with traffic control as ordered
    (D) breaks scrub and mans defibrillator

149. The edges of a wrapper that enclose sterile contents are considered

    (A) sterile
    (B) semisterile
    (C) nonsterile
    (D) surgically clean

150. A ureteral stent catheter is used to

(A) remove ureteral calculi
(B) inject dye through during pyelography
(C) provide long-term drainage in ureteral obstruction
(D) measure bladder pressure

151. Uterotubal insufflation is a

(A) Manchester procedure
(B) Wertheim procedure
(C) Le Fort procedure
(D) Rubin's test

152. An infants average at rest heart rate is _____ beats per minute.

(A) 60
(B) 80
(C) 120
(D) 200

153. Which of the following instruments is not found in a vaginal procedure?

(A) Goodell dilator
(B) Jacobs tenaculum
(C) Auvard speculum
(D) Harrington retractor

154. The operation to correct prolapse of the anterior vaginal wall is

(A) colporrhaphy
(B) Shirodkar
(C) Le Fort
(D) vesicourethral suspension

155. Which nasal sinus can be approached only through an external eyebrow incision?

(A) sphenoid
(B) ethmoid
(C) frontal
(D) maxillary

156. Which sinus is surgically opened in a Caldwell–Luc procedure?

(A) ethmoid
(B) frontal
(C) maxillary
(D) sphenoid

157. Which of the following pieces of hardware will be used in an intramedullary fixation of a fracture of an adult femoral shaft?

(A) Kirschner's wire
(B) Steinmann pin
(C) Kuntschner nail
(D) Jewett nail

158. The second cranial nerve is the

(A) vagus
(B) oculomotor
(C) optic
(D) facial

159. The normal body temperature in centigrade measurement is

(A) 37°C
(B) 56°C
(C) 98°C
(D) 112°C

160. What is the purpose of doing ABGs intra-operatively?

(A) to assess arterial gases
(B) to determine blood volume
(C) to monitor pulmonary artery pressure measurement
(D) to aid in determining antibiotics to use

161. Which tube is used for gastrointestinal decompression?

(A) Penrose
(B) Poole
(C) Ferguson
(D) Levin

162. A tissue expander would be used for

(A) burn debridement
(B) TRAM flap
(C) breast reconstruction
(D) gynecomastia

163. Continuous irrigation of the bladder is necessary during cystoscopy to

    (A) keep the area moistened and thus reduce trauma
    (B) distend the bladder walls for visualization
    (C) act as a viewing medium
    (D) reduce heat from the lighted scope

164. The excision and removal of diseased and necrotic tissue is termed

    (A) desiccation
    (B) decortication
    (C) debridement
    (D) dermabrasion

165. The excision of loose skin and periorbital fat of the eyelids is called

    (A) fasciectomy
    (B) oculoplasty
    (C) rhytidectomy
    (D) blepharoplasty

166. A fleshy encroachment onto the cornea is called

    (A) chalazion
    (B) glaucoma
    (C) pterygium
    (D) strabismus

167. Mandibular fractures are treated by occlusion of the teeth effected by the use of a(n)

    (A) splint
    (B) rigid fixation with plate
    (C) LeFort suspension device
    (D) arch bar

168. Which procedure would require the following instruments: Freer elevator, osteotome, Asch Forcep, Ballinger swivel knife, caliper?

    (A) orthopedic
    (B) arthroscopic
    (C) nasal
    (D) vascular

169. Lacrimal probes are called

    (A) Bowman
    (B) Bakes

    (C) Serrefines
    (D) Swolin

170. The eardrum is also known as the

    (A) external auditory canal
    (B) ear canal
    (C) semicircular canal
    (D) tympanic membrane

171. Which of the following appliances can be used for intramedullary fixation of a femur?

    (A) Smith–Peterson
    (B) Neufeld
    (C) Jewett
    (D) Sampson

172. Bradycardia is

    (A) heartbeat over 100 beats per minute
    (B) irregular heartbeat
    (C) thready, weak heartbeat
    (D) heartbeat less than 60 beats per minute

173. If a needle punctures a sterile team member's glove,

    (A) discard the needle
    (B) change the glove
    (C) place another glove over the punctured one
    (D) A and B

174. A Tenckhoff catheter is placed into

    (A) cephalic vein
    (B) peritoneal cavity
    (C) hepatic vessel
    (D) subclavian artery

175. The needle used for a liver biopsy is

    (A) Silverman
    (B) Charnley
    (C) Chiba
    (D) Dorsey

176. Each of the following treats glaucoma EXCEPT

    (A) trephining
    (B) laser trabeculoplasty
    (C) keratoplasty
    (D) iridectomy

177. An instrument used to incise the eardrum to relieve pressure is called a

   (A) Rosen knife
   (B) Walsh crurotomy knife
   (C) myringotomy knife
   (D) Hough pick

178. In which surgical specialty would a perfusionist be necessary?

   (A) neurologic surgery
   (B) cardiac surgery
   (C) transplant surgery
   (D) microsurgery

179. The preferred method of gloving is _____. In changing during a case, this method _____ be used.

   (A) closed, can
   (B) open, can
   (C) open, cannot
   (D) closed, cannot

180. When a patient goes into hypovolemic shock in the OR, an immediate response would be

   (A) monitor intake and output
   (B) give supplementary oxygen
   (C) raise the head 45°
   (D) restore fluid volume quickly

181. In which surgical wound classification would an appendectomy for ruptured appendix fall?

   (A) clean
   (B) clean contaminated
   (C) contaminated
   (D) dirty or infected

182. The malleus, incus, and stapes are located in the

   (A) middle ear
   (B) outer ear
   (C) inner ear
   (D) external ear

183. Protective goggles are worn during CO_2 laser surgery to

   (A) deflect glare
   (B) prevent corneal damage

   (C) avoid splashing from irrigation
   (D) absorb light rays

184. When gloving a surgeon

   (A) keep the palm of the glove facing the surgeon
   (B) avoid contact by keeping thumbs tucked in
   (C) hold the second glove while doing the first
   (D) glove only over a sterile area

185. After hip joint surgery, immobilization is aided by the use of

   (A) abduction pillow
   (B) Thomas splint
   (C) cast
   (D) traction

186. The blue–green wavelength produced by a laser that is capable of treating retinal detachment, diabetic retinopathy, and macular neovascular lesion is

   (A) krypton
   (B) Ho–YAG
   (C) argon
   (D) Nd–YAG

187. If the patient has a positive breast biopsy, and the surgeon proceeds to do a radical mastectomy

   (A) the same drapes and instruments may be used
   (B) the patient is reprepped, and new drapes and instruments are used
   (C) the drapes may remain, but new instruments are used
   (D) the drapes are replaced, but the same instruments may be used

188. At which artery is the blood pressure taken?

   (A) cephalic
   (B) brachial
   (C) basilar
   (D) axillary

189. The action of white blood cells is to

    (A) transport oxygen
    (B) clot blood
    (C) produce enzymes
    (D) destroy bacteria

190. The function of the endocrine glands is to?

    (A) manufacture sugar
    (B) produce hormones
    (C) maintain acid-base balance
    (D) digest fat

191. Oxygenated blood is returned to the left atrium of the heart from the lungs via the

    (A) pulmonary vein
    (B) pulmonary artery
    (C) carotid artery
    (D) renal vein

192. Bile is manufactured in the _____ and stored in the _____.

    (A) gallbladder, liver
    (B) liver, pancreas
    (C) gallbladder, duodenum
    (D) liver, gallbladder

193. Entrapment of the _____ nerve is relieved by a carpal tunnel release.

    (A) brachial
    (B) radial
    (C) median
    (D) ulnar

194. When intraoperative cultures are obtained, each of the following is true EXCEPT

    (A) tip of swab is placed on back table
    (B) cultures should be refrigerated or sent to lab immediately
    (C) circulator handles tube following appropriate precautions
    (D) cultures are obtained under sterile conditions

195. During vascular surgery, an arteriotomy is executed with a #11 blade and extended by use of a

    (A) Lahey
    (B) Metzenbaum

    (C) Potts–Smith
    (D) Stevens

196. Dehiscence is

    (A) separation of layers of surgical wound
    (B) extrusion of internal organs through a gaping wound
    (C) failure of wound to heal
    (D) infected operative wound

197. The first part of the small intestine is known as the

    (A) jejunum
    (B) pylorus
    (C) duodenum
    (D) ileum

198. What organisms are likely to be found in a surgical wound adjacent to a colostomy?

    (A) *Staphylococcus*
    (B) *Streptococcus*
    (C) *Pseudomonas*
    (D) *Escherichia coli*

199. During a CPR effort, which drug is given to combat metabolic acidosis?

    (A) Xylocaine
    (B) sodium bicarbonate
    (C) Nipride
    (D) Inderal

200. When inserting a Foley catheter, always

    (A) check the integrity of the balloon by inflating it with the correct amount of sterile water prior to insertion
    (B) inflate the balloon immediately after insertion
    (C) connect the catheter to the closed drainage system before the catheter is inserted
    (D) have the scrub nurse hold bag above table level

201. The proper setting for a tourniquet applied to the thigh is about

    (A) 100 mm Hg
    (B) 250 mm Hg

(C)   350 mm Hg

(D)   400 mm Hg

202.   Crushing a urinary calculus in the bladder through the urethra is called

(A)   cystolithotomy

(B)   litholapaxy

(C)   urethrotomy

(D)   urethroplasty

203.   The surgical procedure performed electively as a permanent method of sterilization is

(A)   epididymectomy

(B)   orchiectomy

(C)   vasectomy

(D)   orchiopexy

204.   When doing a skin prep, which includes a draining sinus, the contaminated area is

(A)   done first

(B)   done last or separately

(C)   given no special consideration

(D)   avoided because it is contaminated

205.   The portion of the stomach located at the approach to the small intestine is the

(A)   cardia

(B)   fundus

(C)   pylorus

(D)   antrum

206.   A commonly used diuretic is

(A)   nipride

(B)   lasix

(C)   dobutrex

(D)   adrenalin

207.   The normal bladder capacity is

(A)   100–200 mL

(B)   200–300 mL

(C)   700–800 mL

(D)   800–1000 mL

208.   Rectal surgery preparation is done

(A)   top to bottom

(B)   bottom to top

(C)   surrounding area first, anus last

(D)   anus first, surrounding area last

209.   When changing a gown during a case, the _____ is (are) removed first, the _____ second, and a rescrub is _____.

(A)   gown, gloves, not necessary

(B)   gloves, gown, not necessary

(C)   gown, gloves, necessary

(D)   gloves, gown, necessary

210.   Which piece of equipment is used to make a skin graft larger?

(A)   knife dermatome

(B)   Brown air dermatome

(C)   mesh dermatome

(D)   Reese drum-type dermatome

211.   The item that provides internal drainage of an obstructed ureter is a(n)

(A)   lithotrite

(B)   stone basket

(C)   stent

(D)   extracorporeal shockwave lithotripsy (ESWL)

212.   A way to alleviate a presurgical patient's anxiety is via

(A)   history and physical review

(B)   preoperative visit

(C)   review of charts and records

(D)   visit by hospital social worker

213.   The kidneys are held in place by the

(A)   renal columns

(B)   detrusor muscle

(C)   renal fascia and fat

(D)   tunica fibrosa

214.   A culture and sensitivity is done to

(A)   determine nature of organism and the susceptibility of that organism

(B)   diagnose blood infections

(C)   culture a single organism responsible for infection

(D)   determine if furniture and rooms are being cleaned properly

215. Which of the following is considered the most effective agent for scrubbing?

    (A) povidone–iodine
    (B) glutaraldehyde
    (C) hexachlorophene
    (D) chlorhexidene

216. All of the following would be on the setup for an open thoracotomy EXCEPT

    (A) Alexander's periosteotome
    (B) Duval forceps
    (C) Joseph's saw
    (D) Lebsche knife

217. Transcutaneous electric nerve stimulation (TENS) would be utilized for

    (A) urinary calculi
    (B) soft tissue allograft
    (C) dressing for burns
    (D) antiembolic effort

218. During a basic femoral head fixation, the length and position of the implant is determined by the use of

    (A) guide wire
    (B) compression screw
    (C) tap
    (D) awl

219. Which of the following grafts is not a synthetic vascular graft?

    (A) filamentous velours
    (B) polytetrafluorethylene
    (C) biologic vascular
    (D) exoskeleton prosthesis

220. Fingerlike projections at the end of the Fallopian tubes are called

    (A) fimbriae
    (B) infundibulum
    (C) graphian follicle
    (D) corpus luteum

221. All of the following are true of self-adhering plastic incision drapes EXCEPT

    (A) scrubbed area must be moist at application
    (B) alcohol may be used after iodophor to hasten drying of skin
    (C) drape is smoothed away from incision
    (D) usual skin prep precedes its application

222. An abnormal deposition of collagen that occurs during the healing process is known as

    (A) eschar
    (B) keloid
    (C) contracture
    (D) cicatrix

223. All of the following statements are true during deep vaginal procedures EXCEPT

    (A) suction is part of the setup
    (B) sponges are secured on long forceps
    (C) vaginal packing may be inserted at case end
    (D) count is eliminated

224. The gas introduced into the peritoneum during laparoscopy to create a pneumoperitoneum is

    (A) nitrous oxide
    (B) oxygen
    (C) nitrogen
    (D) carbon dioxide

225. Crutchfield tongs produce skeletal traction to reduce fractures of the

    (A) phalanges
    (B) femoral shaft
    (C) cervical spine
    (D) humeral shaft

226. Which disease could be transmitted via a blood transfusion?

    (A) hepatitis A
    (B) hepatitis B
    (C) infectious hepatitis
    (D) hepatonephritis

227. *Staphylococcus* is usually transmitted by

(A) sexual contact
(B) upper respiratory tract
(C) urine
(D) feces

228. A bacteria with a thick coat that protects it from temperature extremes or strong chemicals is a

(A) parasite
(B) host
(C) saprophyte
(D) spore

229. When a three-way Foley catheter is used, the third lumen is for

(A) drainage
(B) balloon inflation
(C) continuous irrigation
(D) constant suction

230. If a towel clip must be removed during a procedure

(A) the patient must be redraped
(B) discard it from the field and cover the area with another sterile drape
(C) place it near the skin knife
(D) use the same towel clip but cover the area with another sterile drape

231. Constant monitoring of cardiac function, a requirement for vascular surgery is effected by the use of a

(A) Doppler
(B) Swan–Ganz
(C) Greenfield
(D) Fogarty

232. What procedure is accomplished to relieve myasthenia gravis?

(A) mediastinoscopy
(B) pulmonary decortication
(C) adrenalectomy
(D) thymectomy

233. Which specimen would be placed in formalin?

(A) bronchial washings
(B) tonsils
(C) breast biopsy/frozen
(D) kidney stones

234. A legal wrong committed by one person involving injury to another person is called a(n)

(A) tort
(B) default
(C) liability
(D) impressment

235. Scoliosis is surgically treated by the implantation of

(A) Steinmann pins
(B) Rush rods
(C) Lottes nails
(D) Harrington rods

236. An intravenous agent used for anesthesia induction is

(A) lidocaine
(B) Fluothane
(C) sodium pentothal
(D) Demerol

237. A prosthetic implant that requires nonadherence to tissue for the sake of creating normal flexion and extension is

(A) biofixation
(B) methyl–methacrylate fixation
(C) constrained
(D) nonconstrained

238. Unauthorized discussion of a patient's surgery outside of the OR constitutes a lawsuit for

(A) defamation
(B) negligence
(C) assault and battery
(D) invasion of privacy

239. When applying a sterile sheet on the patient,

(A) protect the gloved hands by cuffing the end of the sheet over them
(B) adjust the drape by pulling it toward the sterile area
(C) the gloved hands may touch the painted skin of the patient
(D) unfold from the patient's foot to the operative site

240. A chronic granulomatous inflammation of a meibomian gland in the eyelid is a(n)

(A) entropion
(B) chalazion
(C) blepharochalasis
(D) pterygium

241. A drug given preoperatively that enables the liver to produce clotting factors in blood is

(A) vitamin C
(B) vitamin B$_{12}$
(C) vitamin D
(D) vitamin K

242. When is bowel technique necessary?

(A) when a case is considered septic
(B) when the patient has not had a bowel prep
(C) when the patient has perforated preoperatively
(D) when a contaminated area of the intestinal tract is entered

243. A slowly progressive contracture of the palmar fascia is called

(A) Volkmann's contracture
(B) carpal tunnel syndrome
(C) Dupuytren's contracture
(D) talipes valgus

244. If rubber suction tubing is to be reused

(A) the lumen must be flushed with a detergent–disinfectant before tubing is terminally sterilized
(B) it must be cold-sterilized between uses
(C) it requires no special procedure
(D) the lumen must be flushed with water and sterilized

245. Who is responsible for the final count when reliefs have taken place during the case?

(A) scrub person
(B) scrub person and circulator who do final count
(C) circulator
(D) scrub person and circulator who begin case

246. Which of the following statements is a contraindication to intraocular lens (IOL) implant?

(A) elderly patients with bilateral cataracts
(B) children with traumatic cataracts
(C) patients with occupational vision requirements
(D) children with congenital cataracts

247. Neo-Synephrine is

(A) miotic
(B) retrobulbar blocker
(C) phacoemulsifier
(D) mydriatic

248. The legal doctrine *res ipsa loquitor* applies to

(A) invasion of privacy
(B) an employer's liability for an employee's negligence
(C) damage of personal property
(D) injuries sustained by the patient in the OR due to negligence

249. After a case is completed, the sterile team members

(A) discard gown and gloves before leaving the OR suite
(B) discard gown and keep gloves on to transport soiled equipment
(C) discard gown, gloves, caps, masks, and shoe covers before leaving OR suite
(D) discard gown, gloves, and masks before the room is dismantled

250. Pilocarpine is used to

(A) dilate the pupil
(B) constrict the pupil
(C) keep the eye moist
(D) reduce inflammation

Practice Test
Answers and Explanations

1. **(B)** When an inguinal herniorrhaphy is being performed, the spermatic cord is identified, freed, and a Penrose drain is placed around it for traction, and to prevent injury (Fortunato).

2. **(B)** Polyglycolic acid is a synthetic absorbable suture that is not affected by enzymes but rather by the process of hydrolysis, whereby water in the body acts to break down the polymeric constituents (Meeker and Rothrock).

3. **(D)** Twenty-seven pounds of pressure is necessary for the steam autoclave set at 270°F. The high speed is the flash sterilizer (Meeker and Rothrock).

4. **(A)** The leukocytes (white blood cells) normally range between 5000 and 10,000 cells in each cu mm of whole blood. High white counts may be indicative of an unsuspected inflammatory process that could contraindicate surgery. It would not be contraindicated if surgery were to treat an infectious condition; for example, acute appendicitis (*Mosby's Medical, Nursing, and Allied Health Dictionary*, 5th ed.; Tortora and Grabowski).

5. **(B)** The term distal refers to an area away from the point of origin (body). The hand is distal to the elbow (*Mosby's Medical, Nursing, and Allied Health Dictionary*, 5th ed.).

6. **(C)** Meckel's diverticulum is a congenital sac or blind pouch sometimes found in the lower portion of the ileum. Strangulation may cause an intestinal obstruction (Meeker and Rothrock).

7. **(B)** A Frazier suction would be found on an otologic setup (Meeker and Rothrock).

8. **(D)** Recirculation of filtered air at a rate of no less than 25 air exchanges per hour is considered safe and economical (Fortunato).

9. **(A)** OSHA's main purpose is to ensure safe and healthful working conditions for employees (Fortunato).

10. **(D)** Body heat in pediatric patients is controlled by wrapping the child in plastic materials, a warming blanket, and increasing room temperature. Hot water bottles are not used because they are unsafe (Meeker and Rothrock).

11. **(B)** Telephone, telegram, or written permission is acceptable. If by telephone, two people monitor the conversation and sign the permission form as witnesses (Fortunato).

12. **(A)** Instruments completely unwrapped sterilize at 3 minutes. The autoclave is set at 270°F (Fortunato).

13. **(A)** The tissue through which retention sutures are passed includes the skin, subcutaneous tissue, fascia, and may include the rectus muscle and peritoneum of an abdominal incision (Fortunato).

14. **(B)** Indirect hernias leave the abdominal cavity through the inguinal canal. Consequently, the hernia can often be found in the scrotum (Fortunato).

15. **(B)** Dead space is that space caused by separation of wound edges that have not been closely approximated by sutures (Fortunato).

16. **(D)** Wrapped tubing is autoclaved at 250°F for 30 minutes. A residual of distilled water is left in the lumen (Fortunato).

17. **(B)** Pectus excavatum (funnel chest) and pectus carinatum (pigeon chest) are chest congenital defects (Meeker and Rothrock).

18. **(B)** Hypovolemia means low or decreased blood volume. Hypo means below. Volemia refers to blood volume (*Mosby's Medical, Nursing, and Allied Health Dictionary*, 5th ed.).

19. **(D)** An angiogram is a test in which vessel size, location, and configuration can be studied by injecting dye into intracranial vessels. It is an x-ray procedure (Meeker and Rothrock).

20. **(C)** Instruments alone can be flashed at 270°F. The addition of other items makes the requirement 10 minutes at 270°F (Fortunato).

21. **(A)** Nonabsorbable sutures remain permanently embedded in the body. During the healing process, they become encapsulated with fibrous tissue (Fortunato).

22. **(B)** This procedure is performed to remove a malignant lesion of the right colon and, in some cases, to remove inflammatory lesions involving the ileum, cecum, or right colon (ascending colon) (Meeker and Rothrock).

23. **(D)** Dacryo pertains to tears. The lacrimal sac fills with tears secreted by the lacrimal glands via the lacrimal ducts (*Mosby's Medical, Nursing, and Allied Health Dictionary*, 5th ed.).

24. **(B)** Drainage tubing should be placed so that there is a downward gravity flow. The drainage bag should be below the level of the tubing. This prevents retrograde flow, which could contaminate the bladder (Fortunato).

25. **(C)** Linen packs must not exceed a maximum size of 12 × 12 × 20 inches. Linens are loosely criss-crossed so as not to form a dense mass (Fortunato).

26. **(B)** A retention or stay suture provides a secondary suture line. The purpose is to relieve undue strain on the primary suture line and to help obliterate dead space (Fortunato).

27. **(B)** After complete exposure of the biliary tract, the cystic artery is doubly ligated and divided. The cystic duct is identified, carefully dissected from the common bile duct to the gallbladder neck, then doubly ligated and divided (Meeker and Rothrock).

28. **(B)** The root adeno means gland. Adenitis is inflammation of a gland (*Mosby's Medical, Nursing, and Allied Health Dictionary*, 5th ed.).

29. **(D)** The patient should be lifted or rolled gently and slowly to prevent circulatory depression. A sudden or jarring movement is potentially dangerous to the patient (Fortunato).

30. **(B)** Moist heat and steam under pressure destroy microbial life. Heat destroys microorganisms, but the process is hastened with steam. Pressure is necessary to increase the temperature of the steam for destruction of microbial life (Fortunato).

31. **(A)** Silk suture is used only in the absence of infection (Fortunato; Meeker and Rothrock).

32. **(B)** This surgery is performed for malignant lesions of the lower sigmoid colon, rectum, and anus. It is a two-part procedure that involves resecting the proximal disease-free sigmoid and pulling the diseased portion down through a widely excised anus with total, permanent closure of the anus (Meeker and Rothrock).

33. **(B)** The increased accumulation of cerebrospinal fluid within the ventricles of the brain is hydrocephalus. It results from interference with normal circulation and absorption of fluid and may result from developmental anomalies, infection, injury, or brain tumors. Treatment may be a surgical shunt through which cerebrospinal fluid flows from the ventricles of the brain to a cavity such as the peritoneum (Meeker and Rothrock).

34. **(A)** A patient should never be left on a stretcher or OR table unattended, even though appearing alert and responsible (Fortunato).

35. **(C)** The boiling point of water is 212°F. This is equal to 100°C. 1.0°F is equal to 0.54°C (Fortunato).

36. **(C)** Prednisone has an anti-inflammatory effect useful in reversing early rejection syndrome (Fortunato).

37. **(B)** Congenital hypertrophic pyloric stenosis is an abnormality of the pyloric musculature in which there is alteration of fibrous, gristle-like tissue, causing mechanical obstruction of the distal stomach (Meeker and Rothrock; Tortora and Grabowski).

38. **(B)** A fossa is a basinlike depression, for example, iliac fossa (*Mosby's Medical, Nursing, and Allied Health Dictionary*, 5th ed.).

39. **(C)** Removal of the non-neoplastic thymus gland seems to have equivocal effects on the progression of myasthenia gravis (Fortunato).

40. **(B)** Lidocaine is instilled into the trachea to decrease coughing immediately before insertion of the tracheotomy tube (Meeker and Rothrock; *Mosby's Medical, Nursing, and Allied Health Dictionary*, 5th ed.).

41. **(D)** A temporary colostomy is done to decompress the bowel or give the bowel a rest as in advanced inflammation or trauma (Meeker and Rothrock).

42. **(C)** The Duval lung-grasping forceps is designed to grasp lung tissue firmly while producing minimal tissue trauma (Meeker and Rothrock).

43. **(D)** A sterile processing system that uses peracetic acid, the STERIS system, is appropriate for heat-sensitive items that can be cleaned and completely immersed. The cycle is less than 30 minutes and less damaging than steam (Meeker and Rothrock).

44. **(B)** A general recommendation is that no more than 50 mL of a 1% solution of an anesthetic drug such as Lidocaine be injected per hour for local anesthesia (Meeker and Rothrock).

45. **(B)** Ischemia is local or temporary deficiency of blood supply caused by obstruction of the circulation to a part. A transient ischemic attack (TIA) is a temporary interference with the blood supply to the brain lasting a few moments to several hours (Tortora and Grabowski; *Mosby's Medical, Nursing, and Allied Health Dictionary*, 5th ed.).

46. **(A)** The transporter should be near the patient's head so that he or she can converse with the patient or be available to assist the patient in an emergency, such as vomiting. When the patient is on the stretcher, his or her feet should be pointed down the hallway first (Fortunato).

47. **(D)** Activated glutaraldehyde penetrates into the crevices of items, is noncorrosive, does not damage lenses or cement on lensed instruments, is not absorbed by rubber and plastic, and can be reused throughout the effective activation period (Fortunato).

48. **(D)** A Weitlaner is a self-retaining retractor (Meeker and Rothrock).

49. **(A)** The head of the pancreas is the most common site of a malignant tumor (Fortunato).

50. **(B)** The Verres needle is used to produce pneumoperitoneum. The two-way stopcock at the base controls gas flow (Fortunato).

51. **(B)** A fistula in ano is an abnormal communication between two parts often developing after an I and D or spontaneous drainage of an anorectal abscess (Fortunato).

52. **(A)** Full thickness eschar is excised down to fascia when viable tissues in more superficial layers are not evident. All denuded areas created by the excision are covered with biologic dressing for 3–5 days (Fortunato).

53. **(A)** Solutions are steam sterilized alone and on slow exhaust. This is used so that the solutions do not boil over (Fortunato).

54. **(D)** A medullary canal reamer reams the medullary canal for insertion of a Kuntschner nail (Fortunato).

55. **(C)** Epigastric hernias are located where fatty tissue protrudes through an abdominal wall defect between the xyphoid process and the umbilicus. Surgical repair is simple and successful (Meeker and Rothrock).

56. **(C)** In this position, the entire table is tilted so that the head is higher than the feet. It is used in thyroid surgery to facilitate breathing and decrease blood supply to the operative area. It is used in gallbladder surgery to allow abdominal viscera to fall away from the epigastric area, thus giving better exposure and access (Fortunato).

57. **(A)** Microbial destruction is via a denaturation and coagulation of enzyme–protein in the cell (Fortunato).

58. **(B)** The laparoscope has a trocar that aids in its puncture through the abdominal wall (Fortunato).

59. **(D)** Laminar air flow is an ultraclean air system that filters, dilutes, and distributes air via a controlled unidirectional positive-pressure stream of air. It is used in high-risk procedures to reduce airborne bacterial contamination (Fortunato).

60. **(B)** Rotator cuff tears frequently follow trauma to the shoulder in patients with weakened tendinous fibers who have degenerative changes within the joint. They cannot abduct shoulder (Meeker and Rothrock).

61. **(C)** For pneumonectomy, a posterolateral approach is used, and the patient is placed on the table in the lateral position. A pillow is placed under the head and also between the patient's legs. The bottom leg is flexed, the top straight. The bottom knee is padded. The upper arm is flexed slightly and raised above the head and supported on a raised armboard. Compression of lower arm must be avoided (Meeker and Rothrock).

62. **(B)** In gas sterilization, any tubing or other item with a lumen should be blown out with air to force-dry before packaging because the water combines with the (EO) gas to form a harmful acid, ethylene glycol (Meeker and Rothrock).

63. **(B)** The Doyen is a rib raspatory (Meeker and Rothrock).

64. **(B)** Dissection of the gallbladder from the bed of the liver is accomplished by the use of right-angle (mixter) clamps, blunt peanut dissectors, and Metzenbaum scissors (Meeker and Rothrock).

65. **(A)** A mouthgag used in tonsillectomy and adenoidectomy is a Jennings (Meeker and Rothrock).

66. **(C)** The storage life is 21 to 30 days for muslin-wrapped items. It is longer if it is hermetically sealed in a plastic overwrap (Meeker and Rothrock).

67. **(C)** In kidney position, the knee of the unaffected side is flexed to aid in stabilization, and the upper leg is straight. Legs are separated with a pillow (Fortunato).

68. (D) The closed glove technique cannot be used for glove change during a procedure without contamination of the new glove by the sleeve of the gown or hand by the gown cuff. Preferably another team member regloves another (Fortunato).

69. (C) Humidity should be maintained between 50% and 60%, never less than 45%. This is to reduce the possibility of explosion from static charges A, B, and D are true (Fortunato).

70. (D) There are 12 thoracic, 7 cervical, 5 lumbar, 1 sacrum, and 1 coccyx (Tortora and Grabowski).

71. (B) When in lithotomy position, legs should be raised, positioned, and lowered at the same time slowly, with no sudden movement and good support. Raising the legs simultaneously also prevents strain on the back and possible dislocation of the hips. Slow movements prevent hypotension as blood reenters the legs (Meeker and Rothrock).

72. (A) A sterile muslin-wrapped pack that drops on the floor should be discarded because compression results from the fall and air and dust could enter the package. It can no longer be considered sterile (Fortunato).

73. (D) A Yankauer suction tip is used in a T&A and has a small hole at the end for directed suctioning. It is frequently used in general surgery when a limited amount of suctioning is to be done (Fortunato).

74. (D) The eye is the most susceptible organ to laser injury, thus safety glasses or goggles must be worn. Each type of laser requires specific types of lenses (Fortunato).

75. (C) Great care must be taken in ligating the splenic artery and vein because they are friable. Hemorrhage is the principal hazard encountered in surgery (Fortunato).

76. (A) One must handle the cast with flat, open hands, never the fingers, which would cause finger pressure areas. The plaster bandage is held under water vertically to allow bubbles to escape. Water is 70–75° so the patient will not be burned. Rolls are soaked one at a time, keeping just ahead to avoid plaster hardening and waste (Fortunato).

77. (C) Thromboembolism is the most common postoperative complication of orthopedic surgery, particularly if a patient must be immobilized for an extended period (Fortunato).

78. (D) If a solution must be poured into a sterile receptacle on a sterile field, the scrub nurse holds the receptacle away from the table or sets it near the edge of a waterproof-draped table. The circulating nurse may not pour by reaching over the sterile field. She also must be careful not to drip any solution from outside of bottle onto sterile field (Meeker and Rothrock).

79. (D) Peroneal concerns the fibula (bone in the lower leg) and the common peroneal (lateral popliteal) nerve. Inadequately padded or improperly placed legs can cause pressure on the peroneal nerve (Fortunato; Meeker and Rothrock).

80. (D) The ultrasonic vibrating nature of irrigation with a phaecoemulsification unit may cause injury to cells because of the substantial amount of anterior chamber irrigation. Corneal cells are very sensitive to manipulation. The short convalescence and small incision are both advantages (Fortunato).

81. (C) The epiglottis is the lidlike cartilaginous structure overhanging the entrance to the larynx, guarding it during swallowing (*Mosby's Medical, Nursing, and Allied Health Dictionary*, 5th ed.).

82. (D) Ringer's lactate solution, a physiologic salt solution, may be infused when the body's supply of sodium, calcium, and potassium have been depleted or for the improvement of circulation and stimulation of renal activity (Fortunato).

83. **(C)** A precautionary measure in the lateral chest position is to place a sandbag under the weightbearing thorax at axillary level to relieve pressure and ensure uninhibited infusion therapy (Fortunato).

84. **(A)** Healon, a viscous jelly, occupies space to prevent damage and adhesion formation, when opening the anterior capsule of the eye (Fortunato).

85. **(A)** An adhesive spray or collodian is adequate over a small incision and is especially desirable under diapers, unless dressings are needed to absorb drainage (Fortunato).

86. **(A)** Marcaine, a local anesthetic, is used for epidurals, spinals, or local infiltration. It is long acting and provides good relaxation (Meeker and Rothrock).

87. **(D)** The direction of the cervical canal and the depth of the uterine cavity are determined by means of a graduated uterine sound (Meeker and Rothrock).

88. **(D)** A popular method of treating patients with ulcers is by cutting the vagus nerve. The vagus nerve stimulates gastric acid. This procedure reduces gastric acid secretions (Meeker and Rothrock).

89. **(C)** Antiembolic stockings or elastic bandages may be applied to the lower extremities to prevent embolic phenomena or venous stasis. It also helps maintain blood pressure (Fortunato).

90. **(A)** The OR staff should remask between patients (Meeker and Rothrock).

91. **(B)** Benzoin may be sprayed on the skin before applying tape to increase its adhesion (Fortunato).

92. **(C)** A Shirodkar operation is the placement of a collar-type ligature of mersilene or Dacron at the level of the internal os to close it and prevent premature cervical dilation in a pregnancy (Meeker and Rothrock).

93. **(B)** To produce pneumoperitoneum, a Verres needle is introduced infraumbilically into the peritoneal cavity. The gas is slowly introduced into the cavity under controlled flow and pressure (Meeker and Rothrock).

94. **(A)** Hemostatic agents usually are packed into extremely vascular prostatic fossa to help control bleeding. Pressure from the Foley catheter balloon inserted after the closure of the urethra also helps obtain hemostasis (Fortunato; Meeker and Rothrock).

95. **(C)** Electrical connection of the patient to the conductive floor is provided by a conductive strap in contact with the patient's skin, with one end of the strap fastened to the metal frame of the OR table (Fortunato).

96. **(A)** Paddle switches are pressed simultaneously. The operator should have dry hands and stand on dry floor. Operator should not touch the OR table or the patient while current is applied to prevent self-electrocution (Fortunato).

97. **(B)** Given IV, heparin is effective immediately and is used as a flush to keep IV lines open or to flush blood vessel lumens, 1 mL heparin in 100 mL normal saline (Fortunato).

98. **(A)** Tattooing may complete the reconstruction of the nipple after breast reconstruction surgery. Tissue to create the new nipple is harvested from the groin, auricular area, or contralateral nipple (*Mosby's Medical, Nursing, and Allied Health Dictionary*, 5th ed.).

99. **(B)** The adrenal glands are located above each kidney (Tortora and Grabowski).

100. **(D)** Anterior–posterior repairs are more easily accomplished when done with a vaginal hysterectomy and are not contraindicated (Fortunato; Meeker and Rothrock).

101. **(B)** Potentially contaminated instruments used on the cervix and vagina are placed in a discard basin and removed from the field after surgery (Meeker and Rothrock).

102.   **(D)**   Adrenalin is a potent stimulant. When combined with an anesthetic agent, it causes vasoconstriction to slow the uptake and absorption, thus prolonging the anesthetic and decreasing bleeding (Fortunato).

103.   **(B)**   Prescription glasses are not considered appropriate eye protection because the lens material may not stop the transmission of the laser beam. Each of the other policies provides eye protection (Ball).

104.   **(C)**   There are four parathyroid, tiny bodies located behind the thyroid gland, embedded in its capsule (Tortora and Grabowski).

105.   **(A)**   A Hemovac is used for constant closed suction. The suction is maintained by a plastic container with a spring inside that tries to force apart the lids, thereby producing suction that is transmitted through plastic tubing. It is left in for about 3 days (Meeker and Rothrock).

106.   **(B)**   The ileocecal sphincter or valve joins the large intestine to the small intestine (Tortora and Grabowski).

107.   **(B)**   Hepatitis B (HBV) has a risk factor for physicians, nurses, dentists, medical technologists, and others who are in contact with blood daily (Tortora, Funke, and Case).

108.   **(A)**   Methylene blue is used for gynecologic diagnostic procedures such as to test tubal patency (Fortunato).

109.   **(B)**   When surgical wounds are characterized by tissue loss with an inability to approximate wound edges, healing occurs through secondary intention. The area of tissue loss gradually fills in with granulation tissue (Meeker and Rothrock).

110.   **(B)**   Normally a small amount of clear fluid is contained in the tunica vaginalis, a sac in the scrotum. When the amount increases, it is known as a hydrocele. A varicocele is a congested vein; a cystocele is a herniation of the bladder through the vaginal mucosa of a female; a spermatocele is a cystic mass attached to the upper pole of the epididymis (Fortunato; Meeker and Rothrock).

111.   **(D)**   Periosteal elevators are used to lift the periosteum from the surface of the bone. The size ranges in width and choice is dependent on the width of the surface to be removed (Fortunato).

112.   **(B)**   Cranioplasty is the repair of a skull defect resulting from trauma, malformation, or a surgical procedure (Fortunato).

113.   **(C)**   To minimize the risk of needle stick, needles should not be resheathed and should be placed in a puncture-proof container for sterilization and disposal (Tortora, Funke, and Case).

114.   **(B)**   Hepatitis B is caused by a virus and a vaccination for it is available (Tortora, Funke, and Case).

115.   **(A)**   Insertion of a cannula directly into the bladder through a suprapubic incision (suprapubic cystostomy) provides an alternative indwelling drainage system (Fortunato).

116.   **(D)**   Renographin is a radiopaque contrast medium used intraoperatively (Fortunato).

117.   **(A)**   Chest drainage prevents outside air from being drawn into the pleural space during expiration. Water in the collection units seals off outside air to maintain a negative pressure within the pleural cavity. Fluids drain by gravity from the chest into the water. This system ensures complete lung expansion postoperatively (Fortunato).

118.   **(B)**   Extreme flexion of the thighs in lithotomy position impairs respiratory function by increasing intraabdominal pressure against the diaphragm (Fortunato).

119.   **(C)**   After a vertical incision is made and extended along the medial aspect of the thigh over the femoral artery, a Weitlaner retractor is inserted into the incision (Meeker and Rothrock).

120. **(C)** The Ellik evacuator is a double-bowl-shaped glass evacuator. It contains a trap for fragments so they cannot be washed back into the sheath of the endoscope while irrigating with pressure on the rubber-bulb attachment (Fortunato).

121. **(C)** Universal precautions are designed to prevent transmission of AIDS and hepatitis in health care settings (Tortora and Grabowski).

122. **(B)** A PSA test measures prostate-specific antigen in blood. The amount of PSA is elevated in cancer of the prostate (Tortora and Grabowski).

123. **(C)** Granulation tissue in third-intention healing usually forms a wide, fibrous scar. Suturing is delayed because of much tissue removal (Fortunato).

124. **(D)** *Staphylococcus aureus* is a cause of suppurative conditions. It is pathogenic, Gram-positive, and is transmitted because of its presence on skin and mucous membrane. The others are Gram-negative (Fortunato).

125. **(B)** Mannitol is a most effective osmotic diuretic and is valuable in reducing intercranial pressure or edema. It may be given prophylactically to prevent renal failure. It also reduces intraocular pressure (Fortunato).

126. **(A)** Hepatitis is an inflammation of the liver. Viral hepatitis is the second most frequently reported infectious disease in the United States. There are at least five different viruses causing hepatitis. Hepatitis B is caused by the hepatitis B virus (HBV) (Tortora, Funke, and Case).

127. **(A)** Cortisone is used as an anti-inflammatory. It is used to reduce resistance to the invasion of bacteria (Fortunato).

128. **(B)** The clinical manifestations of hemorrhage are pulse increase, fall in temperature, rapid and deep respirations, and fall in blood pressure. The patient is apprehensive and restless. He or she may be thirsty. The skin is cold, moist, and pale (Fortunato).

129. **(C)** All flammable gases and vapors except ethylene are heavier than air and settle to the floor when released. Electrical fixtures and outlets located less than 5 feet above the ground must meet rigid explosion code requirements (Fortunato).

130. **(B)** Carpal tunnel syndrome is a disease of the hand resulting in compression of the median nerve within the carpal tunnel. The necessary surgery is release of the bound down nerve and relief of pressure (Fortunato).

131. **(B)** Strict guidelines regarding implants by the FDA include documentation (patient and operative records), tracking, and registering (data returned to manufacturer includes lot, serial number, size, type, position of use, patient's name, etc.) (Meeker and Rothrock).

132. **(C)** Phimosis is a condition in which the foreskin is narrowed so that it cannot be retracted over the glans (head of the penis) (*Mosby's Medical, Nursing, and Allied Health Dictionary*, 5th ed.).

133. **(B)** Second-degree burns include all epidermis and varying degrees or depths of corium. It is characterized by blister, pain, and redness. Hair follicles and sebaceous glands may be destroyed (Fortunato).

134. **(D)** Anaerobes are those microbes that prefer to live without oxygen (Fortunato).

135. **(D)** The islets of Langerhans are dispersed throughout the pancreas (Tortora and Grabowski).

136. **(B)** The master gland is the pituitary located in the brain (Tortora and Grabowski).

137. **(C)** Osteomyelitis develops from hematogenous spread, gross bone contamination, or improper technique. A breakdown in aseptic technique, sterility, or inappropriate traffic patterns may also result in osteomyelitis (Meeker and Rothrock).

138. **(B)** Drugs that exert a selective action on the smooth muscled uterus to promote contractions are called oxytocics. They exert a stronger effect on the fundus than they do on the cervix (Fortunato).

139. **(C)** After an opening is made into the anterior bladder and the opening is extended with scissors, a Mason–Judd self-retaining bladder retractor is inserted and the bladder is explored (Meeker and Rothrock).

140. **(D)** During a lumbar laminectomy, one or two Beckman–Adson self-retaining retractors are used to expose the bone structure of the spinal column (Meeker and Rothrock).

141. **(C)** Adhesions are a common development after previous abdominal or pelvic surgery. Also acute appendicitis or peritonitis can cause adhesion formation (Fortunato).

142. **(D)** A Hakim valve system is used to direct the flow of cerebrospinal fluid and regulate ventricular fluid pressure by opening within a preset range and draining excess fluid into the atrium or the peritoneum (Meeker and Rothrock).

143. **(C)** Spinal fusion may be effected by use of an autogenous graft from the crest of the patient's ilium (Fortunato).

144. **(D)** All are complications of orthopedic surgery (Meeker and Rothrock).

145. **(A)** Electrical stimulation can induce or influence osteogenesis (growth or repair of bone) for treatment of nonunion, delayed union, and bone defects (Meeker and Rothrock).

146. **(D)** Repairs in certain cases may be done in stages or series, for example, hypospadias repair, reconstruction using expanders (Meeker and Rothrock).

147. **(A)** Nosocomial infections are hospital-acquired infections. These are infections the patient did not have before admission in the hospital (Fortunato).

148. **(B)** The scrub nurse remains sterile and keeps tables sterile, keeping track of all surgical items being used, keeping his or her attention on surgical field, and also attending to surgeon's needs (for example, syringes of medications filled) (Fortunato).

149. **(C)** The edges of anything that encloses sterile contents are considered unsterile (Fortunato).

150. **(C)** An indwelling stent catheter is inserted for long-term drainage in a wide variety of benign and malignant diseases causing ureteral obstruction (Fortunato).

151. **(D)** The Rubin's test (uterotubal insufflation) may be used to test patency of the fallopian tubes (Fortunato).

152. **(C)** An infant's (4 weeks to 18 months) average at rest heart rate is 120 per minute (Fortunato).

153. **(D)** A Harrington retractor is used in deep abdominal surgery. All of the others can be found in a dilation and curettage (Meeker and Rothrock).

154. **(A)** Anterior colporrhaphy is performed to correct prolapse of the anterior vaginal vault and repair herniation of the bladder into the vaginal canal (Fortunato).

155. **(C)** The frontal sinus is approached by making an incision above the eyebrow on the affected side. Diseased tissue is then removed, the sinus cavity is cleansed, and drainage is instituted (Fortunato).

156. **(C)** An incision is made under the upper lip in a Caldwell–Luc procedure. An opening is created into the maxillary sinus, after which the infected contents of the sinus are removed. To promote good drainage, a large nasoantral window is created (Fortunato).

157. **(C)** A Kuntschner or Schneider nail can be used to immobilize a fracture of the femoral shaft (Fortunato).

158. **(C)** The second cranial nerve is the optic (Tortora and Grabowski).

159. **(A)** The under-the-tongue normal body temperature is 98.6°F. This is 37°C. Rectal temperature degree reading is likely to be 0.5–1.0° above the oral (Tortora and Grabowski).

160. **(A)** Arterial gas measurements (ABGs) are analyzed and measured when arterial or venous catheters are in place (Fortunato).

161. **(D)** The Levin tube is a common rubber or plastic nasogastric tube. It is inserted through the nostril down into the stomach or small intestine to remove flatus, fluids, or other contents (Fortunato).

162. **(C)** Breast reconstruction using tissue expanders stretches normal tissue by weekly injections into the expander until maximum stretch has been achieved (Meeker and Rothrock).

163. **(B)** Continuous irrigation of the bladder is necessary during cystoscopy to distend the walls for visualization and to wash out blood, tissue, and stone fragments (Fortunato).

164. **(C)** Debridement, the excision of necrotic tissue, is accomplished with a scalpel, an electrosurgical knife, a dermatome, or a laser beam. After a good vascular supply is located, a full-thickness or split-thickness graft can be used to preserve and cover the area (Fortunato).

165. **(D)** The aging process causes a sagging or relaxation of eyelid skin and the orbital septum. As the latter becomes weaker, it allows periorbital fat to bulge. These changes are perceived as baggy eyelids. The surgical repair of this condition is blepharoplasty (Meeker and Rothrock).

166. **(C)** A pterygium is a fleshy, triangular encroachment onto the cornea. It occurs nasally and tends to be bilateral. If it encroaches on the visual axis it is removed surgically (Meeker and Rothrock).

167. **(D)** An arch bar treats a mandibular fracture by placing teeth in occlusion to achieve adequate immobilization for healing. Scissors or wire cutters stay with the patient to prevent aspiration should the patient vomit (Meeker and Rothrock).

168. **(C)** Nasal instrumentation would include these items (Meeker and Rothrock).

169. **(A)** Bowmans are lacrimal duct probes that also may be used in fallopian tube reconstruction (Meeker and Rothrock).

170. **(D)** At the end of the auditory canal is the tympanic membrane (Tortora and Grabowski).

171. **(D)** An intramedullary nail, rod, or pin is driven into the medullary canal through the site of the fracture. Sampson rods, straight and curved, are a good choice for femurs. All of the others are used for intertrochanteric fractures of the head of the femur (Fortunato).

172. **(D)** Bradycardia is slowness of the heartbeat, less than 60 beats per minute. Sinus bradycardia is seen normally in athletes or secondary to certain drugs (digitalis or morphine) (*Mosby's Medical, Nursing, and Allied Health Dictionary,* 5th ed.).

173. **(D)** If a glove is pricked by a needle or snagged by an instrument, the glove should be changed at once and the needle or instrument discarded (Fortunato).

174. **(B)** A Tenckhoff catheter is inserted into the peritoneal cavity for chemotherapeutic instillation or peritoneal dialysis (Fortunato).

175. **(A)** A Silverman needle is used to biopsy a liver (Fortunato).

176. **(C)** A keratoplasty is a corneal transplant for a diseased cornea. Iridectomy, iridotomy, trephining, and trabeculectomy are used to treat glaucoma. Cyclodialysis, cyclodiathermy, and cyclocryotherapy are also used to diminish aqueous secretions. Optical lasers offer an alternative with laser trabeculoplasty (Fortunato).

177. **(C)** Through microscopic visualization, the aural speculum is inserted in the canal. Using a sharp myringotomy knife, a small curved incision is made in the posteroinferior quadrant or the pars tina, and the thickened membrane is cut (Meeker and Rothrock).

178. **(B)** A perfusionist aids in temperature, arterial and venous pressure, and blood gas monitoring, as well as peripheral tissue perfusion (passing of fluid) monitoring during a cardiopulmonary bypass (Fortunato).

179. **(D)** The closed glove method is preferred because it affords assurance against contamination. This technique cannot be safely used for glove change during an operation (Fortunato).

180. **(D)** Hypovolemic shock is the most common. Fluid volume must be restored quickly so that there can be a rapid return of oxygenated blood to the tissues. Supplemental oxygen should also be administered (*Mosby's Medical, Nursing, and Allied Health Dictionary*, 5th ed.).

181. **(C)** Contaminated wounds occur in operations with major breaks in aseptic technique. An example is appendectomy for ruptured appendix (Meeker and Rothrock).

182. **(A)** The middle ear consists of an air-filled space in the temporal bone called the tympanic cavity. This separates the external and inner ears. Three small bones or auditory ossicles—the malleus (hammer), incus (anvil), and stapes (stirrup)—are attached to the wall of the tympanic cavity by tiny ligaments (Meeker and Rothrock).

183. **(B)** During CO_2 laser use, goggles are worn to protect the cornea and resulting corneal opacification (Meeker and Rothrock).

184. **(A)** The right glove is usually done first. The palm of the glove is held toward the person, stretching the cuff and holding thumbs out so as to avoid touching the hand. The everted cuff is unfolded over the cuff of the sleeve (Fortunato).

185. **(A)** Abduction pillow aids in immobilizing hip joints after surgery. This prevents leg adduction, internal rotation, and hip flexion (Meeker and Rothrock).

186. **(C)** The color or wavelength of a laser determines which part of the eye it can best treat. The blue–green argon laser is used for retinal detachment, diabetic retinopathy, and other retinal problems. All of the others treat various portions of the eye (Fortunato).

187. **(B)** When a patient has a breast biopsy and immediate extended operation, two separate prepping, draping, and instrument sets are necessary (Fortunato).

188. **(B)** Blood pressure sounds are heard over the brachial artery. The bell of the stethoscope is placed over the brachial artery below the blood pressure cuff. The first sound heard is the systolic pressure. The time at which the sound is no longer heard is the diastolic (*Mosby's Medical, Nursing, and Allied Health Dictionary*, 5th ed.).

189. **(D)** Leukocytes (white blood cells) are phagocytic, which is a response to tissue destruction by bacteria. They ingest bacteria and dispose of dead matter (*Mosby's Medical, Nursing, and Allied Health Dictionary*, 5th ed.).

190. **(B)** Ductless glands or endocrine glands secrete hormones internally discharged into blood or lymph and are circulated to all parts of the body. Hormones, the active principals of the glands, produce effects on tissues (pituitary, thyroid, parathyroid, adrenals, pineal, and thymus) (Tortora and Grabowski).

191. **(A)** One of the two pairs of large vessels that return oxygenated blood from each lung to the left atrium of the heart is the pulmonary vein (*Mosby's Medical, Nursing, and Allied Health Dictionary*, 5th ed.).

192. **(D)** Bile is manufactured in the liver. One pint of bile is produced daily. The gallbladder stores and concentrates bile until it is needed in the small intestine (Tortora and Grabowski).

193. **(C)** Carpal tunnel syndrome results from entrapment of the median nerve on the volar surface of the wrist resulting in pain, tingling of the fingers, and weakness of the thumb muscles. This surgery relieves the compression of the median nerve (Meeker and Rothrock).

194. **(A)** Cultures should be refrigerated or sent to the lab immediately. They are obtained under sterile conditions. Tips of swabs must not be contaminated by any other source. The circulating nurse receives the tube in a bag or container (Fortunato).

195. **(C)** With vascular forceps and a #11 blade, an arteriotomy is effected and extended with a Potts–Smith vascular scissor (Meeker and Rothrock).

196. **(A)** Dehiscence is the separation of layers of a surgical wound. In evisceration, the internal organs protrude through the wound (Meeker and Rothrock).

197. **(C)** The first 10 or 12 inches of the small intestine is called the duodenum. It joins with the jejunum, which is 8 feet long. The jejunum joins with the ileum, which is 12 feet long (Meeker and Rothrock).

198. **(D)** *Escherichia coli* live in the colon or large intestine. A colostomy is an opening of some portion of the colon on the abdominal surface. An adjacent wound could be contaminated with *E. coli.* (Fortunato).

199. **(B)** Sodium bicarbonate reverses acidosis. It should not be mixed with any other drug in the IV line (Fortunato).

200. **(A)** Urinary catheterization requires aseptic technique. The integrity of the balloon is checked by inflating it with the correct amount of sterile water or air before insertion. After insertion, the bladder is drained, and the balloon is then inflated (Fortunato).

201. **(C)** The tourniquet pressure for the average adult arm is 250–300 mm Hg. An adult requires about 350 mm Hg on the thigh. Thin adults and children may require less; whereas, the muscular and obese may require more (Fortunato).

202. **(B)** Crushing a urinary calculus with a lithotrite is referred to as litholapaxy. A lithotrite is introduced through the urethra, and the stone is crushed and removed. A cystoscope is introduced into the urethra for introduction of the lithotrite (Fortunato).

203. **(C)** A vasectomy is the excision of the vas deferens performed electively as a permanent method of sterilization (Meeker and Rothrock).

204. **(B)** Draining sinuses, skin ulcers, vagina, anus, etc., are considered contaminated areas. The general rule of scrubbing the most contaminated area last or with separate sponges is followed (Fortunato).

205. **(C)** Below the fundus of the stomach, the region narrows as it approaches the junction to the small intestine. This is the pylorus or distal portion of the stomach (*Mosby's Medical, Nursing, and Allied Health Dictionary*, 5th ed.).

206. **(B)** Lasix (furosemide) is a diuretic. A diuretic increases the secretion of urine (Fortunato).

207. **(C)** The average capacity of the bladder is 700–800 mL. When the amount of urine in the bladder exceeds 200–400 mL, impulses are transmitted that initiate a conscious desire to expel urine. Although emptying of the bladder is controlled by reflex, it may be initiated voluntarily and stopped at will (Tortora and Grabowski).

208. **(C)** The anus is considered a contaminated (dirty) area. The prep is done of the surrounding area first. The anus itself is last (Fortunato).

209. **(A)** When changing a gown during an operation, the gown is always removed first with the circulator pulling the gown off inside out. The gloves are removed using glove-to-glove then skin-to-skin technique. A rescrub is not necessary (Fortunato).

210. **(C)** Skin meshers cut small slits in the graft. When expanded, the slits become diamond-shaped openings. This permits expansion of the graft to cover three times as large an area as the original graft obtained from the donor site (Fortunato).

211. **(C)** A ureteral stent provides internal drainage of an obstructed ureter. It is attached to a sterile closed urinary drainage system, and an adapter must be used because they are small in diameter (Fortunato).

212. **(B)** The patient's level of anxiety and fear is reduced by the preoperative visit because it supplies the patient with factual information and allows the opportunity for him or her to express feelings and concerns (Fortunato).

213. **(C)** The kidneys are held in position by connective tissue (renal fascia) and masses of adipose tissue (renal fat) that surround them. Inadequate renal fascia may cause ptosis or floating kidney (Tortora and Grabowski).

214. **(A)** A culture identifies the suspected organism causing infection. Sensitivity determines the susceptibility of the patient's bacterial infection to antibiotics or antibacterials (Fortunato).

215. **(A)** The most frequently used scrub agent is povidine–iodine (an iodophor) (Fortunato).

216. **(C)** A Joseph's saw is bayonet-like in design and is used for nasal procedures. The Alexander, Duval, and Lebsche are used for chest procedures (Meeker and Rothrock).

217. **(A)** Transcutaneous electric nerve stimulation (TENS) is shockwave energy generated electromagnetically, which fragments calculi. It is verified by fluoroscopy or x-ray. It is tubeless lithotripsy (Fortunato).

218. **(A)** A guide wire or pin is placed in the neck and head of the proximal fragment of the fracture. This determines the final position and length of the implant to be used (Meeker and Rothrock).

219. **(C)** Biologic or synthetic prosthetic grafts are required to bypass vascular obstruction. The biologic vascular is a natural graft and may be either an autograft, homograft, or heterograft. All of the others are synthetic (Fortunato).

220. **(A)** Fallopian tubes (oviducts) have a funnel-shaped portion (infundibulum), which ends in a fringe of fingerlike projections called fimbriae (Tortora and Grabowski).

221. **(A)** The scrubbed area must be dried after application of iodophors. Alcohol may be used to hasten drying or excess can be blotted or wiped off with a sterile towel (Fortunato).

222. **(B)** Keloid formation, an abnormal deposition of collagen in healing skin wounds, presents a particularly difficult problem for plastic surgeons. Keloids may require excision and grafting (Fortunato).

223. **(D)** Sponges are secured on sponge forceps in deep areas. All counts are very important in these procedures. Suction and vaginal packing may be used (Fortunato).

224. **(D)** In laparoscopy, carbon dioxide is introduced via a Verres needle to create a pneumoperitoneum (Fortunato).

225. **(C)** Skeletal traction, applied by Crutchfield tongs inserted in the parietal eminence of the skull, is generally used for reduction of fractures and dislocations of the cervical vertebrae (Fortunato).

226. **(B)** Hepatitis is an inflammation of the liver. Hepatitis A, infectious hepatitis, is spread by the oral–intestinal route and is caused by hepatitis A virus. Common modes are contaminated food, water, and shellfish from contaminated water. Hepatitis B, serum hepatitis, is associated with the blood. Common transmission modes are blood transfusions and contaminated equipment, such as syringes (Fortunato).

227. **(B)** *Staphylococcus* is transmitted by the skin and mucous membrane. It is especially common to the nose and mouth (Fortunato; Meeker and Rothrock).

228. **(D)** Spores remain dormant while the conditions for its growth are unfavorable. Its thick coating protects it from temperature extremes or strong chemicals. Spores are extremely resistant to any disinfectant but are killed by steam and gas sterilization (Meeker and Rothrock; Fortunato).

229. **(C)** Three-way Foley catheters are available in 30- or 50-cc balloons. The third lumen can be used for irrigation. Following some types of genitourinary (GU) surgery, it is important to irrigate any clots or debris from the bladder (Fortunato).

230. **(B)** If a towel clip must be removed, discard it from the sterile setup without touching the points because they are considered contaminated. The area from which it was removed is covered with another sterile drape (Fortunato).

231. **(B)** Constant monitoring of cardiac function with a Swan–Ganz pulmonary artery catheter is important in vascular patients. Patients may require frequent blood gas determination. Doppler is an ultrasound. Greenfield is a vena caval device for catching venous emboli. Fogarty is for thrombectomy and embolectomy (Fortunato).

232. **(D)** Thymectomy without en bloc dissection may be done to relieve myasthenia gravis. It may be done through a median sternotomy incision or through a transverse cervical incision (Fortunato).

233. **(B)** Breast biopsy usually requires frozen section that is not placed in formalin. Kidney stones are sent dry so the chemical composition is not altered. Bronchial washings are sent down in the specimen collection unit as soon as possible, and formalin is not used on them. Tonsils would be sent in formalin (Meeker and Rothrock).

234. **(A)** A tort is a legal wrong committed by one person involving injury to another person or loss of or damage to personal property. When a tort has been committed, a patient or family member may institute a civil action against the person or persons who caused the injury, loss, or damage (Fortunato).

235. **(D)** Harrington rods are implanted into the spine by clips that hold onto the laminae. They are used in combination with (rather than as a replacement for) the external methods of scoliosis support (Meeker and Rothrock).

236. **(C)** Pentothal sodium is a barbiturate. It is a short-acting drug used for induction before administration of more potent anesthetics, such as inhalants. It can also be used for short procedures not requiring relaxation (Fortunato).

237. **(D)** Silastic nonconstrained prosthetics allow for normal range of motion postoperatively (Fortunato).

238. **(D)** Legally, the patient's condition is confidential information. The case should not be discussed outside of the OR. The patient's right to privacy exists either by statutory or common law (Fortunato).

239. **(A)** Protect the gloved hands by cuffing the end of the sheet over them (Fortunato).

240. **(B)** Located in the tarsal plate of the eyelid, the meibomian gland may inflame and require surgical removal. It is known as a chalazion (Meeker and Rothrock).

241. **(D)** Vitamin K enables the liver to produce clotting factors in blood, including prothrombin. To reduce the possibility of intra-operative hemorrhage, patients who have been receiving anticoagulant therapy are given it preoperatively (Fortunato).

242. **(D)** Bowel technique is utilized when a contaminated area of the intestinal tract is entered and may be discontinued when the bowel has been anastomosed (Fortunato).

243. **(C)**   Dupuytren's contracture is a progressive contracture of the palmar fascia. It causes flexion of the little finger, the ring finger, and frequently the middle fingers, rendering them useless (Meeker and Rothrock).

244. **(A)**   Disposable suction tubing is recommended. If tubing is reused, however, special care must be given to cleaning the lumen before placing tubing with instruments for terminal sterilization. Suction a detergent–disinfectant solution through the lumen (Fortunato).

245. **(B)**   If either the scrub person or circulating nurse is relieved by another person during an operation, the incoming person should verify all counts before the person being relieved leaves the room. Persons who take final counts are held accountable and must sign the records (Fortunato).

246. **(D)**   Young patients with congenital cataracts present a condition that contraindicates the use of implants. Children with traumatic cataracts are good candidates for IOLs (Fortunato).

247. **(D)**   Neosynephrine (phenylephrine HCl) is a mydriatic. It dilates the pupil thereby facilitating examination of the retina and also lens removal (Meeker and Rothrock).

248. **(D)**   *Res ipsa loquitor* means "the thing speaks for itself" and is frequently applied to injuries sustained by the patient while in the OR. Three conditions must exist: 1) the type of injury does not ordinarily occur without a negligent act; 2) the injury was caused by the conduct within the control of the person or persons being sued; 3) the injured person could not have contributed to the negligence or voluntarily assumed the risk (Fortunato).

249. **(C)**   The sterile team members discard gown, gloves, caps, masks, and shoe covers because these items should remain in the contaminated area (Fortunato).

250. **(B)**   Pilocarpine is used to constrict the pupil to reduce intraocular pressure. In cataract surgery, it is used to help prevent the loss of vitreous (Meeker and Rothrock).

REFERENCES

Ball KA. *Lasers, The Perioperative Challenge*, 2nd ed. St. Louis: Mosby-Year Book, 1995.

Fortunato N. *Berry and Kohn's Operating Room Technique*, 9th ed. St. Louis: Mosby, 2000.

Meeker M, Rothrock J. *Alexander's Care of the Patient in Surgery*, 11th ed. St. Louis: Mosby-Year Book, 1999.

Mosby's Medical, Nursing, and Allied Health Dictionary, 5th ed. St. Louis: Mosby-Year Book, 1998.

Tortora G, Funke B, Case C. *Microbiology, An Introduction*, 7th ed. Menlo Park, CA: Benjamin Cummings, 2001.

Tortora G, Grabowski S. *Principles of Anatomy and Physiology*, 9th ed. New York: John Wiley & Sons, 2000.

Practice Test
Subject Listing

NAME_____
          Last   First   Middle

ADDRESS_____
          Street

_____
  City   State   Zip

S O C S E C	N U M B E R	0 1 2 3 4 5 6 7 8 9
		0 1 2 3 4 5 6 7 8 9
		0 1 2 3 4 5 6 7 8 9
		0 1 2 3 4 5 6 7 8 9
		0 1 2 3 4 5 6 7 8 9
		0 1 2 3 4 5 6 7 8 9
		0 1 2 3 4 5 6 7 8 9
		0 1 2 3 4 5 6 7 8 9
		0 1 2 3 4 5 6 7 8 9

DIRECTIONS Mark your social security number from top to bottom
in the appropriate boxes on the right.
Use No. 2 lead pencil only.
Mark one and only one answer for each item.
Make each mark black enough to obliterate the letter
within the parentheses.
Erase clearly any answer you wish to change.

1. (A) (B) (C) (D)
2. (A) (B) (C) (D)
3. (A) (B) (C) (D)
4. (A) (B) (C) (D)
5. (A) (B) (C) (D)
6. (A) (B) (C) (D)
7. (A) (B) (C) (D)
8. (A) (B) (C) (D)
9. (A) (B) (C) (D)
10. (A) (B) (C) (D)
11. (A) (B) (C) (D)
12. (A) (B) (C) (D)
13. (A) (B) (C) (D)
14. (A) (B) (C) (D)
15. (A) (B) (C) (D)
16. (A) (B) (C) (D)
17. (A) (B) (C) (D)
18. (A) (B) (C) (D)
19. (A) (B) (C) (D)
20. (A) (B) (C) (D)
21. (A) (B) (C) (D)
22. (A) (B) (C) (D)
23. (A) (B) (C) (D)

24. (A) (B) (C) (D)
25. (A) (B) (C) (D)
26. (A) (B) (C) (D)
27. (A) (B) (C) (D)
28. (A) (B) (C) (D)
29. (A) (B) (C) (D)
30. (A) (B) (C) (D)
31. (A) (B) (C) (D)
32. (A) (B) (C) (D)
33. (A) (B) (C) (D)
34. (A) (B) (C) (D)
35. (A) (B) (C) (D)
36. (A) (B) (C) (D)
37. (A) (B) (C) (D)
38. (A) (B) (C) (D)
39. (A) (B) (C) (D)
40. (A) (B) (C) (D)
41. (A) (B) (C) (D)
42. (A) (B) (C) (D)
43. (A) (B) (C) (D)
44. (A) (B) (C) (D)
45. (A) (B) (C) (D)
46. (A) (B) (C) (D)

47. (A) (B) (C) (D)
48. (A) (B) (C) (D)
49. (A) (B) (C) (D)
50. (A) (B) (C) (D)
51. (A) (B) (C) (D)
52. (A) (B) (C) (D)
53. (A) (B) (C) (D)
54. (A) (B) (C) (D)
55. (A) (B) (C) (D)
56. (A) (B) (C) (D)
57. (A) (B) (C) (D)
58. (A) (B) (C) (D)
59. (A) (B) (C) (D)
60. (A) (B) (C) (D)
61. (A) (B) (C) (D)
62. (A) (B) (C) (D)
63. (A) (B) (C) (D)
64. (A) (B) (C) (D)
65. (A) (B) (C) (D)
66. (A) (B) (C) (D)
67. (A) (B) (C) (D)
68. (A) (B) (C) (D)
69. (A) (B) (C) (D)

70. (A) (B) (C) (D)
71. (A) (B) (C) (D)
72. (A) (B) (C) (D)
73. (A) (B) (C) (D)
74. (A) (B) (C) (D)
75. (A) (B) (C) (D)
76. (A) (B) (C) (D)
77. (A) (B) (C) (D)
78. (A) (B) (C) (D)
79. (A) (B) (C) (D)
80. (A) (B) (C) (D)
81. (A) (B) (C) (D)
82. (A) (B) (C) (D)
83. (A) (B) (C) (D)
84. (A) (B) (C) (D)
85. (A) (B) (C) (D)
86. (A) (B) (C) (D)
87. (A) (B) (C) (D)
88. (A) (B) (C) (D)
89. (A) (B) (C) (D)
90. (A) (B) (C) (D)
91. (A) (B) (C) (D)
92. (A) (B) (C) (D)

93. (A) (B) (C) (D)	124. (A) (B) (C) (D)	155. (A) (B) (C) (D)	186. (A) (B) (C) (D)
94. (A) (B) (C) (D)	125. (A) (B) (C) (D)	156. (A) (B) (C) (D)	187. (A) (B) (C) (D)
95. (A) (B) (C) (D)	126. (A) (B) (C) (D)	157. (A) (B) (C) (D)	188. (A) (B) (C) (D)
96. (A) (B) (C) (D)	127. (A) (B) (C) (D)	158. (A) (B) (C) (D)	189. (A) (B) (C) (D)
97. (A) (B) (C) (D)	128. (A) (B) (C) (D)	159. (A) (B) (C) (D)	190. (A) (B) (C) (D)
98. (A) (B) (C) (D)	129. (A) (B) (C) (D)	160. (A) (B) (C) (D)	191. (A) (B) (C) (D)
99. (A) (B) (C) (D)	130. (A) (B) (C) (D)	161. (A) (B) (C) (D)	192. (A) (B) (C) (D)
100. (A) (B) (C) (D)	131. (A) (B) (C) (D)	162. (A) (B) (C) (D)	193. (A) (B) (C) (D)
101. (A) (B) (C) (D)	132. (A) (B) (C) (D)	163. (A) (B) (C) (D)	194. (A) (B) (C) (D)
102. (A) (B) (C) (D)	133. (A) (B) (C) (D)	164. (A) (B) (C) (D)	195. (A) (B) (C) (D)
103. (A) (B) (C) (D)	134. (A) (B) (C) (D)	165. (A) (B) (C) (D)	196. (A) (B) (C) (D)
104. (A) (B) (C) (D)	135. (A) (B) (C) (D)	166. (A) (B) (C) (D)	197. (A) (B) (C) (D)
105. (A) (B) (C) (D)	136. (A) (B) (C) (D)	167. (A) (B) (C) (D)	198. (A) (B) (C) (D)
106. (A) (B) (C) (D)	137. (A) (B) (C) (D)	168. (A) (B) (C) (D)	199. (A) (B) (C) (D)
107. (A) (B) (C) (D)	138. (A) (B) (C) (D)	169. (A) (B) (C) (D)	200. (A) (B) (C) (D)
108. (A) (B) (C) (D)	139. (A) (B) (C) (D)	170. (A) (B) (C) (D)	201. (A) (B) (C) (D)
109. (A) (B) (C) (D)	140. (A) (B) (C) (D)	171. (A) (B) (C) (D)	202. (A) (B) (C) (D)
110. (A) (B) (C) (D)	141. (A) (B) (C) (D)	172. (A) (B) (C) (D)	203. (A) (B) (C) (D)
111. (A) (B) (C) (D)	142. (A) (B) (C) (D)	173. (A) (B) (C) (D)	204. (A) (B) (C) (D)
112. (A) (B) (C) (D)	143. (A) (B) (C) (D)	174. (A) (B) (C) (D)	205. (A) (B) (C) (D)
113. (A) (B) (C) (D)	144. (A) (B) (C) (D)	175. (A) (B) (C) (D)	206. (A) (B) (C) (D)
114. (A) (B) (C) (D)	145. (A) (B) (C) (D)	176. (A) (B) (C) (D)	207. (A) (B) (C) (D)
115. (A) (B) (C) (D)	146. (A) (B) (C) (D)	177. (A) (B) (C) (D)	208. (A) (B) (C) (D)
116. (A) (B) (C) (D)	147. (A) (B) (C) (D)	178. (A) (B) (C) (D)	209. (A) (B) (C) (D)
117. (A) (B) (C) (D)	148. (A) (B) (C) (D)	179. (A) (B) (C) (D)	210. (A) (B) (C) (D)
118. (A) (B) (C) (D)	149. (A) (B) (C) (D)	180. (A) (B) (C) (D)	211. (A) (B) (C) (D)
119. (A) (B) (C) (D)	150. (A) (B) (C) (D)	181. (A) (B) (C) (D)	212. (A) (B) (C) (D)
120. (A) (B) (C) (D)	151. (A) (B) (C) (D)	182. (A) (B) (C) (D)	213. (A) (B) (C) (D)
121. (A) (B) (C) (D)	152. (A) (B) (C) (D)	183. (A) (B) (C) (D)	214. (A) (B) (C) (D)
122. (A) (B) (C) (D)	153. (A) (B) (C) (D)	184. (A) (B) (C) (D)	215. (A) (B) (C) (D)
123. (A) (B) (C) (D)	154. (A) (B) (C) (D)	185. (A) (B) (C) (D)	216. (A) (B) (C) (D)

217. (A) (B) (C) (D)   226. (A) (B) (C) (D)   235. (A) (B) (C) (D)   243. (A) (B) (C) (D)

218. (A) (B) (C) (D)   227. (A) (B) (C) (D)   236. (A) (B) (C) (D)   244. (A) (B) (C) (D)

219. (A) (B) (C) (D)   228. (A) (B) (C) (D)   237. (A) (B) (C) (D)   245. (A) (B) (C) (D)

220. (A) (B) (C) (D)   229. (A) (B) (C) (D)   238. (A) (B) (C) (D)   246. (A) (B) (C) (D)

221. (A) (B) (C) (D)   230. (A) (B) (C) (D)   239. (A) (B) (C) (D)   247. (A) (B) (C) (D)

222. (A) (B) (C) (D)   231. (A) (B) (C) (D)   240. (A) (B) (C) (D)   248. (A) (B) (C) (D)

223. (A) (B) (C) (D)   232. (A) (B) (C) (D)   241. (A) (B) (C) (D)   249. (A) (B) (C) (D)

224. (A) (B) (C) (D)   233. (A) (B) (C) (D)   242. (A) (B) (C) (D)   250. (A) (B) (C) (D)

225. (A) (B) (C) (D)   234. (A) (B) (C) (D)